INSURANCE IN THE
MEDICAL OFFICE

From Patient to Payment **Seventh Edition**

Cynthia Newby, CPC, CPC-P

Nikita Carr, CPC

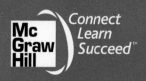

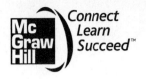

INSURANCE IN THE MEDICAL OFFICE: FROM PATIENT TO PAYMENT, SEVENTH EDITION

Published by McGraw-Hill, a business unit of The McGraw-Hill Companies, Inc., 1221 Avenue of the Americas, New York, NY, 10020. Copyright © 2014 by The McGraw-Hill Companies, Inc. All rights reserved. Printed in the United States of America. Previous editions © 2010, 2008, and 2005. No part of this publication may be reproduced or distributed in any form or by any means, or stored in a database or retrieval system, without the prior written consent of The McGraw-Hill Companies, Inc., including, but not limited to, in any network or other electronic storage or transmission, or broadcast for distance learning.

Some ancillaries, including electronic and print components, may not be available to customers outside the United States.

This book is printed on acid-free paper.

2 3 4 5 6 7 8 9 0 QVS/QVS 1 0 9 8 7 6 5

ISBN   978-0-07-337459-8
MHID   0-07-337459-8

Senior Vice President, Products
    & Markets: *Kurt L. Strand*
Vice President, General Manager,
    Products & Markets: *Martin J. Lange*
Vice President, Content Production &
    Technology Services: *Kimberly Meriwether David*
Managing Director: *Michael S. Ledbetter*
Executive Brand Manager: *Natalie J. Ruffatto*
Director of Development: *Rose Koos*
Managing Development
    Editor: *Michelle L. Flomenhoft*
Development Editor: *Raisa Priebe Kreek*
Digital Product Analyst: *Katherine Ward*
Director of Marketing: *Chad Grall*

Executive Marketing Manager: *Roxan Kinsey*
Project Manager: *Marlena Pechan*
Senior Buyer: *Sandy Ludovissy*
Senior Designer: *Srdjan Savanovic*
Cover Designer: *Matt Backhaus*
Cover Image: *Tetra Images/Getty Images/Paul Burns/*
    Image Source/JGI/Tom Grill
Content Licensing Specialist: *Joanne Mennemeier*
Manager, Digital Production: *Janean A. Utley*
Media Project Manager: *Brent dela Cruz*
Media Project Manager: *Cathy L. Tepper*
Typeface: *11.5/13 Janson*
Compositor: *Aptara®, Inc.*
Printer: *Quad/Graphics*

All credits appearing at the end of the book are considered to be an extension of the copyright page.

Library of Congress Cataloging-in-Publication Data

Newby, Cynthia.
    Insurance in the medical office : from patient to payment / Cynthia Newby, Nikita Carr.—7th ed.
        p.; cm.
    Rev. ed. of: From patient to payment / Cynthia Newby. 6th ed. c2010.
    Includes bibliographical references and index.
    ISBN 978-0-07-337459-8 (alk. paper)—ISBN 0-07-337459-8 (alk. paper)
    I. Carr, Nikita. II. Newby, Cynthia. From patient to payment. III. Title.
    [DNLM: 1. Insurance Claim Reporting—United States. 2. Fees and Charges—United States.
    3. Medical Records—United States. 4. Practice Management—economics—United States. W 100]
    610.68—dc23

                                                                                    2012039186

The Internet addresses listed in the text were accurate at the time of publication. The inclusion of a website does not indicate an endorsement by the authors or McGraw-Hill, and McGraw-Hill does not guarantee the accuracy of the information presented at these sites.

Medisoft® is a registered trademark of McKesson Corporation and/or one of its subsidiaries. Screenshots and material pertaining to Medisoft® Software used with permission of McKesson Corporation. © 2012 McKesson Corporation and/or one of its subsidiaries. All Rights Reserved.

The illustrations, instructions, and exercises in *Insurance in the Medical Office* are compatible with the Medisoft Advanced Version 17 Patient Accounting software available at the time of publication.

All brand or product names are trademarks or registered trademarks of their respective companies.

CPT five-digit codes, nomenclature, and other data are copyright 2012 American Medical Association. All Rights Reserved. No fee schedules, basic units relative values, or related listings are included in CPT. The AMA assumes no liability for the data contained herein.

CPT codes are based on CPT 2013.

ICD-9-CM codes are based on ICD-9-CM 2013.

ICD-10-CM codes are based on ICD-10-CM 2013.

All names, situations, and anecdotes are fictitious. They do not represent any person, event, or medical record.

www.mhhe.com

Brief Contents

Contents

Preface

Medical insurance plays an important role in the financial well-being of every health care business. The regulatory environment of medical insurance is evolving faster than ever. Changes due to health care reform require medical office professionals to acquire and maintain an in-depth understanding of compliance, electronic health records, medical coding, and more.

The seventh edition of *Insurance in the Medical Office: From Patient to Payment* emphasizes the medical billing cycle—ten steps that clearly identify all the components needed to successfully manage the medical insurance claims process. Studying this cycle shows how administrative medical assistants must first collect accurate patient information and then be familiar with the rules and guidelines of each health plan in order to submit proper documentation and follow up on payments. This ensures that offices receive maximum, appropriate reimbursement for services provided. Without an effective administrative staff, a medical office would have no cash flow!

So, why is studying medical insurance especially important for Medical Assisting students? Medical Assistants (MAs) have the ability to work both clinically and administratively in the physician practice. This flexibility makes them valuable members of the health care team. With the unpredictable nature of the economy, many practices are doing more with less. This means that MAs may find themselves in a position where they are working in a clinical capacity and also asked to assist with billing tasks. Furthermore, knowing about insurance, billing, and reimbursement is not only important for MAs in the workforce, but this knowledge is also required for certification. *Insurance in the Medical Office* is specifically targeted to Medical Assisting students and addresses the role they play in contributing to the financial success of the medical office.

Organization of *Insurance in the Medical Office, 7e*

Here is an overview of the chapters, including how they relate to the steps of the medical billing cycle:

Chapter	Coverage
Chapters 1, 2, 3	Covers Steps 1 through 4 of the medical billing cycle by introducing the major types of medical insurance, payers, and regulators, as well as the medical billing cycle. Also covers HIPAA/HITECH Privacy, Security, and Electronic Health Care Transactions/Code Sets/Breach Notification rules.
Chapters 4, 5, 6	Covers Steps 5 and 6 of the medical billing cycle, while building skills in correct coding procedures, use of coding references, and compliance with proper linkage guidelines.
Chapters 7, 8, 9, 10, 11, 12	Covers Step 7 of the medical billing cycle and the general procedures for calculating reimbursement, how to bill compliantly, and preparing and transmitting claims. Describes the major third-party private and government sponsored payers' procedures and regulations, along with specific filing guidelines.
Chapter 13	Covers Steps 8 through 10 of the medical billing cycle by explaining how to handle payments from payers, follow up and appeal claims, and correctly bill and collect from patients.
Chapter 14	Provides necessary background in hospital billing, coding, and payment methods.
Chapter 15 (available at www.mcgrawhillcreate.com)	Covers dental insurance for those programs that include it.
Chapter 16 (available at www.mcgrawhillcreate.com)	Covers ICD-9 and ICD-10 as an alternative to Chapter 4 for those programs still early in their transition from ICD-9 to ICD-10.

New to the Seventh Edition

One of the first things you may notice, if you are familiar with earlier editions of *From Patient to Payment*, is that the seventh edition has been tailored to the specific needs of medical assistants as they handle office administration tasks. Content and coverage are updated and refocused to provide a practical, targeted overview of medical insurance and billing. To that end, the title has been updated to better reflect the new content of the book. The new title is thus *Insurance in the Medical Office: From Patient to Payment.*

The new seventh edition has benefited from the extensive teaching experience with Medical Assisting students that new co-author Nikita Carr brings to the project.

The new edition is now designed around the current medical billing cycle that follows the overall medical billing and documentation cycle used in Practice Management and Electronic Health Records environments and applications. Groups of chapters sequentially cover the major sections of that cycle, followed by exercises to apply the skills needed in each section.

Because of the mandate to the health care industry to adopt ICD-10-CM/PCS on October 1, 2014, students must work toward expertise using this coding system. For this reason, with the seventh edition of this book, ICD-10 is the primary diagnostic coding system taught and exemplified in *Insurance in the Medical Office*. An alternate to Chapter 4 on ICD-9-CM (Chapter 16) is provided through McGraw-Hill's *Create* system for additional study if the instructor elects to cover it in more depth.

Starting in Chapter 3, in-chapter Exercises give students the opportunity to get hands-on experience with key Practice Management Program tasks through simulations of real software. Completing on-the-job tasks relating to PMPs is an important aspect of a medical assistant's work. *Insurance in the Medical Office* offers options for completing these tasks:

- **Connect Plus** Connect Plus provides simulated Medisoft® exercises in four modes: Demo, Practice, Test, and Assessment. The exercises simulate usage of Medisoft Advanced Version 17. The simulated exercises, offered online, cover key practice management tasks to provide experience in working with patient, insurance, procedure, diagnosis, claims, and transaction databases. If assigned this option, students should read Appendix A, *Guide to Medisoft*, as the first step, and then follow the instructions that are printed in each chapter's Connect Plus Exercises, indicated with the connect (plus) logo.

Many of the exercises involve insurance claims. These specific exercises may be completed one of three ways:

- **Paper Claim Form** If you are gaining experience by completing a paper CMS-1500 claim form, use the blank form supplied to you (from the back of *Insurance in the Medical Office* or printed out from a PDF file on the book's Online Learning Center, www.mhhe.com/newbycarr), and follow the instructions in the text chapter that is appropriate for the particular payer to fill in the form by hand.
- **Electronic CMS-1500 Form** If you are assigned to use the electronic CMS-1500 form, access either the HTML or Adobe Form Filler form at the book's Online Learning Center, www.mhhe.com/newbycarr. See Appendix B, *The Interactive Simulated CMS-1500 Form*, for further instructions.
- **Connect Plus** If you are assigned to use Connect Plus for these exercises, Connect Plus also provides simulated CMS-1500 exercises in four modes: Demo, Practice, Test, and Assessment. In this version, some data may be pre-populated to allow the students to focus on the key tasks of each exercise. These simulations are auto-graded.

Key Content Changes

Pedagogy

- Learning Outcomes are restated to reflect the revised version of Bloom's Taxonomy and the range of difficulty levels to teach and assess critical thinking about medical insurance and coding concepts.
- Major chapter heads are now structured to reflect the numbered Learning Outcomes.
- In addition to the listing of learning outcomes and the listing of key terms, each chapter opener displays the Medical Billing Cycle, with the steps relevant to that chapter highlighted.
- Key terms are now defined in the margins for easy reference, while also being listed in the Glossary toward the end of the book.
- Billing Tips and Compliance Guidelines highlight key concepts or provide additional tips to help students navigate through the material.
- "Thinking It Through" questions have been added at the end of each section to assess each Learning Outcome.
- New Chapter Summaries have been created in a tabular, step-by-step format with page references to help with review of the material.
- End-of-chapter elements are now tagged with Learning Outcomes.
- The Chapter Review section includes:

    Using Terminology—matching questions with key terms and definitions.

    Checking Your Understanding—multiple choice and short answer questions.

    Applying Your Knowledge—cases.

Chapter-by-Chapter

- **Chapter 1:** New key terms—accounts payable (AP), cash flow, certification, coding, documentation, electronic health record (EHR), health information technology (HIT), medical assistant, medical billing cycle, medical documentation and billing cycle, out of pocket, PM/EHR, revenue cycle management (RCM), statement, third-party payer. Chapter now focuses on the medical assistant's role in revenue cycle management and clinical workflow; new coverage of health information technology and practice management programs; updated medical billing cycle; chapter now highlights the importance of certification and continuing education.
- **Chapter 2:** New key terms—abuse, audit, breach, breach notification, business associate (BA), Centers for Medicare and Medicaid Services (CMS), code set, covered entity (CE), designated record set (DRS), electronic data interchange (EDI), encounter, encryption, medical standards of care, Office of E-Health Standards and Services (OESS), Office of Inspector General (OIG), password, transaction. New coverage and discussion on the Affordable Care Act and the Health Information Technology for Economic and Clinical Act (HITECH).
- **Chapter 3:** New to this edition, this chapter focuses on the patient encounter and billing information. Simulated chapter exercises include creating a new patient account, updating an existing patient account, verifying patient eligibility, and entering a patient's insurance information.
- **Chapter 4:** (Chapter 3 in the previous edition) Updated for ICD-10. New Key terms—combination code, diagnostic statement, eponym, exclusion notes, GEM, ICD-10-CM, ICD-10-CM Official Guidelines for Coding and Reporting, inclusion notes, Index to External Causes, laterality, manifestation, NEC (not elsewhere classified), Neoplasm Table, nonessential modifier, NOS (not otherwise specified), outpatient, placeholder character (x) sequelae, seventh-character extension, Table of Drugs and Chemicals, Z Code. Simulated chapter exercise covers entering a patient's diagnosis.

- **Chapter 5:** (Chapter 4 in the previous edition) New key terms—eponym, key component, moderate sedation, place of service (POS), resequenced, section guidelines, separate procedure. Updated steps for locating correct CPT codes. Simulated chapter exercise covers entering a patient's procedure and charge.
- **Chapter 6:** (Chapter 5 in the previous edition) New key terms—accept assignment, adjustment, bundled payment, conversion factor, financial policy, flexible saving account (FSA), health reimbursement account (HRA), health savings account (HSA), high-deductible health plan (HDHP), independent practice association (IPA), meaningful use, Medicare Physician Fee Schedule (MPFS), partial payment, per member per month (PMPM), real-time claims adjudication (RTCA), self-pay patient. Chapter is focused on check-out procedures. Simulated chapter exercises cover entering a patient's copayment in the PMP, billing for supplies, and creating a walkout receipt.
- **Chapter 7:** (Chapter 6 in the previous edition) New key terms—5010 format, CMS-1500 (02/12), secondary claim, tertiary claim. Expanded coverage of electronic claims transmission. Coverage of secondary claims transmission. Simulated chapter exercises cover completing a CMS-1500 form, submitting claims electronically, and completing a secondary claim.
- **Chapter 8:** New key terms—carve out, Consolidated Omnibus Budget Reconciliation Act (COBRA), credentialing, elective surgery, Employee Retirement Income Security Act of 1974 (ERISA), family deductible, group health plan (GHP), individual deductible, individual health plan (IHP), late enrollee, maximum benefit limit, monthly enrollment list, open enrollment period, precertification, rider, self-insured health plan, stop loss provision, utilization review, utilization review organization (URO), waiting period. Simulated chapter exercises cover completing a primary payer claim and completing a Blue Cross Blue Shield primary payer claim.
- **Chapter 9:** New key terms—health insurance claim number (HICN), Internet-Only Manuals (IOM), Medicare Integrity Program (MIP), Medicare Learning Network (MLN), Medicare Secondary Payer (MSP), Physician Quality Reporting System (PQRS), urgently needed care. Step by step instructions on filling out the ABN. Simulated chapter exercise covers completing a Medicare claim.
- **Chapter 10:** New discussion on the expected impact of the Affordable Care Act on the Medicaid program. Simulated chapter exercises cover completing a Medicaid claim.
- **Chapter 11:** New key terms—catchment area, Civilian Health and Medical Program of the Uniformed Services (CHAMPUS). Simulated chapter exercise covers completing a TRICARE claim.
- **Chapter 12:** New coverage of automobile and disability insurance. New key terms—Admission of Liability, automobile insurance policy, disability compensation programs, independent medical examination (IME), lien, Notice of Contest, Occupational Safety and Health Administration (OSHA). Simulated chapter exercise covers completing a workers' compensation claim.
- **Chapter 13:** (Chapter 7 in the previous edition) New key terms—adjustment code, aging, autoposting, bad debt, collections, cycle billing, day sheet, development, electronic remittance advice (ERA), Equal Credit Opportunity Act (ECOA), explanation of benefits (EOB), Fair Debt Collection Practices Act (FDCPA) of 1977, guarantor billing, NSF checks, overpayment, patient refund, reconciliation, Telephone Consumer Protection Act of 1991, Truth in Lending Act, upcoding. Expanded coverage of collection regulations and procedures. Coverage of NSF checks. Simulated chapter exercises cover posting an insurance payment, generating a patient statement, and writing off an uncollectible account.
- **Chapter 14:** (Chapter 15 in the previous edition) New key terms—comorbidities, complications, ICD-10-PCS. Expanded coverage of the Medicare Inpatient and Outpatient payment systems.

For a detailed transition guide between the sixth and seventh editions, visit www.mhhe.com/newbycarr.

Insurance in the Digital World—Supplementary Materials for the Instructor and Student

Instructors, McGraw-Hill knows how much effort it takes to prepare for a new course. Through focus groups, symposia, reviews, and conversations with instructors like you, we have gathered information about what materials you need in order to facilitate successful courses. We are committed to providing you with high-quality, accurate instructor support. Knowing the importance of flexibility and digital learning, McGraw-Hill has created multiple assets to enhance the learning experience no matter what the class format: traditional, online or hybrid. This revision is designed to help instructors and students be successful with digital solutions proven to drive student success.

A one-stop spot to present, deliver, and assess digital assets available from McGraw-Hill: McGraw-Hill Connect® Insurance in the Medical Office

McGraw-Hill Connect®—Insurance in the Medical Office provides online presentation, assignment, and assessment solutions. It connects your students with the tools and resources they'll need to achieve success. With Connect you can deliver assignments, quizzes, and tests online. A robust set of questions and activities, including all of the end-of-section and end-of-chapter questions, interactives, the in-chapter exercise simulations and Testbank questions, are presented and aligned with the textbook's learning outcomes. As an instructor, you can edit existing questions and author entirely new problems. Track individual student performance—by question, assignment, or in relation to the class overall—with detailed grade reports. Integrate grade reports easily with Learning Management Systems (LMS), such as Blackboard, DesiretoLearn, or eCollege—and much more. **Connect Plus—Insurance in the Medical Office** provides students with all the advantages **of Connect®—Medical Assisting** *plus* 24/7 online access to an eBook. This media-rich version of the book is available through the McGraw-Hill Connect® platform and allows seamless integration of text, media, and assessments. To learn more, visit http://connect.mcgraw-hill.com.

A single sign-on with Connect® and your Blackboard course: McGraw-Hill Higher Education and Blackboard

Blackboard®, the Web-based course management system, has partnered with McGraw-Hill to better allow students and faculty to use online materials and activities to complement face-to-face teaching. Blackboard features exciting social learning and teaching tools that foster active learning opportunities for students. You'll transform your closed-door classroom into communities where students remain connected to their educational experience 24 hours a day. This partnership allows you and your students access to McGraw-Hill's Connect® and McGraw-Hill Create™ right from within your Blackboard course—all with one single sign-on. Not only do you get single sign-on with Connect and Create, you also get deep integration of McGraw-Hill content and content engines right in Blackboard. Whether you're choosing a book for your course or building Connect assignments, all the tools you need are right where you want them—inside of Blackboard. Gradebooks are now seamless. When a student completes an integrated Connect assignment, the grade for that assignment automatically (and instantly) feeds your Blackboard grade center. McGraw-Hill and Blackboard can now offer you easy access to industry leading technology and content, whether your campus hosts it or we do. Be sure to ask your local McGraw-Hill representative for details.

Looking for more material on coding? The *Medical Coding Workbook for Physician Practices & Facilities, ICD-10 Edition* (0073511048, 9780073513713) provides practice and instruction in coding and compliance skills. The coding workbook reinforces and enhances skill development by applying the coding principles introduced in *Insurance in the Medical Office, 7e* and extending knowledge through additional coding guidelines, examples, and compliance tips.

Create™ a textbook organized the way you teach: McGraw-Hill Create™

With **McGraw-Hill Create™,** you can easily rearrange chapters, combine material from other content sources, and quickly upload content you have written, like your course syllabus or teaching notes. Find the content you need in Create by searching through thousands of leading McGraw-Hill textbooks. Arrange your book to fit your teaching style. Create even allows you to personalize your book's appearance by selecting the cover and adding your name, school, and course information. Order a Create book and you'll receive a complimentary print review copy in 3–5 business days or a complimentary electronic review copy (eComp) via e-mail in minutes. Go to www.mcgrawhillcreate.com today and register to experience how McGraw-Hill Create empowers you to teach *your* students *your* way. Create is your resource for including Chapters 15 and/or 16 in your book. Visit the website or contact your sales rep for more information. **www.mcgrawhillcreate.com**

Record and distribute your lectures for multiple viewing: My Lectures—Tegrity®

McGraw-Hill Tegrity® records and distributes your class lecture with just a click of a button. Students can view anytime/anywhere via computer, iPod, or mobile device. It indexes as it records your PowerPoint® presentations and anything shown on your computer so students can use keywords to find exactly what they want to study. **Tegrity®** is available as an integrated feature of **McGraw-Hill Connect®— Insurance in the Medical Office** and as a standalone.

Instructors' Resources

You can rely on the following materials to help you and your students work through the material in the book, all of which are available on the book's website, www.mhhe.com/newbycarr (instructors can request a password through their sales representative):

Supplement	Features
Instructor's Manual (organized by Learning Outcomes)	• Lesson Plans • Answer Keys for all exercises • Documentation of Steps and Screenshots for Simulated Medisoft and CMS-1500 Exercises
PowerPoint Presentations (organized by Learning Outcomes)	• Key Terms • Key Concepts • Teaching Notes
Electronic Testbank	• EZ Test Online (Computerized) • Word Version • Questions have tagging for Learning Outcomes, Level of Difficulty, Level of Bloom's Taxonomy, Feedback, ABHES, CAAHEP, CAHIIM, and Estimated Time of Completion.
Tools to Plan Course	• Correlations of the Learning Outcomes to Accrediting Bodies such as ABHES CAAHEP, and CAHIIM • Sample Syllabi • Conversion Guide between sixth and seventh editions • Asset Map—re-cap of the key instructor resources, as well as information on the content available through Connect Plus
Medisoft Exercises Resources	• *McGraw-Hill Guide to Success for Insurance in the Medical Office* • Technical Support Information • Steps for those students completing the simulated exercises in Connect Plus
CMS-1500 and UB-04 Forms	• Electronic versions of both forms

Need help? Contact McGraw-Hill's Customer Experience Group (CXG). Visit the CXG website at www.mhhe.com/support. Browse our FAQs (Frequently Asked Questions), product documentation, and/or contact a CXG representative. CXG is available Sunday through Friday.

Want to learn more about this product? Attend one of our online webinars. To learn more about the webinars, please contact your McGraw-Hill sales representative. To find your McGraw-Hill representative, go to www.mhhe.com and click Find My Sales Rep.

About the Authors

Cynthia Newby, CPC, CPC-P, has worked with educational programming across her career, first with the McGraw-Hill Community College Division, then moving to a business/industry information technology training firm, and currently as founder and president of Chestnut Hill Enterprises, Inc., a textbook development company with over twenty years of proven programs. Cynthia is the author or managing director of many McGraw-Hill programs, including *Medical Insurance, Insurance in Medical Offices, Medical Coding Workbook, Hospital Billing,* and *Computers in the Medical Office.* Interests include community-based volunteering and gardening; Cynthia's *Lagniappe Garden* in Roxbury, CT, has been featured on the national Garden Conservancy Open Garden Days tour and in national magazines.

Nikita Carr, CPC, has instructed and developed curricula for medical assisting and medical billing and coding programs in a variety of academic settings. Nikita has taught in the Adult Education program for Chesterfield County Public Schools and coordinated the Medical Billing and Coding Specialist program at the Centura College, Midlothian, Virginia, campus. Nikita has worked with the Allied Health Division of McGraw-Hill in the production of several billing, insurance, and coding titles. Prior to her educational career Nikita worked over fifteen years in health care clinically and administratively for hospitals, long-term care facilities, and physician practices.

Acknowledgments

Suggestions have been received from faculty and students throughout the country. This is vital feedback that is relied upon with each edition. Each person who has offered comments and suggestions has our thanks. The efforts of many people are needed to develop and improve a product. Among these people are the reviewers and consultants who point out areas of concern, cite areas of strength, and make recommendations for change. In this regard, the following instructors provided feedback that was enormously helpful in preparing the seventh edition.

Book Reviews

Many instructors reviewed the sixth edition once it was published and/or the seventh edition manuscript, providing valuable feedback that directly impacted the book.

Stephanie Bernard, AA, CMA, AHI
Sanford-Brown Institute

Amy L. Blochowiak, MBA/HR, CPC, CCA, CMAA, CBCS
Northeast Wisconsin Technical College

Gerry A. Brasin, CMA (AAMA), CPC
Premier Education Group

Robin Dukart
Institute of Technology

Christine Dzoga, CMA, RMA, RPT, AHI, CPCT, CPT, CECGT, CECGI, CPI, CPCTI, CPR (AHA)
Illinois School of Health Careers

Terri Gilbert, CMAA, CEHRS, BSBA, AS
Medical Careers Institute College of Health ECPI University

Debbie Kosydar, LPN
McCann School of Business and Technology

Amy Lawrence, MBA, ACS, AIAA, AIRC, ARA, FLHC, FLMI, HCSA, HIA, HIPAA, MHP, PCS, SILA-F
Ultimate Medical Academy

Karen McAbee, CMA (AAMA), CPC
Miami-Jacobs Career College

Laura Melendez, BS, RMA, RT BMO
Keiser Career College

Tatyana Pashnyak, MEd, COI
Bainbridge College

Karen Patton
Stautzenberger College

Shauna Phillips, CMA, CPT, CET, CMT
Fortis College

Jodi Taylor, A.A.S., LPN, RMA, NCIS,
Terra State Community College

Tiffany Vercillo, AS, HIT
Great Lakes Institute of Technology

Market Surveys

Multiple instructors participated in a survey to help guide the revision of the book and related materials.

Dr. Amer Alata, M.D.
Detroit Business Institute-Downriver

Yvonne Beth Alles, DHA
Davenport University

Yvonne Denise Arnold-Jenkins, NRCMA, CMRS, CPC
Remington College

Amber Barba, NCMA
The Learning Pad LLC

Joey L. Brown, CMA
Great Lakes Institute of Technology

Adelia M. Cooley, CPC, BBA, MSHA
Sanford Brown College

Patricia Cormier, MA, CMA
Acadiana Technical College

Vicki Davis, MLT (ASCP), BS, CHI
Duluth Business University

Laurie Dennis, CBCS
Florida Career College

Patricia Dudek, RN, RMA
McCann School
of Business and Technology

Lynnette Garetz, MS
Heald College

Deborah S.Gilbert, RHIA,
CMA
Dalton State College

Donna Gittler, RN
Pace Institute Medical
Instructor

Katie Goffard
Fox Valley Technical
College

Pauletta D. Gullett, RN,
CRRN, BSN
Lincoln Trail College

Glenda Hatcher, BSN,
RN, CMA (AAMA)
Southwest Georgia
Technical College

Kate Hickey
OfficeStar Training

Cynthia Holliday, CMA
Sanford Brown
Ft. Lauderdale, Fl

Traci Hotard, RHIA
SCLTC Young Memorial

Judy Hurtt, MEd
East Central Community
College

Debi Kenney, NCMA,
NCBCS, As, Ed.
Harris School of Business

Zia Khan, CBCS, CCMA
Florida Career College

Sharon Kibbe, BA, MSM,
NSCA-CPT
Brown Mackie College

Jody Kirk, BS, CCS-P
Cambria-Rowe Business
College

Jan Klawitter, AS in
Medical Assisting, CMA
(AAMA), and CPC
San Joaquin Valley
College

Diana Lee-Greene, RMA
(AMT), MT (ASCP)
Columbia Gorge
Community College

Barbara Marchelletta,
CMA (AAMA), CPC,
CPT
Beal College

Nikki Marhefka, MT
(ASCP), MS
Central Penn College

Pamela McNutt, Ed M,
MT (ASCP), CMA
(AAMA)
Wright Career College

Chris Metcalfe, EMT
The Learning Pad LLC

Lori Mikell, RMA
Ridley Lowell Business
and Technical Institute

Tamara E. Mottler, CMA
(AAMA)
Daytona State College

Karen Nelson, RN
Iowa Western Community
College

Tina Nolen, CMA
(AAMA), RMA (AMT)
Ben Franklin Career
Center

Marion D. Odom, AHI,
RMA, NCMA, CPCT,
CPT, CEKGT
Illinois School of Health
Careers

Julie Pepper, CMA, BS
Chippewa Valley
Technical College

Gail Piscaglia, BS, CMA-
AAMA, CPC, CMRS
Midstate College

Dr. Azam Rahman, M.D.,
CBCS, CPT, CET,
CPCT, BCLS
Dover Business College

Sheba Schlaikjer, RHIT,
ICD-10 Certification
Colorado Technical
University Campus and
Online

Wendy Schmerse,
Certified Medical
Reimbursement Specialist,
Certified Postsecondary
Instructor
Charter College

Lorraine Schoenbeck, MS,
CMA(AAMA), CAHI
Lone Star College–North
Harris

Wanda D. Strayhan,
CCMA, CBCS, MS
Florida Career College

Patti Sweeney, RN-CBN
Wisconsin Indianhead
Technical College

Marilyn M. Turner, R.N.,
C.M.A. (AAMA)
Ogeechee Technical
College

Anthony Vollmer,
RMA, AS
Dorsey School of Business

William Warner, BSN
Howard College

Kari Williams, DC
Front Range Community
College

Barbara Worley, DPM, BS,
RMA
Kings College

Nancy Worsinger
Nash Community College

Sandra Wright, RMA,
Ph.D.
Atlanta Medical Academy

Carole Zeglin, MS, MT,
RMA
Westmoreland County
Community College

Susan Zolvinski, (CCA)
with AHIMA
Brown Mackie College

Technical Editing/Accuracy Panel

A panel of instructors completed a technical edit and review of all the content in the book page proofs to verify its accuracy.

Stephanie Bernard, AA, CMA, AHI
Sanford-Brown Institute

Debi Kenney, NCMA, NCBCS, AS, Ed.
Harris School of Business

Jan Klawitter, AS in Medical Assisting, CMA (AAMA), and CPC
San Joaquin Valley College

Amy Lawrence, MBA, ACS, AIAA, AIRC, ARA, FLHC, FLMI, HCSA, HIA, HIPAA, MHP, PCS, SILA-F
Ultimate Medical Academy

Barbara Marchelletta, CMA (AAMA), CPC, CPT
Beal College

Barbara Worley, DPM, BS, RMA
Kings College

Acknowledgments from the Authors

To the students and instructors who use this book, your feedback and suggestions have made it a better learning tool for all.

Thank you to the key supplements contributors: Tatyana Pashnyak, Bainbridge College; Terri Gilbert, Medical Careers Institute; and Laura Melendez, Keiser Career College. Thank you to the various reviewers and Melinda Bilecki for providing feedback on those supplements.

Thank you to the instructors who helped with the material for Connect Plus, including Judith Hurtt, East Central Community College; and Sharon Turner, Brookhaven College.

Hats off to the Customer Experience Group at McGraw-Hill for providing outstanding technical assistance to students and instructors. Thank you to Katie Ward for her help on the digital front, as well as Tim Goodell for his guidance and efforts on the simulations. The content production staff was also outstanding; senior designer Srdj Savanovic and designer Matt Backhaus created a terrific updated interior design and fantastic cover design, which was implemented through the production process by Marlena Pechan, project manager; Sandy Ludovissy, senior buyer; and Brent dela Cruz and Cathy Tepper, media project managers.

Cynthia Newby

Appreciation to my new co-author, Nikita Carr, for sharing her insights into the essential administrative skills medical assistants must acquire and helping to guide the revision to ensure careful coverage. Her wisdom and knowledge have been invaluable.

Nikita Carr

Nikita would like to thank the McGraw-Hill team of Natalie Ruffatto, Michelle Flomenhoft, Raisa Kreek, Jessica Dimitrijevic and Roxan Kinsey, and the Chestnut Hill team of co-author Cynthia Newby and Susan Sanderson for their support and encouragement. These guys are such a wonderful group to work with.

Nikita would like to thank her family for their patience during the development of this text. You guys are the best! Thanks for cheering for mom!

A COMMITMENT TO ACCURACY

You have a right to expect an accurate textbook, and McGraw-Hill invests considerabletime and effort to make sure that we deliver one. Listed below are the many steps we take to make sure this happens.

OUR ACCURACY VERIFICATION PROCESS

First Round—Development Reviews

STEP 1: Numerous health professions instructors review the draft manuscript and report on any errors that they may find. The authors make these corrections in their final manuscript.

Second Round—Page Proofs

STEP 2: Once the manuscript has been typeset, the authors check their manuscript against the page proofs to ensure that all illustrations, graphs, examples, and exercises have been correctly laid out on the pages.

STEP 3: An outside panel of peer instructors completes a review of content in the page proofs to verify its accuracy. The authors add these corrections to their review of the page proofs.

STEP 4: A proofreader adds a triple layer of accuracy assurance in pages by looking for errors; then a confirming, corrected round of page proofs is produced.

Third Round—Confirming Page Proofs

STEP 5: The author team reviews the confirming round of page proofs to make certain that any previous corrections were properly made and to look for any errors they might have missed on the first round.

STEP 6: The project manager, who has overseen the book from the beginning, performs another proofread to make sure that no new errors have been introduced during the production process.

Final Round—Printer's Proofs

STEP 7: The project manager performs a final proofread of the book during the printing process, providing a final accuracy review. In concert with the main text, all supplements undergo a proofreading and technical editing stage to ensure their accuracy.

RESULTS

What results is a textbook that is as accurate and error-free as is humanly possible. Our authors and publishing staff are confident that the many layers of quality assurance have produced books that are leaders in the industry for their integrity and correctness. Please view the Acknowledgments section for more details on the many people involved in this process.

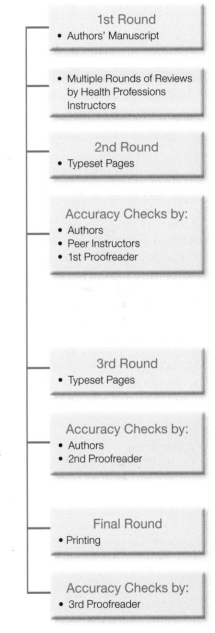

1st Round
- Authors' Manuscript

- Multiple Rounds of Reviews by Health Professions Instructors

2nd Round
- Typeset Pages

Accuracy Checks by:
- Authors
- Peer Instructors
- 1st Proofreader

3rd Round
- Typeset Pages

Accuracy Checks by:
- Authors
- 2nd Proofreader

Final Round
- Printing

Accuracy Checks by:
- 3rd Proofreader

FROM PATIENT TO PAYMENT: UNDERSTANDING MEDICAL INSURANCE

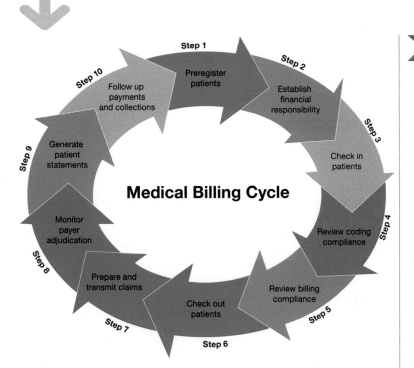

Medical Billing Cycle

- Step 1 — Preregister patients
- Step 2 — Establish financial responsibility
- Step 3 — Check in patients
- Step 4 — Review coding compliance
- Step 5 — Review billing compliance
- Step 6 — Check out patients
- Step 7 — Prepare and transmit claims
- Step 8 — Monitor payer adjudication
- Step 9 — Generate patient statements
- Step 10 — Follow up payments and collections

KEY TERMS

accounts payable (AP)
accounts receivable (AR)
benefits
cash flow
certification
coding
coinsurance
copayment
covered services
deductible
diagnosis
documentation
electronic claim (e-claim)
electronic health record (EHR)
fee-for-service
health care claim
health information technology (HIT)
health plan
indemnity plan
managed care
managed care organization (MCO)
medical assistant
medical billing cycle
medical documentation and billing cycle
medical insurance
medically necessary
noncovered (excluded) services
out-of-pocket
PM/EHR
policyholder
practice management program (PMP)
preauthorization
premium
procedures
provider
remittance advice (RA)
revenue cycle management (RCM)
statement
third-party payer

Learning Outcomes

After studying this chapter, you should be able to:

1.1 Explain how healthy practice finances depend on correctly accomplishing administrative tasks in the medical office.

1.2 Compare coinsurance and copayment requirements for health plan benefits.

1.3 Identify the key steps in the medical billing cycle.

1.4 Discuss the impact of electronic health records on clinical and billing workflow.

1.5 Evaluate the importance of professional certification and of medical liability insurance for career advancement.

Patients who come to physicians' practices for medical care are obligated to pay for the services they receive. Some patients pay these costs themselves, while others have medical insurance to help them cover medical expenses. Administrative staff members help collect the maximum appropriate payments by handling patients' financial arrangements, billing insurance companies, and processing payments to ensure both top-quality service and profitable operation.

1.1 Working with Medical Insurance

The trillion-dollar health care industry—including pharmaceutical companies, hospitals, doctors, medical equipment makers, nursing homes, assisted-living centers, and insurance companies—is a fast-growing and dynamic sector of the American economy.

Spending on health care in the United States continues to rise. Advances in medical technology improve health care delivery but are expensive. Health care reform legislation requires insurance coverage for a growing number of people. Perhaps most importantly, the aging American population requires more health care services. Average life expectancy is increasing and a larger percentage of the population is over age 65. Older people need more health care services than do younger people. Two-thirds of Americans over 65 and three-quarters of those over 80 have multiple chronic diseases, such as diabetes, hypertension, osteoporosis, and arthritis.

Since medical costs are rising faster than the overall economy is growing, more of everyone's dollars are spent on health care. Federal and state government budgets increase to pay for medical services, employers pay more each year for medical services for their employees, and patients also pay higher costs. These rising costs increase the financial pressure on physicians' practices. To remain profitable, physicians must carefully manage the business side of their practices. Knowledgeable administrative medical office employees are in demand to help.

medical assistant Administrative medical employee.

Medical administration tasks in medical offices may be handled by employees who have various educational backgrounds and work experience, such as administrative medical assistants, medical assistants, medical billers, patient services specialists, and receptionists. (In this text, for simplicity, the term **medical assistant** includes all of these administrative medical employees.) Their effective and efficient work is critical for the satisfaction of the patients—the physician's customers—and for the financial success of the practice.

cash flow Movement of monies into or out of a business.

To maintain a regular **cash flow**—the movement of monies into or out of a business—specific tasks must be completed on a regular schedule before, during, and after a patient visit. Managing cash flow means making sure that sufficient monies flow into the practice from patients and insurance companies paying for medical services, referred to as **accounts receivable (AR),** to pay the practice's operating expenses, such as for overhead, salaries, supplies, and insurance—called **accounts payable (AP).** Tracking AR and AP is an accounting job. *Accounting,* often referred to as "the language of business," is a financial information system that records, classifies, reports on, and interprets financial data. Its purpose is to analyze the financial condition of a business following generally accepted accounting principles. The practice accountant sets up accounts such as AR, AP, and Patient Accounts for all aspects of running the practice and then prepares financial statements that show whether the cash flow is adequate. These statements are monitored regularly to see if revenues are sufficient or need improving.

accounts receivable (A/R) Monies owed to a medical practice.

accounts payable (AP) Practice's operating expenses.

revenue cycle management (RCM) Actions that help to ensure the provider receives maximum appropriate payment.

For this reason, **revenue cycle management (RCM)**—acting to ensure that the practice receives all appropriate payments from both insurance companies and patients, and gets them on time—is critical to practice success. Medical assistants have an important role in revenue cycle management. They help to ensure financial success by (1) carefully following procedures, (2) communicating effectively, and (3) using health information technology—medical billing software, electronic health records, Microsoft Office, and the Internet—to improve efficiency and contribute to better health outcomes.

Following Procedures

Medical administrative work requires following a set of procedures. Some procedures involve administrative duties, such as entering data, updating patients' records, and billing insurance companies. Other procedures are done to comply with government regulations, such as keeping computer files secure from unauthorized viewing. In most offices, policy and procedure manuals are available that describe how to perform major duties.

For most procedures, medical assistants work in teams with both licensed medical professionals and other administrative staff members. Providers include physicians and nurses as well as physician assistants (PAs), nurse-practitioners (NPs), clinical social workers, physical therapists, occupational therapists, audiologists, and clinical psychologists. Administrative staff may be headed by an office manager, practice manager, or practice administrator to whom medical assistants, patient services representatives or receptionists, and billing, insurance, and collections specialists report.

Communicating with Physicians and Patients

Communication skills are as important as knowing about specific forms and regulations. Using a pleasant tone, a friendly attitude, and a helpful manner when gathering information increases patient satisfaction. Having interpersonal skills enhances the billing and reimbursement process by establishing professional, courteous relationships with people of different backgrounds and communication styles. Patients may need help with their questions about insurance reimbursement and the health care claim process. Patients also need assistance when problems with payments arise. Effective communicators have the skill of empathy; their actions convey that they understand the feelings of others.

Equally important are effective communications with physicians, other professional staff members, and all members of the administrative team. Conversations must be brief and to the point, showing that the speaker values the provider's time. People are more likely to listen when the speaker is smiling and has an interested expression, so speakers should be aware of their facial expressions and should maintain moderate eye contact. In addition, good listening skills are important.

Using Health Information Technology

Medical assistants use **health information technology (HIT)**—computer hardware and software information systems that record, store, and manage patient information—in almost all physician practices.

Practice Management Programs

A good example of HIT is **practice management programs (PMPs)**, specialized accounting software programs used in almost all medical offices for tracking charges for patients' services and treatments, billing insurance companies and patients, recording payments, and collecting overdue accounts. Most programs also have the ability to schedule patient appointments. Since PMPs can send information electronically, rather than just on paper, cash flow is improved because physicians receive payment in less time than when they send in paper claims and wait for checks to arrive in the mail.

Practice management programs facilitate the day-to-day financial operations of a medical practice. Before PMPs became so universally used, manual accounting systems logged all of this information by hand, a time-consuming and cumbersome process. Now PMPs automate that work, so staff members can work more efficiently and in a timely manner.

Not all medical offices use the same PMP, but most programs operate in a similar manner. Initially, the program is prepared for use by entering basic facts about

health information technology (HIT) Computer information systems that record, store, and manage patient information.

practice management program (PMP) Business software that organizes and stores a medical practice's financial information.

documentation Recording of a patient's health status in a patient medical record.

electronic health record (EHR) Computerized lifelong health care record with data from all sources.

PM/EHR Software program that combines both a PMP and an EHR.

the practice. Often a computer consultant or an accountant helps set up these records. Information about many aspects of the business is entered, including:

▶ *Patient data* Information about each patient, such as name, address, contact numbers, and insurance coverage.
▶ *Provider data* Information about each provider, including facts about providers, referring providers, and outside providers such as labs, radiology, and ambulatory surgery centers.
▶ *Health plan data* Details about the companies that insure the practice's patients.
▶ *Transaction data* The dates of patients' past visits along with records of their illness and treatments, as well as payments collected.

Once the initial setup and data entry are complete, the PMP is ready to be used to accomplish many of the daily tasks of a medical practice.

Electronic Health Records

Another HIT application is rapidly becoming critical in physician practices: electronic health records, or EHRs. While patients' financial records have been electronic for over a decade, clinical records—the **documentation** of a patient's health entered by doctors, nurses, and other health care professionals—until recently, have been stored in paper charts. An **electronic health record (EHR)** is a computerized lifelong health care record for an individual that incorporates data from all sources that provide treatment for the individual. EHR systems are set up to gather patients' clinical information using the computer rather than paper. Most EHR systems are designed to exchange information with—"to talk to"—the PMP and to cut out the need for many paper forms.

PM/EHRs

Some software programs combine both a PMP and an EHR in a single product called an integrated **PM/EHR.** Data entered in either the PMP or the EHR can be used in all applications, such as scheduling, billing, and clinical care. For example, if a receptionist enters basic information about a patient in the electronic health record during the patient's first visit to the practice, that data is automatically available for the medical assistant to use in the billing program. Facts such as the patient's identifying information, type of health insurance, and previous health care records must be entered only once, rather than in both programs. PM/EHRs greatly improve administrative efficiency.

A Note of Caution: What Health Information Technology Cannot Do
Although computers increase efficiency and reduce errors, they are not more accurate than the individual who is entering the data. If people make mistakes while entering data, the information the computer produces will be incorrect. Computers are very precise and also very unforgiving. While the human brain knows that *flu* is short for *influenza*, the computer regards them as two distinct conditions. If a computer user accidentally enters a name as *ORourke* instead of *O'Rourke*, a human might know what is meant; the computer does not. It might respond with the message "No such patient exists in the database."

THINKING IT THROUGH 1.1

1. The Internet is a valuable source of information about many topics of interest to those who will be working in the health care industry. Explore career opportunities by studying the job statistics for medical assistants in the *Occupational Outlook Handbook* of the Bureau of Labor Statistics at www.bls.gov/oco. Based on your research, would you say the prospects were favorable or unfavorable for growth in this profession?

1.2 Paying for Medical Services

People need preventive care, such as routine checkups and vaccinations, to stay healthy. They also need treatment for sicknesses, accidents, and injuries. A person who receives medical care is charged for the medical services and supplies that are involved. To be able to afford the charges, many people in the United States have **medical insurance,** which is an agreement between a person, who is called the **policyholder,** and a **health plan.** Health plans, also called *insurance companies*, are organizations that offer financial protection in case of illness or accidental injury.

There are actually three participants in the medical insurance relationship. The patient (policyholder) is the first party, and the physician is the second party. Legally, a patient–physician contract is created when a physician agrees to treat a patient who is seeking medical services. Through this unwritten contract, the patient is legally responsible for paying for services. The patient may have a policy with a health plan, the third party, which agrees to carry some of the risk of paying for those services and therefore is called a **third-party payer,** often referred to just as a *payer*. The physician usually sends the **health care claim**—a formal insurance claim in either electronic or hard copy format that reports data about the patient and the services provided by the physician—to the payer on behalf of the patient.

medical insurance Financial plan that covers the cost of hospital and medical care.

policyholder Person who buys an insurance plan.

health plan Individual or group plan that provides or pays for medical care.

third-party payer Private or government organization that insures or pays for health care on behalf of beneficiaries.

health care claim Electronic transaction or paper document filed to receive benefits.

Insured versus Noninsured Patients

Medical insurance helps pay for the policyholder's medical treatment. Nearly 250 million people in the United States have medical coverage through commercial payers or are eligible for government programs. Nearly 50 million people—about 16 percent of the population—have no insurance. Many of the uninsured people work for employers that either do not offer health benefits or do not cover certain employees, such as temporary workers or part-time employees. People without insurance are responsible for their own bills without benefit of insurance.

Insurance Basics

A person who buys medical insurance pays a **premium** to a health plan. In exchange for the premium, the health plan agrees to pay amounts, called **benefits,** for medical services. Most health plans require the beneficiary to pay an annual amount called a deductible before they make any payments on the patient's behalf. Medical services include the care supplied by **providers**—hospitals, physicians, and other medical staff members and facilities.

The health plan issues the policyholder an insurance policy that contains a list of **covered services** that is called a schedule of benefits. Benefits commonly include payment of medically necessary medical treatments received by policyholders and their dependents. The Health Insurance Association of America defines the insurance term **medically necessary** as "medical treatment that is appropriate and rendered in accordance with generally accepted standards of medical practice." The place of service must also be appropriate for the diagnosis and care provided. In general, the procedure must meet these conditions to be considered necessary:

premium Money the insured pays to a health plan for a policy.

benefits Health plan payments for covered services.

provider Person or entity that supplies medical or health services and bills for, or is paid for, the services.

covered services Medical procedures and treatments included as benefits in a health plan.

medically necessary Medical treatment that is appropriate and rendered in accordance with generally accepted standards of medical practice.

▶ Procedures or services match the patient's illness.
▶ Procedures are not elective (that is, they are required to treat a condition, rather than being elected to be done by the patient).
▶ Procedures are not experimental. The procedures must be approved by the appropriate federal regulatory agency, such as the Food and Drug Administration.
▶ Procedures are furnished at an appropriate level. Simple diagnoses need simple procedures; complex or time-consuming procedures are reserved for complex conditions.

Typical covered medical services include surgical, primary care, emergency care, and specialists' services. Other medically related expenses, such as hospital-based services,

Table 1.1 Types of Insurance	
Basic Health (Medical)	Covers treatments and procedures other than surgery by providers; may also cover pathology, radiology, and laboratory fees
Major Medical Insurance	Covers expenses resulting from very expensive or prolonged illnesses and injuries
Hospital Insurance	Covers the hospital charges for room, board, and special services
Surgical Insurance	Covers physicians' fees for surgical procedures in medical offices and hospitals
Dental Insurance	Covers dental procedures
Vision Insurance	Pays for costs of eye examinations and glasses/lenses
Liability Insurance	Covers injuries in cars or homes, such as homeowners', business, and automobile policies
Workers Compensation Insurance	State or federal plan that covers medical care and other benefits for job-related illnesses and injuries
Disability Insurance	Covers loss of income resulting from illness
Life Insurance	Pays benefits in the case of the loss of the policyholder's life

noncovered (excluded) services Medical procedures not included in a plan's benefits.

are usually included. Many health plans also cover *preventive* medical services, such as annual physical examinations, pediatric and adolescent immunizations, prenatal care, and routine cancer screening procedures such as mammograms. Policies list treatments that are covered at different rates and medical services that are not covered. For example, a plan may pay 80 percent of most physically related treatments but a smaller percentage of the charges for drugs and medications. The medical insurance policy also describes **noncovered (excluded) services**—what it does not pay for. For example, dental care is generally not included. (However, separate dental insurance plans are available for purchase.) Table 1.1 shows the basic types of insurance that can be bought.

Private Insurance

Private (also known as *commercial*) health plans offer a variety of types of medical insurance coverage. Most people enrolled in private insurance are covered under group contracts—policies that cover people who work for the same employer or belong to the same organization, such as school employees and labor unions. Other plans are offered as individual contracts, which are policies purchased by people who do not qualify as members of a group.

Some employers have established themselves as self-insured health plans. Rather than paying a premium to an insurance carrier, the organization assumes the risk of paying directly for medical services, establishes contracts with local physician practices, and sets up a fund with which it pays for claims. The organization itself establishes the benefit levels and the plan types it will offer.

People may also have medical coverage through their liability insurance and automobile insurance. For example, people injured in automobile accidents may be insured through the medical benefit of their or another party's automobile policy. Coverage varies by state.

Government Plans

The most common government plans in effect in the United States are:

▶ Medicare—Medicare is a federal health plan that covers most citizens aged 65 and over, people with disabilities, end-stage renal disease (ESRD), and dependent widows.

- Medicaid—Individuals with low income who cannot afford medical care are covered by Medicaid, which is cosponsored by federal and state governments. (Medicaid is a state-run program; there are matching federal dollars available for states that satisfy certain requirements, such as providing prenatal care and child vaccinations.) Qualifications and benefits vary by state.
- Workers' Compensation—People with job-related illnesses or injuries are covered under workers' compensation insurance through their employer. Workers' compensation benefits vary according to state law.
- TRICARE—Covers expenses for dependents of active-duty members of the uniformed services and for retired military personnel. It also covers dependents of military personnel who were killed while on active duty.
- CHAMPVA—The Civilian Health and Medical Program of the Department of Veterans Affairs is for the dependents of veterans with permanent service-related disabilities. It also covers surviving spouses and dependent children of veterans who died from service-related disabilities.

Indemnity Plans

In the last century, most medical insurance policies in the United States were **indemnity plans.** Under an indemnity plan, the medical costs policyholders incur when they receive treatment for accidents and illnesses are paid by the insurance carrier. If a policyholder or a covered *dependent* (a spouse, child, or other relative specified in the insurance policy) gets sick, the health plan pays most of the bill. Benefits are determined on a **fee-for-service** basis. In other words, benefits are based on the fees physicians charge for the services.

For each claim, four conditions must be met before the payer makes a payment:

1. The medical charge must be for medically necessary services and covered by the insured's health plan.
2. The insured's payment of the premium must be up-to-date. Unless the premium is current, the insured is not eligible for benefits and the insurance company will not make any payment.
3. If part of the policy, a **deductible**—the amount that the insured pays on covered services before benefits begin—must have been met (paid). Deductibles range widely, usually from $200 to thousands of dollars annually. Higher deductibles generally mean lower premiums.
4. Any **coinsurance**—the percentage of each claim that the insured pays—must be taken into account. The coinsurance rate states the health plan's percentage of the charge, followed by the insured's percentage, such as 80/20. This means that the payer pays 80 percent of the covered amount and the patient pays 20 percent after the premiums and deductibles are paid.

indemnity plan Health plan that offers protection from loss.

fee-for-service Charging method based on each service performed.

deductible Amount the insured must pay for health care services before a health plan's payment begins.

coinsurance Portion of charges an insured person must pay for health care services after the deductible.

The formula is as follows:

$$\text{Charge} - \text{Deductible} - \text{Patient Coinsurance} = \text{Health Plan Payment}$$

Example

An indemnity policy states that the deductible is the first $200 in covered annual medical fees and that the coinsurance rate is 80/20. A patient whose first medical charge of the year was $2,000 would owe $560:

Charge	$2,000
Patient owes the deductible	200
Balance	$1,800
Patient also owes coinsurance (20% of the balance)	$360
Total balance due from patient	$200 + $360 = $560

In this case, the patient must pay an **out-of-pocket** expense of $560 this year before benefits begin. The health plan will pay $1,440, or 80 percent of the balance:

Charge	$2,000
Patient payment	−560
Health plan payment	$1,440

If the patient has already met the annual deductible, the patient's benefits apply to the charge, as in this example:

Charge	$2,000
Patient coinsurance (20%)	−400
Health plan payment (80%)	$1,600 ◄

Managed Care Plans: PPOs, HMOs, and CDHPs

Under indemnity plans, it is difficult for insurance carriers to control costs because there have been few restrictions on providers' charges, especially for new technology, drugs, and procedures. To counter this trend, the concept of **managed care** was introduced. Managed care is a way of supervising medical care with the goal of ensuring that patients get needed services in the most appropriate, cost-effective setting.

To accomplish managed care goals, the financing and management of health care are combined with the delivery of services. **Managed care organizations (MCOs)** establish links among provider, patient, and payer. Instead of only the patient's having a policy with the health plan, under managed care both the patient and the provider have agreements with the MCO. The patient agrees to the payments for the services, and the provider agrees to accept the fees the MCO offers for services. This arrangement gives the managed care plan more control over the services the provider performs and the fees the plan pays.

Managed care is the leading type of health plan, and many different kinds of managed care programs are available. The basic types are introduced below.

Preferred Provider Organizations

The most common type of managed care health plan is a *preferred provider organization (PPO)*. A PPO is a network of providers under contract with a managed care organization to perform services for plan members at discounted fees. Usually, members may choose to receive care from other doctors or providers outside the network, but they pay a higher cost.

Health Maintenance Organizations

Another common type of managed care system is a *health maintenance organization (HMO)*. In one typical arrangement, providers are paid fixed rates at regular intervals, such as monthly, to provide necessary contracted services to patients who are plan members. This fixed payment is referred to as *capitation*.

The rate the provider is paid is based on several factors, including the number of plan members in the insured pool and their ages. The capitated rate per enrollee is paid to the provider even if the provider does not provide any medical services to the patient during the time period covered by the payment. Similarly, the provider receives the same capitated rate if a patient is treated more than once during the time period. In other plans, negotiated per-service fees are paid. These fees are less than the regular rate for a service that the provider normally charges.

Consumer-Driven Health Plans

A *consumer-driven health plan (CDHP)* is a type of managed care insurance in which a high-deductible low-premium insurance plan is combined with a pretax savings account to cover out-of-pocket medical expenses. These plans typically include two elements. The first is an insurance plan, usually a PPO, with a high deductible (such as $2,500), for which the policyholder pays a lower premium than for a plan with a lower deductible.

The second element is a designated health savings account (HSA) that is used to pay medical bills before the deductible has been met. The savings account, similar to an individual retirement account (IRA), lets people set aside untaxed wages to cover their out-of-pocket medical expenses. Some employers contribute to employees' accounts as a benefit. If money is left in the account at the end of a plan year, it rolls over to help cover the next year's health expenses.

Cost Containment

Most health plans, including indemnity plans, now have cost-containment practices to help control costs. For example, patients may be required to choose from a specific group of physicians and hospitals for all medical care. A visit to specialists may require a referral from the patient's primary care physician. A second physician's opinion may be required before surgery can be reimbursed. Also, many services that previously involved overnight hospital stays are now covered only if done during daytime hospital visits, with patients recuperating at home.

In some cases, patients pay fixed premiums at regular time periods, such as monthly. A patient may also pay a **copayment**—a small fixed fee, such as $10, for each office visit. In some plans, this "copay" is a percentage of the amount the provider receives. In either case, the copayment must always be paid by the patient at the time of service. This is considered to encourage patients to use medical services more carefully.

copayment Amount a beneficiary must pay at the time of a health care encounter.

Preauthorization is another example of a cost-containment practice. If preauthorization is required, the health plan must approve a procedure before it is done in order for the procedure to be covered. For example, many nonemergency services must be approved before patients are admitted to the hospital. Also, shorter hospital stays are encouraged, and weekend hospital admissions for Monday services may not be permitted.

preauthorization Prior authorization from a payer for services to be provided.

THINKING IT THROUGH 1.2

1. A patient has a health plan with a 70/30 *coinsurance* requirement. The patient has met the annual deductible for the plan. If today's fees are $800, what amount is billed on a health care claim and what amount does the patient owe?

1.3 The Medical Billing Cycle

It is clear that teamwork is essential in the medical office. The administrative staff members work closely with the professional staff of physicians and nonphysician practitioners. An overall focus is smoothing the way for payments from health plans and from patients. Managing revenue includes much more than entering data in a billing program to complete a health care claim. It requires knowledge of the billing and reimbursement process and the ability to work with a variety of complex insurance plans.

In small physician practices, medical assistants handle a variety of billing and collections tasks. In larger medical practices, duties may be more specialized. Billing, insurance, and collections duties may be separated, or one individual may work exclusively with claims sent to just one of many payers, such as Medicare or workers'

BILLING TIP

Administrative Complexity

The average practice works with nearly twenty different health plans, and some with over eighty of them.

Table 1.2	Steps in the Medical Billing Cycle
Before the encounter	Step 1: Preregister patients
During the encounter	Step 2: Establish financial responsibility Step 3: Check in patients Step 4: Review coding compliance Step 5: Review billing compliance Step 6: Check out patients
After the encounter	Step 7: Prepare and transmit claims Step 8: Monitor payer adjudication Step 9: Generate patient statements Step 10: Follow up payments and collections

compensation. The administrative functions in larger groups or networks are usually headed by a practice manager, office manager, or administrator to whom the administrative staff, such as clinical/administrative medical assistants, transcriptionists, receptionists, accounting personnel, and billers, report.

The physicians and, often, the practice manager determine the medical assistant's administrative job duties. Examples include gathering patient information and signatures, filing health care claims, reviewing payments, and helping patients understand insurance procedures. These medical billing tasks, as shown in Table 1.2 and in the inner circle of Figure 1.2 on page 17, require knowledge of the office workflow relating to claims and skills in using the medical billing program, accurately entering data, and carefully proofreading data.

Step 1: Preregister Patients

medical billing cycle Process that results in timely payment for medical services.

The first step in the **medical billing cycle** is to gather information to preregister patients before their office visits. This information includes

▶ The patient's name.
▶ The patient's contact information; at the minimum, address and phone number.
▶ The patient's reason for the visit, such as a medical complaint or a need for an immunization. (The visit reason is used to calculate an estimated visit length for scheduling appointments, often done at this time as well.)
▶ Whether the patient is new or returning to the practice (different information is gathered in these two situations).

The information is obtained over the telephone or via the Internet, if the practice has a website.

Step 2: Establish Financial Responsibility for Visit

The second step is very important: determine financial responsibility for the visit. For insured patients, these questions must be answered:

▶ What services are covered under the plan? What medical conditions establish medical necessity for these services?
▶ What services are not covered?
▶ What are the billing rules of the plan?
▶ What is the patient responsible for paying?

Knowing the answers to these questions is essential to correctly billing payers for patients' covered services. This knowledge also helps medical assistants ensure that patients will pay their bills when benefits do not apply.

To determine financial responsibility, these procedures are followed:

▶ Verify patients' eligibility for their health plan.
▶ Check the health plan's coverage.
▶ Determine the first payer if more than one health plan covers the patient (this is the payer to whom the first claim will be sent).
▶ Meet payers' conditions for payment, such as preauthorization, ensuring that the correct procedures are followed to meet them.

The practice's financial policy—when bills have to be paid—is explained so that patients understand the medical billing cycle. Patients are told that they are responsible for paying charges that are not covered under their health plans. Uninsured patients are informed of their responsibility for the entire charge. Payment options are presented if the bill will be substantial.

Step 3: Check In Patients

The third step is to check in individuals as patients of the practice. When new patients arrive for their appointments, detailed and complete demographic and medical information is collected at the front desk (the common term for the reception area). Returning patients are asked to review the information that is on file for them, making sure that demographics and medical data are accurate and up-to-date. Their financial records are also checked to see if balances are due from previous visits.

Both the front and back of insurance cards and other identification cards such as driver's licenses are scanned or photocopied and stored in the patient's record. If the health plan requires a copayment, the correct amount is noted for the patient. Copayments should always be collected at the time of service. Some practices collect copayments before the patient's encounter with the physician; others collect them after the visit.

Also, during the office visit, a physician evaluates, treats, and documents a patient's condition. The notes taken at this time include the procedures performed and treatments provided, as well as the physician's determination of the patient's complaint or condition.

Steps 1–3 are covered in Chapters 2 and 3 of this text.

Step 4: Review Coding Compliance

Office visit physician notes contain two very important pieces of information—the **diagnosis,** which is the physician's opinion of the nature of the patient's illness or injury, and the **procedures,** which are the services and treatments performed. When diagnoses and procedures are reported to health plans, code numbers are used in place of descriptions. **Coding** is the process of translating a description of a diagnosis or procedure into a standardized code. Standardization allows information to be shared among physicians, office personnel, health plans, and so on, without losing the precise meaning.

diagnosis Physician's opinion of the nature of the patient's illness or injury.

procedures Services and treatments performed by a practice.

coding Translating a description of a diagnosis or procedure into a standardized code.

Visit Coding

The patient's primary complaint (the illness or condition that is the reason for the visit) is assigned a *diagnosis code* from the International Classification of Diseases (see Chapter 4). Until October 1, 2014, these codes are taken from the International Classification of Diseases, Ninth Revision, Clinical Modification (ICD-9-CM). Beginning on October 1, 2014, the International Classification of Diseases, Tenth Revision, Clinical Modification (ICD-10-CM) will be used for diagnosis coding.

BILLING TIP

ICD-9-CM

Chapter 16, available at the text's Online Learning Center, www. mhhe.com/newbycarr, covers ICD-9-CM coding basics.

Examples of ICD-10-CM Codes

The ICD-10-CM code for Alzheimer's disease is G30.9 [F02.80].

The ICD-10-CM code for influenza with other respiratory manifestations is J11.1. ◄

Similarly, each procedure the physician performs is assigned a *procedure code* that stands for the particular service, treatment, or test. This code is selected from the Current Procedural Terminology (CPT). A large group of codes covers the physician's evaluation and management of a patient's condition during office visits or visits at other locations, such as nursing homes. Other codes cover groups of specific procedures, such as surgery, pathology, and radiology. Yet another group of codes covers supplies and other services.

Examples of CPT Codes

99460 is the CPT code for the physician's examination of a normal newborn infant in a hospital or birthing center.

27130 is the CPT code for a total hip replacement operation. ◄

Visit Data

The physician identifies the patient's diagnoses and procedures. This information is used by the medical assistant after the visit to update the patient's account. The transactions for the visit, which include both the charges and any payment the patient made, are entered in the PMP and the patient's balance is updated. Following is an example of a manual account for one patient's recent series of visits:

Date/Procedure	Charge	Payment	Balance
7/2/16 OV	200.00	200.00	—
7/3/16 OV	150.00		
7/4/16 INS	—	—	150.00
7/13/16 PMT	Insurance	120.00	30.00
7/25/16 STM	—	—	30.00
7/30/16 PMT	Patient	30.00	0.00

This formula is followed to calculate the current balance:

$$\text{Previous Balance} + \text{Charge} - \text{Payment} = \text{Current Balance}$$

In this example, on 7/2 the patient's office visit (OV) resulted in a $200 charge. The patient paid this bill, so there is no current balance. The patient's next office visit, 7/3, resulted in a charge of $150. The medical assistant sent a health care claim to the health plan (INS for insurance) the next day, and the payer paid $120 (PMT) on 7/13. This payment is subtracted from the charge to equal the current balance of $30.

Step 5: Review Billing Compliance

Medical practices bill numerous health plans and government payers. The provider's fees for services are listed on the medical practice's fee schedule. A *fee schedule* is a listing of standard charges for procedures. Each charge, or fee, is related to a specific procedure code. However, the fees listed on the master fee schedule are not necessarily the amount the provider will be paid. Instead, each of the health plans and government payers reimburses the practice according to its own negotiated or government-mandated fee schedule. Many providers enter into contracts with health plans that require a discount from standard fees. In addition, although there is a separate fee associated with each code, each code is not necessarily billable. Whether it can be billed depends on the payer's particular rules. Following these rules when preparing claims results in billing compliance.

Steps 4 and 5 are covered in Chapters 4 and 5 of this text.

Step 6: Check Out Patients

Checkout is the last step that occurs while the patient is still in the office. The medical codes have been assigned and checked, and the amounts to be billed have also been verified according to payers' rules. The charges for the visit are calculated, and payment for these types of charges is usually collected at time of service:

> Previous balances
>
> Copayments
>
> Coinsurance
>
> Noncovered or overlimit fees
>
> Charges of nonparticipating providers
>
> Charges for self-pay patients
>
> Deductibles for patients with certain types of health plans
>
> Billing for supplies

A receipt is prepared for the payments made by the patients, and follow-up work is scheduled as ordered by the physician.

Step 6 is covered in Chapter 6 of this text.

Step 7: Prepare and Transmit Claims

A major step in the medical billing cycle is the preparation of accurate, timely health care claims. Most practices prepare claims for their patients and send them electronically; these are **electronic claims** or **e-claims.** A claim communicates information about the diagnosis, procedures, and charges to a payer. The practice has a schedule for transmitting claims, such as daily or every other day, which is followed. When a patient is covered by more than one health plan, the second and any other plans must be sent claims after the primary payer sends a payment on the account.

electronic claim (e-claim)
Health care claim sent electronically.

General information on claims is found in Chapter 7. Chapters 8 through 12 explain how to prepare correct claims for each major payer group:

► Private payers/Blue Cross and Blue Shield
► Medicare
► Medicaid
► TRICARE and CHAMPVA
► Workers' compensation and disability/liability insurance

A related topic, hospital billing, is covered in Chapter 14.

Step 7 is covered in Chapters 7–12 of this text.

Step 8: Monitor Payer Adjudication

When the payer receives the claim, it goes through a series of steps designed to determine whether the claim should be paid, a process called *adjudication*. Claims may be paid in full, partially paid, or denied. Payments from insurance companies are listed on a remittance advice, which is sent to the provider along with the payment. The **remittance advice (RA)** lists the transactions included on the claims, states the amount billed and the amount paid, and provides an explanation of why certain charges were not paid in full or were denied entirely. The remittance advice provides details about each patient transaction, such as

remittance advice (RA)
Health plan document describing a payment resulting from a claim adjudication.

► Date of service
► Services provided
► Patient name and control number
► Provider identifier number
► Amount allowed by contract
► Amount paid to provider
► Amount owed by patient

When the RA arrives at the provider's office, it is reviewed for accuracy by the medical assistant, who compares each payment and explanation with the claim to check that:

▶ All procedures that were listed on the claim also appear on the payment transaction.
▶ Any unpaid charges are explained.
▶ The codes on the payment transactions match those on the claim.
▶ The payment listed for each procedure is as expected.

If any discrepancies are found, a request for a review of the claim is filed with the payer. If no issues are discovered, the amount of the payment is recorded in the PMP program. The payment is usually an electronic payment transmitted from the payer to the practice's bank, called an *electronic funds transfer (EFT)*, or, occasionally, a paper check that must be deposited. Depending on the rules of the health plan, the patient may be billed for an outstanding balance. In other circumstances, an adjustment is made and the patient is not billed. Occasionally, an overpayment may be received, and a refund check is issued by the medical practice.

Step 9: Generate Patient Statements

statement Shows services provided to a patient, total payments made, total charges, adjustments, and balance due.

Payers' payments are applied to the appropriate patients' accounts and patient **statements** are generated. In most cases, payer payments do not fully pay the bills, and patients will be billed for the rest. The amount paid by all payers (the primary insurance and any other insurance) plus the amount to be billed to the patient should equal the expected fee. Bills that are mailed to patients list the dates and services provided, any payments made by the patient and the payer, and the balances now due.

Step 10: Follow Up Patient Payments and Collections

Practice management programs (PMPs) are used to track accounts receivable (AR) and to produce financial reports that are used to manage the revenue cycle by following up on late or reduced payments.

Day Sheets

One key report is a day sheet, produced at the end of each day. This report lists all charges, payments, and adjustments that occurred during that day for each patient (see Figure 1.1). To balance out a day, all transactions and totals from bank deposit entries are compared against an end-of-day report.

Monthly Report

A monthly report summarizes the financial activity of the entire month. This report lists charges, payments, adjustments, and the total accounts receivable for the month. It is possible to balance out the month by totaling the daily charges, payments, and adjustments and then comparing the totals to the amounts listed on the monthly report.

Outstanding Balances

It is also good practice to print reports that list the outstanding balances owed to the practice by insurance companies and by patients. Regularly printing and reviewing the reports can alert medical assistants to accounts that require action to collect the amount due. A collection process is often started when patient payments are later than permitted under the practice's financial policy.

Overdue accounts require diligent follow-up to maintain the practice's cash flow. Insurance claims that are not paid in a timely manner also require follow-up to determine the reason for the nonpayment and to resubmit or appeal as appropriate.

Steps 8, 9, and 10 are covered in Chapter 13 of this text.

Orchard Hill Medical Center
Patient Day Sheet
Show all data where the Date From is between 9/6/2016, 9/6/2016

Entry	Date	Document	POS	Description	Provider	Code	Amount
FITZWJO0		**Fitzwilliams, John**					
380	09/06/2016	1009070000	11		2	CHVCPAY	-15.00
471	09/06/2016	0506020000	11		2	99211	36.00
472	09/06/2016	0506020000	11		2	84478	29.00
				Patient Charges	Patient Receipts	Adjustments	Patient Balance
				$65.00	-$15.00	$0.00	$50.00
FITZWSA0		**Fitzwilliams, Sarah**					
563	09/06/2016	1010040000	11		1	90471	15.00
565	09/06/2016	1009070000	11		1	90703	29.00
566	09/06/2016	1009070000	11		1	CHVCPAY	-15.00
				Patient Charges	Patient Receipts	Adjustments	Patient Balance
				$44.00	-$15.00	$0.00	$29.00
GARDIJO0		**Gardiner, John**					
385	09/06/2016	1009070000	11		1	99211	36.00
387	09/06/2016	1009070000	11		1	OHCCPAY	-20.00
				Patient Charges	Patient Receipts	Adjustments	Patient Balance
				$36.00	-$20.00	$0.00	$0.00
KLEINRA0		**Klein, Randall**					
388	09/06/2016	1009070000	11		2	99212	54.00
389	09/06/2016	1009070000	11		2	29540	121.50
390	09/06/2016	1009070000	11		2	99070	20.00
				Patient Charges	Patient Receipts	Adjustments	Patient Balance
				$195.50	$0.00	$0.00	$0.00

FIGURE 1.1 Sample Page from a Patient Day Sheet Report

THINKING IT THROUGH 1.3

1. In your opinion, is each of the following procedures likely to be considered medically necessary by a payer's health care claims examiner? Why?

   A. Diagnosis: deviated septum
   Procedure: nasal surgery

   B. Diagnosis: mole on a female patient's cheek, questionable nature
   Procedure: surgical removal and biopsy

   C. Diagnosis: male syndrome hair loss
   Procedure: implant hair plugs on scalp

   D. Diagnosis: probable broken wrist
   Procedure: comprehensive full-body examination, with complete set of lab tests, chest X-ray, and ECG

1.4 Using PM/EHRs: The Integrated Medical Documentation and Billing Cycle

Every time a patient is treated by a health care provider, documentation of the visit is created. This chronological medical record, or chart, includes information that the patient provides, such as medical history, as well as the physician's assessment, diagnosis, and treatment plan. Records also contain laboratory test results, X-rays and other diagnostic images, a list of medications prescribed, and reports that indicate the results of operations and other medical procedures. They contain information from a number of different physicians as well as from pharmacies, laboratories, hospitals, insurance carriers, and so on. Patients today use several providers to meet their health care needs, and each physician maintains a separate medical record for each patient. Unless the patient volunteers information, providers do not know whether the patient is being treated by another physician or what medications might have been prescribed. With an EHR, information is added to the record by health care professionals working in a variety of settings, and the record can be accessed by other professionals when needed.

Features of EHRs

While paper and electronic health records serve many of the same purposes, the electronic record is much more than a computerized version of a paper record. The Institute of Medicine has suggested that an EHR should include eight core functions (*Key Capabilities of an Electronic Health Record System*, 2003):

1. Health information and data elements
2. Results management
3. Order management
4. Decision support
5. Electronic communication and connectivity
6. Patient support
7. Administrative support
8. Population reporting and management

Electronic health records also save valuable time for health care providers by reducing the time needed to enter information about patients. Currently, physicians spend almost 40 percent of their time documenting patient cases. EHRs provide tools that make documentation more efficient, such as entering notes by typing or voice recognition, or completing templates during the patient examination.

With EHRs, physicians are finished entering notes when the patient leaves the examination room or shortly after. Nurses and medical assistants record information directly into the computer, so there is no need to copy information to a paper chart. EHRs also

▶ Improve the overall efficiency of the workflow.
▶ Speed the delivery of diagnostic test results to the physician and the patient through electronic transmission.
▶ Allow two or more people to work with a patient's record at the same time.
▶ Eliminate the need to search for a misplaced or lost patient chart.
▶ Reduce the time it takes to refill a prescription through electronic prescribing.
▶ Organize all information in one place, including in-house messages, telephone messages, requests for information, and referral letters.
▶ Enable physicians to receive payment for services more quickly because patient visit information is automatically transferred to the billing software.

Integrated Workflow

The increased use of electronic health records in physician practices has changed office workflow. In a medical office, a flow of work must be in place that provides medical care to patients and collects payment for these services. When integrated PM/EHRs are used, previous paper-based tasks, such as pulling file folders and making photocopies, are replaced by efficient electronic processes.

medical documentation and billing cycle Combination of the billing cycle and medical documentation cycle of a practice.

The **medical documentation and billing cycle** explains how using EHRs is integrated with practice management programs as the 10-step billing process is performed. This cycle is illustrated in Figure 1.2. The inner circle represents the billing cycle, as explained in the previous section; the outer circle contains the medical documentation cycle.

Medical Documentation and Billing Cycle

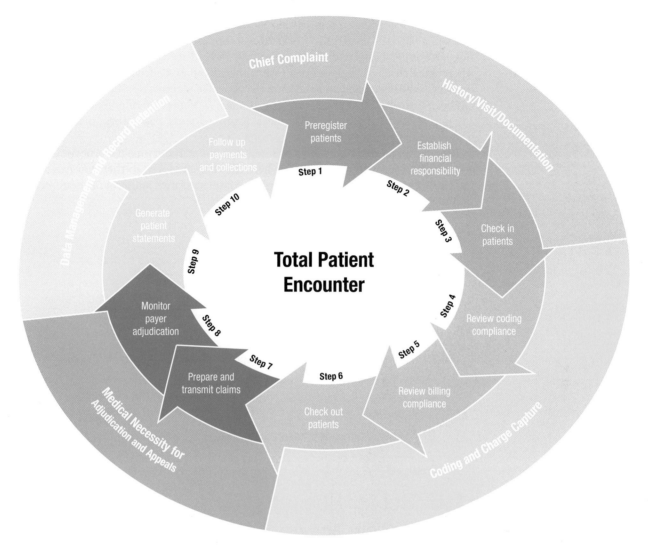

FIGURE 1.2 The Medical Documentation and Billing Cycle

As the illustration shows, the two cycles are interrelated. For example, during preregistration, a new patient phones for an appointment. Both billing and clinical information must be collected during the phone call. From a billing perspective, the office wants to know whether the patient has insurance that will cover some or all of the cost of the visit, or whether the patient will pay for the visit. From a health or medical perspective, the staff wants to know the reason the person needs to see the doctor, known as the *chief complaint*.

Following the billing steps that establish financial responsibility and handle check-in, the professional medical staff gather clinical information. Often, a medical assistant measures and inputs vital signs, such as the patient's temperature, pulse, respirations, and blood pressure, as well as height and weight, in the EHR. The physician then documents the results of the physical examination, relevant history, and planned treatments.

As the medical documentation and billing cycle continues, so does the interaction between the two types of information. The physician or a medical coder assigns medical codes to the patient's diagnosis and procedures, and the charges for those procedures are determined. Based on this information, the biller reviews coding and billing compliance, after which the patient is checked out. When the biller then prepares and transmits claims, documentation may be studied to support medical necessity during claim creation and later during adjudication, if a payer requires it. During the steps of claim follow-up, patients' statements, and payment and collections, on the documentation side, the process of managing and retaining patient data according to regulations is carried out.

Even a partially electronic workflow is more efficient than a paper-based workflow. In a paper-based workflow, the coding and billing process normally takes anywhere from three to 14 days. As a result, there is an extended lag between the time the service was provided and the time the provider receives reimbursement. Also, it has been estimated that physicians lose as much as 10 percent of potential revenue as a result of forgetting to bill for services, losing patients' paperwork, making errors when preparing claims, and other reasons.

Medical assistants become knowledgeable about the connection between PMs and EHRs in the medical practices where they are employed so that they can access the clinical information they need as they complete claims and provide documentation in support of their medical necessity.

THINKING IT THROUGH 1.4

1. Which program, a PMP or an EHR, do you think would handle each of the following tasks?

A. The medical assistant verifies and documents a patient's medications and allergies during an examination.

B. A patient's payment of coinsurance is entered.

C. A physician enters needed prescriptions and orders tests following a patient's examination.

D. A medical assistant sends a claim for the encounter to the patient's health plan.

E. A payment from the health plan is received via EFT and checked.

1.5 Set for Success

Personal Skills and Attributes

A number of skills and attributes are required for successful mastery of the tasks of a medical assistant.

Skills

▶ *Knowledge of medical terminology, anatomy, physiology, and medical coding:* Medical assistants must analyze physicians' descriptions of patients' conditions and treatments and relate these descriptions to the systems of diagnosis and procedure codes used in the health care industry.

▶ *Communication skills:* The job of a medical assistant requires excellent communication skills, both oral and written. For example, patients often need explanations of insurance benefits or clarification of instructions such as how to obtain referrals. Courteous, helpful answers to questions strongly influence patients' desire to continue to use the practice's services. Memos, letters, the telephone, and e-mail are used to research and follow up on changes in health plans' billing rules. These skills also are needed to send claim attachments that explain special conditions or treatments to obtain maximum reimbursement from payers, and to create and send effective collection letters.

▶ *Attention to detail:* Many aspects of the job involve paying close attention to detail, such as correctly completing health care claims, filing patients' medical records, recording preauthorization numbers, calculating the correct payments, and posting payments for services.

- *Flexibility:* Working in a changing environment requires the ability to adapt to new procedures, multitask to handle varying kinds of problems and interactions during a busy day, and work successfully with different types of people with various cultural backgrounds.
- *Health information technology (HIT) skills:* Most medical practices use computers to handle billing and to process claims. Many also use computers to keep patients' medical records. General computer literacy, including a working knowledge of (1) the Microsoft Windows operating system, (2) Microsoft office, (3) a PMP, and (4) Internet-based research, is essential. Data-entry skills are also necessary. Many human errors occur during data entry, such as pressing the wrong key on the keyboard. Other errors are a result of a lack of computer literacy—not knowing how to use a program to accomplish tasks. For this reason, proper training in data-entry techniques so that errors are caught, as well as knowing how to use computer programs, are both essential for medical assistants.
- *Honesty and integrity:* Medical assistants work with patients' medical records and with finances. It is essential to maintain the confidentiality of patient information and communications, as well as to act with integrity when handling these tasks.
- *Ability to work as a team member:* Patient service is a team effort. To do their part, medical assistants are cooperative and focus on the best interests of patients and the practice.

Attributes

A number of attributes are also very important for success as a medical assistant. Most have to do with the quality of professionalism, which is key to getting and keeping employment. These factors include:

- Appearance: A neat, clean, professional appearance increases confidence in your skills and abilities. Being well-groomed, with clean hair, nails, and clothing, presents a businesslike demeanor to patients and other staff members.
- Attendance: Being on time for work demonstrates that you are reliable and dependable.
- Initiative: Being able to start a course of action and stay on task is an important quality to demonstrate.
- Courtesy: Treating patients and fellow workers with dignity and respect is an interpersonal quality that helps build good professional relationships at work.

Ethics and Etiquette in the Medical Office

Licensed medical staff members and other employees working in physicians' practices share responsibility for observing a code of ethics and for following correct etiquette.

Ethics

Medical *ethics* are standards of behavior requiring truthfulness, honesty, and integrity. Ethics guide the behavior of physicians, who have the training, the primary responsibility, and the legal right to diagnose and treat human illnesses and injuries. All medical office employees and those working in health-related professions share responsibility for observing the ethical code.

Each professional organization has a code of ethics that is to be followed by its members. In general, this code states that information about patients, other employees, and confidential business matters should not be discussed with anyone not directly concerned with them. Behavior should be consistent with the values of the profession. For example, it is unethical for an employee to take money or gifts from a company in exchange for giving them business.

Etiquette

Professional *etiquette* is also important for medical assistants. Correct behavior in the office is generally covered in the practice's employee policy and procedure manual.

For example, guidelines establish which types of incoming calls must go immediately to a physician or to a nurse or assistant, and which require a message to be taken.

Certification and Continuing Education

Completion of a medical insurance specialist program, coding specialist program, or medical assisting or health information technology program at a postsecondary institution provides an excellent background for many types of positions in the medical insurance field. Another possibility is to earn an associate degree or a certificate of proficiency by completing a program in a curriculum area such as health care business services. Further baccalaureate and graduate study enables advancement to managerial positions.

Moving ahead in a career is often aided by membership in professional organizations that offer certification in various areas. **Certification** by a professional organization provides evidence to prospective employers that the applicant has demonstrated a superior level of skill on a national test. Certification is the process of earning a credential through a combination of education and experience followed by successful performance on a national examination.

certification Recognition of a superior level of skill by an official organization.

CMA

American Association of Medical Assistants
20 N. Wacker Drive, Suite 1575
Chicago, IL 60606-2903
312-899-1500
www.aama-natl.org

RMA

American Medical Technologists
10700 West Higgins, Suite 150
Rosemont, IL 60018
847-823-5169
www.AmericanMedTech.org

RHIT, RHIA, CCS, CCS-P, CCS-A

American Health Information Management Association (AHIMA)
233 N. Michigan Ave., Suite 2150
Chicago, IL 60601-5809
800-335-5535
www.ahima.org

CPC, CPC-H, CPC, CPC-A

American Academy of Professional Coders
2480 South 3850 West, Suite B
Salt Lake City, Utah 84120
800-626-2633
www.aapc.com

Medical Assisting Certification

Two organizations offer tests in the professional area of medical assisting. After earning a diploma in medical assisting from an accredited school (or having a year's work experience for the RMA only), medical assistants may sit for the Certified Medical Assistant (CMA) titles from the American Association of Medical Assistants or the Registered Medical Assistant (RMA) designation from the American Medical Technologists.

Health Information Certification

Students who are interested in the professional area of health information (also known as medical records) may complete an associate degree from an accredited college program and pass a credentialing test to be certified as a Registered Health Information Technician, or RHIT. An RHIT examines medical records for accuracy, reports patient data for reimbursement, and helps with information for medical research and statistical data.

Also offered is the Registered Health Information Administrator (RHIA), requiring a baccalaureate degree and national certification. RHIAs are skilled in the collection, interpretation, and analysis of patient data. Additionally, they receive the training necessary to assume managerial positions related to these functions. RHIAs interact with all levels of an organization—clinical, financial, and administrative—that use patient data in decision making and everyday operations.

Coding Certification

Medical coders are expert in classifying medical data. They assign codes to physicians' descriptions of patients' conditions and treatments. For employment as a medical coder, employers typically prefer—or may require—certification. AHIMA offers three coding certifications: the Certified Coding Associate (CCA), intended as a starting point for entering a new career as a coder; the Certified Coding Specialist (CCS); and the Certified Coding Specialist-Physician-based (CCS-P). The American Academy of Professional Coders (AAPC) grants the Certified Professional Coder (CPC); the CPC-A, an apprentice level for those who do not yet have medical coding work experience; and a number of advanced specialty coding certifications.

Continuing Education

Most professional organizations require certified members to keep up-to-date by taking annual training courses to refresh or extend their knowledge. Continuing education sessions are assigned course credits by the credentialing organizations, and satisfactory completion of a test on the material is often required for credit. Employers often approve attendance at seminars that apply to the practice's goals and ask the person who attends to update other staff members.

Medical Liability Insurance

Because of the risk of liability, medical practices must be sure that treatment and billing rules are followed by all staff members. In addition to responsibility for their own actions, physicians are liable for the professional actions of employees they supervise. This responsibility is a result of the law of *respondeat superior*, which states that an employer is responsible for an employee's actions. Physicians are held to this doctrine, so they can be charged for the fraudulent behavior of any staff member.

Medical liability cases for fraud often result in lawsuits. Physicians purchase professional liability insurance to cover such legal expenses. Although they are covered under the physician's policy, other medical professionals often purchase their own liability insurance. Those who perform clinical or administrative tasks are advised to have professional liability insurance called error and omission (E&O) insurance, which protects against financial loss due to intentional or unintentional failure to perform work correctly.

THINKING IT THROUGH 1.5

1. Why is it important for administrative medical office employees to become certified in their area of expertise? At this point, what are your personal goals relating to certification?

Chapter Summary

Learning Outcomes	Key Concepts/Examples
1.1 Explain how healthy practice finances depend on correctly accomplishing administrative tasks in the medical office. Pages 2–3	• Cash flow must be monitored and managed to make sure that sufficient money comes into the practice from patients and insurance companies. • To remain profitable physicians must carefully manage the business side of their practice by employing knowledgeable administrative medical office employees. • Medical assistants ensure financial success by carefully following procedures, communicating effectively, and using health information technology to improve efficiency.
1.2 Compare coinsurance and copayment requirements for health plan benefits. Pages 3–9	• Insurance is based on one of two types of plans, indemnity and managed care. • Coinsurance, the amount that the payer and the insured pay on a claim, is based on a percentage. • Copayment, the fixed amount that the patient pays, must always be paid at the time of service.
1.3 Identify the key steps in the medical billing cycle. Pages 9–15	• The ten steps in the billing cycle are 1. Preregister patients 2. Establish financial responsibility for visits 3. Check in patients 4. Review coding compliance 5. Review billing compliance 6. Check out patients 7. Prepare and transmit claims 8. Monitor payer adjudication 9. Generate patient statements 10. Follow up patient payments and handle collections

Learning Outcomes	Key Concepts/Examples
1.4 Discuss the impact of electronic health records on clinical and billing workflow. Pages 15–18	• Improve the overall efficiency of workflow. • Speed the delivery of diagnostic test results to the physician and the patient. • Allow two or more people to work with a patient's record at the same time. • Eliminate the need to search for a misplaced or lost patient chart. • Reduce the time it takes to refill a prescription. • Organize all information in one place. • Enable physicians to receive payment for services quickly.
1.5 Evaluate the importance of professional certification and of medical liability insurance for career advancement. Pages 18–21	• Certification by a professional organization provides evidence to prospective employers that an applicant has demonstrated a superior level of skill. • Professional liability insurance can protect administrative and clinical medical assistants against financial loss due to intentional or unintentional failure to perform work correctly.

Using Terminology

Match the key terms in the left column with the definitions in the right column.

_____ 1. **[LO 1.2]** Third-party payer

_____ 2. **[LO 1.2]** Copayment

_____ 3. **[LO 1.2]** Managed care

_____ 4. **[LO 1.1]** Accounts receivable (AR)

_____ 5. **[LO 1.2]** Indemnity plan

_____ 6. **[LO 1.2]** Coinsurance

_____ 7. **[LO 1.2]** Premium

_____ 8. **[LO 1.2]** Benefits

_____ 9. **[LO 1.2]** Deductible

_____ 10. **[LO 1.2]** Fee-for-service

A. Monies owed to a medical practice by its patients and third-party payers.

B. The amount of money a health plan pays for services covered in an insurance policy.

C. The portion of charges that an insured person must pay for health care services after payment of the deductible amount; usually stated as a percentage.

D. An amount that a health plan requires a beneficiary to pay at the time of service for each health care encounter.

E. An amount that an insured person must pay, usually on an annual basis, for health care services before a health plan's payment begins.

F. Method of charging under which a provider's payment is based on each service performed.

G. Type of medical insurance that reimburses a policyholder for medical services under the terms of its schedule of benefits.

H. System that combines financing and the delivery of appropriate, cost-effective health care services to its members.

I. Money the insured pays to a health plan for a health care policy.

J. Private or government organization that insures or pays for health care on the behalf of beneficiaries.

Checking Your Understanding

Write the letter of the choice that best completes the statement or answers the question.

1. **[LO 1.1]** Monies used by the physician practice to pay for operating expenses such as salaries, supplies, and utilities are called _____.
   - **A.** Accounts receivable
   - **B.** Accounts payable
   - **C.** Purchase order
   - **D.** Accounting

2. **[LO 1.1]** Which of the following data is stored in a practice management program? _____
   - **A.** Transaction data
   - **B.** Provider data
   - **C.** Health plan data
   - **D.** All of these

3. **[LO 1.1]** A system used to gather a patient's clinical information is a(n) _____.
   - **A.** Practice management program
   - **B.** Revenue cycle management
   - **C.** Electronic health record
   - **D.** Electronic claim

4. **[LO 1.2]** Participants in the medical insurance relationship include _____.
   - **A.** Provider
   - **B.** Patient
   - **C.** Health plan
   - **D.** All of these

5. **[LO 1.2]** Health plans pay for _____ services.
   - **A.** Indemnity
   - **B.** Covered
   - **C.** Coded
   - **D.** Out-of-network

6. **[LO 1.2]** Coinsurance is calculated based on _____.
   - **A.** The number of policyholders in a plan
   - **B.** A fixed charge for each visit
   - **C.** A capitation rate
   - **D.** A percentage of a charge

7. **[LO 1.2]** The major government-sponsored health programs are _____.
   - **A.** Medicare, Medicaid, TRICARE, and CHAMPVA
   - **B.** HEDIS, Medicare, Medicaid, and CHAMPUS
   - **C.** Blue Cross and Blue Shield
   - **D.** Medicare, Medicaid, and Coventry

8. **[LO 1.3]** If a patient's payment is later than permitted under the financial policy of the practice, the _____ may be started.
   - **A.** Copayment process
   - **B.** Appeal process
   - **C.** Coding process
   - **D.** Collection process

9. **[LO 1.3]** When a patient has insurance coverage for which the practice will create a claim, the patient bill is usually done _____.
   - **A.** Before the patient encounter
   - **B.** During the patient encounter
   - **C.** After the health claim has been transmitted and the payer's payment is posted
   - **D.** When the health claim is transmitted

10. **[LO 1.5]** Insurance that protects against financial loss as a result of unintentional failed work performance is _____.
    - **A.** Errors and omissions
    - **B.** Workers' compensation
    - **C.** Medical liability
    - **D.** Workplace insurance

Define the following abbreviations:

1. **[LO 1.1]** AP _____
2. **[LO 1.1]** AR _____
3. **[LO 1.1]** EHR _____
4. **[LO 1.1]** HIT _____
5. **[LO 1.2]** MCO _____
6. **[LO 1.1]** PM _____
7. **[LO 1.3]** RA _____
8. **[LO 1.1]** RCM _____

Answer the following questions:

1. **[LO 1.3]** List the ten steps in the billing cycle.

2. **[LO 1.5]** List at least four important skills of a medical assistant.

Applying Your Knowledge

Case 1.1   Abstracting Insurance Information

A patient shows the following insurance identification card to the medical assistant.

Connecticut HealthPlan

I.D.#:	1002.9713
Employee:	DANIEL ANTHONY
Group #:	A0000323
Eff. date:	03/01/2016
Status:	Dependent Coverage? F
In-network:	$10 Co-Pay
Out-of-network:	$250 Ded; 80%/20%

Front of card

IMPORTANT INFORMATION
Notice to Members and Providers of Care

To avoid a reduction in your hospital benefits, you are responsible for obtaining certification for hospitalization and emergency admissions. The review is required regardless of the reason for hospital admission. For specified procedures, Second Surgical Opinions may be mandatory.
For certification, call Utilization Management Services at 800-837-8808:
• At least 7 days in advance of Scheduled Surgery of Hospital Admissions.
• Within 48 hours after Emergency Admissions or on the first business day following weekend or holiday Emergency Admissions.

CONNECTICUT HEALTHPLAN C/O

WEISS   Robert S. Weiss
& Company
Silver Hill Business Center
500 S. Broad Street
P.O. Box 1034
Meriden, CT 06450
(800) 466-7900

THIS CARD IS FOR IDENTIFICATION ONLY AND DOES NOT ESTABLISH ELIGIBILITY FOR COVERAGE BY CONNECTICUT HEALTH PLAN. Please refer to your insurance booklet for further details.

Back of card

A. [LO 1.2] What copayment is due when the patient sees a network physician?

B. [LO 1.2] What payment rules apply when the patient sees an out-of-network physician?

C. [LO 1.2] What rules apply when the patient needs to be admitted to the hospital?

Case 1.2   Calculating Insurance Math

Calculate the payment(s) billed in each of the following situations.

A. [LO 1.2] The patient's health plan has a $100 annual deductible. At the first visit of the year, the charges are $95. What does the patient owe?

B. [LO 1.2] The patient's coinsurance percentage is stated as 75-25 in the insurance policy. The deductible for the year has been met. If the visit charges are $1,000, what payment should the medical assistant expect from the payer? What amount will the patient be billed?

C. [LO 1.2] The patient's coinsurance percentage is stated as 80-20 in the insurance policy. The deductible for the year has been met. If the visit charges are $420, what payment should the medical assistant expect from the payer? What amount will the patient be billed?

D. [LO 1.2] The patient is enrolled in a capitated HMO with a $10 copayment for primary care physician visits and no coinsurance requirements. After collecting $10 from the patient, what amount can the medical assistant bill the payer for an office visit?

E. [LO 1.2] The patient has a policy that requires a $20 copayment for an in-network visit, due at the time of service. The policy also requires 30 percent coinsurance from the patient. Today's visit charges total $785. After subtracting the copayment collected from the patient, the medical assistant expects a payment of what amount from the payer? What amount will the patient be billed?

connect plus+

Enhance your learning at mcgrawhillconnect.com!
• Practice Exercises   • Worksheets
• Activities   • Integrated eBook

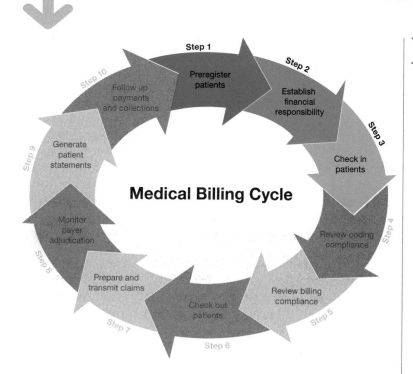

KEY TERMS

abuse
Affordable Care Act (ACA)
audit
authorization
breach
breach notification
business associate (BA)
Centers for Medicare and Medicaid Services (CMS)
clearinghouse
code set
compliance plan
covered entity (CE)
designated record set (DRS)
electronic data interchange (EDI)
encounter
encryption
fraud
Health Insurance Portability and Accountability Act (HIPAA) of 1996
Health Information Technology for Economic and Clinical Health (HITECH) Act
HIPAA Electronic Health Care Transactions and Code Sets (TCS)
HIPAA Privacy Rule
HIPAA Security Rule
medical records
medical standards of care
minimum necessary standard
National Provider Identifier (NPI)
Notice of Privacy Practices (NPP)
Office for Civil Rights (OCR)
Office of E-Health Standards and Services (OESS)
Office of the Inspector General (OIG)
password
protected health information (PHI)
retention schedule
transaction
treatment, payment, and health care operations (TPO)

Learning Outcomes

After studying this chapter, you should be able to:

2.1 Explain the importance of accurate documentation when working with medical records.

2.2 Compare the major regulations affecting patient records in medical offices.

2.3 Discuss the purpose of the HIPAA Privacy Rule.

2.4 Briefly state the purpose of the HIPAA Security Rule and the HITECH Breach Notification Rule.

2.5 Describe the HIPAA Electronic Health Care Transactions and Code Sets Standards.

2.6 Explain how to guard against potentially fraudulent situations.

2.7 Discuss the purpose of compliance plans.

Medical assistants work with important clinical data as well as demographic data. Health plans need patient clinical information to assess the medical necessity of claims sent for payment. Other physicians need to know the results of tests and examinations patients have already had to provide the right level of care. Keeping all this patient data safe and secure is the job of everyone on the health care team. But it is no longer a job of managing stacks of paper files. Like shopping, buying tickets, banking and sharing photos online, health care records are moving to a digital platform. Working in this environment requires knowledge of electronic health records and of the federal rules that regulate access to them.

2.1 Medical Records and the Need for Accurate Documentation

medical records Files containing the documentation of a patient's medical history and related information.

Patients' **medical records** contain all facts, findings, and observations about their health history. The medical record also contains all communications with and about the patient. The medical record in the medical office begins with a patient's first contact and continues through all treatments and services. The record provides continuity and communication among physicians and other health care professionals who are involved in a patient's care. Patient medical records are also used in research and for education.

Patient medical records are legal documents. Physicians own the physical record (although patients own the information about themselves), and properly documented patient care is part of a physician's defense against accusations that patients were not treated correctly. Medical records should clearly state who performed what service and describe why, where, when, and how it was done. Physicians document the rationale behind their treatment decisions. This rationale is the basis for the proof of medical necessity to payers—establishing a clinically logical link between a patient's condition and the treatment provided. For example, when a test or drug is ordered for a patient, the physician documents the diagnosis or condition that is being confirmed or ruled out.

Documentation Standards and Content

medical standards of care State-specified performance measures for the delivery of health care.

encounter Office visit between a patient and a medical professional.

Documentation means organizing a patient's medical record in chronological order using a systematic, logical, and consistent method. A patient's health history, examinations, tests, and results of treatments are all documented. Complete and comprehensive documentation is important to show that physicians have followed the **medical standards of care** that apply in their state. Health care providers are liable (that is, legally responsible) for providing this level of care to their patients. The term *medical professional liability* describes this responsibility of licensed health care professionals.

Every patient **encounter**—the face-to-face meeting between a patient and a provider in a medical office, clinic, hospital, or other location—should be documented with the following information:

▶ Patient's name
▶ Encounter date and reason
▶ Appropriate history and physical examination, such as the patients' vital signs
▶ Review of all tests that were ordered
▶ Diagnosis
▶ Plan of care, or notes on procedures or treatments that were given
▶ Instructions or recommendations that were given to the patient
▶ Signature of the provider who saw the patient

In addition, a patient's medical record must contain:

▶ Biographical and personal information, including the patient's full name, Social Security number, date of birth, full address, marital status, home and work telephone numbers, and employer information as applicable.

- Records of all communications with the patient, including letters, telephone calls, faxes, and e-mail messages; the patient's responses; and a note of the time, date, topic, and physician's response to each communication.
- Records of prescriptions and instructions given to the patient, including refills.
- Scanned or original documents that the patient has signed, such as an authorization to release information and an advance directive.
- Medical allergies and reactions, or their absence.
- Up-to-date immunization record and history if appropriate, such as for a child.
- Previous and current diagnoses, test results, health risks, and progress.
- Records of referral or consultation letters.
- Hospital admissions and release documents.
- Records of any missed or canceled appointments.
- Requests for information about the patient (from a health plan or an attorney, for example), and a detailed log of to whom information was released.

Evaluation and Management Services Reports

When providers evaluate a patient's condition and decide on a course of treatment to manage it, the service is called *evaluation and management (E/M)* (see Chapter 5). Evaluation and management services may include a complete interview and physical examination for a new patient or for a new problem presented by a person who is already a patient. There are many other types of E/M encounters, such as a visit to decide whether surgery is needed or to follow up on a patient's problem. An E/M service is usually documented with chart notes.

History and Physical Examination A complete history and physical (H&P) is documented with four types of information: (1) the chief complaint (CC), (2) the history and physical examination, (3) the diagnosis, and (4) the treatment plan. The provider documents the patient's reason for the visit, often using the patient's own words to describe the symptom, problem, condition, diagnosis, or other factor. For clarity, the provider may restate the reason as a "presenting problem," using medical terminology.

The provider also documents the patient's relevant medical history. The extent of the history is based on what the provider considers appropriate. It may include the history of the present illness (HPI), past medical history (PMH), and family/social history. There is usually also a review of systems (ROS), in which the provider asks questions about the function of each body system considered appropriate to the problem.

The provider performs a physical examination and documents the diagnosis—the interpretation of the information that has been gathered—or the suspected problem if more tests or procedures are needed for a diagnosis. The treatment plan, or plan of care, is described. It includes the treatments and medications that the provider has ordered, specifying dosage and frequency of use. The H&P is illustrated in Figure 2.1.

Other Chart Notes Many other types of chart notes appear in patients' medical records. *Progress reports* document a patient's progress and response to a treatment plan. They explain whether the plan should be continued or changed. *Discharge summaries* are prepared during a patient's final visit for a particular treatment plan or hospitalization. Discharge summaries include:

- The final diagnosis
- Comparisons of objective data with the patient's statements
- Whether goals were achieved
- Reason for and date of discharge
- The patient's current condition, status, and final prognosis
- Instructions given to the patient at discharge, noting any special needs such as restrictions on activities and medications

> **BILLING TIP**
>
> **SOAP Format**
>
> A common documentation structure is the *problem-oriented medical record (POMR)* that contains *SOAP* notes—Subjective information from the patient, and three elements the provider enters: Objective data such as examination and/or test results, Assessment of the patient's diagnosis, and Plan, the intended course of treatment, such as surgery or medication.

James E. Ribielli
5/19/2016

CHIEF COMPLAINT: This 79-year-old male presents with sudden and extreme weakness. He got up from a seated position and became light-headed.

PAST MEDICAL HISTORY: History of congestive heart failure. On multiple medications, including Cardizem, Enalapril 5 mg qd, and Lasix 40 mg qd.

PHYSICAL EXAMINATION: No postural change in blood pressure. BP, 114/61 with a pulse of 49, sitting; BP, 111/56 with a pulse 50, standing. Patient denies being light-headed at this time.

HEENT: Unremarkable.

NECK: Supple without jugular or venous distension.

LUNGS: Clear to auscultation and percussion.

HEART: S1 and S2 normal; no systolic or diastolic murmurs; no S3, S4. No dysrhythmia.

ABDOMEN: Soft without organomegaly, mass, or bruit.

EXTREMITIES: Unremarkable. Pulses strong and equal.

LABORATORY DATA: Hemoglobin, 12.3. White count, 10.800. Normal electrolytes. ECG shows sinus bradycardia.

DIAGNOSIS: Weakness on the basis of sinus bradycardia, probably Cardizem induced.

TREATMENT: Patient told to change positions slowly when moving from sitting to standing, and from lying to standing.

John R. Ramirez, MD

FIGURE 2.1 Example of Physical Examination Documentation

Procedural Services Documentation

Specific procedures, done either in the office or elsewhere, are documented. Examples are:

▶ Procedure or operative reports for simple or complex surgery
▶ Laboratory reports for laboratory tests
▶ Radiology reports for the results of X-rays
▶ Forms for a specific purpose, such as immunization records, preemployment physicals, and disability reports

Advantages of Electronic Health Records

Because of their advantages over traditional paper records, electronic health records are now used by nearly 60 percent of physician practices (National Center for Health

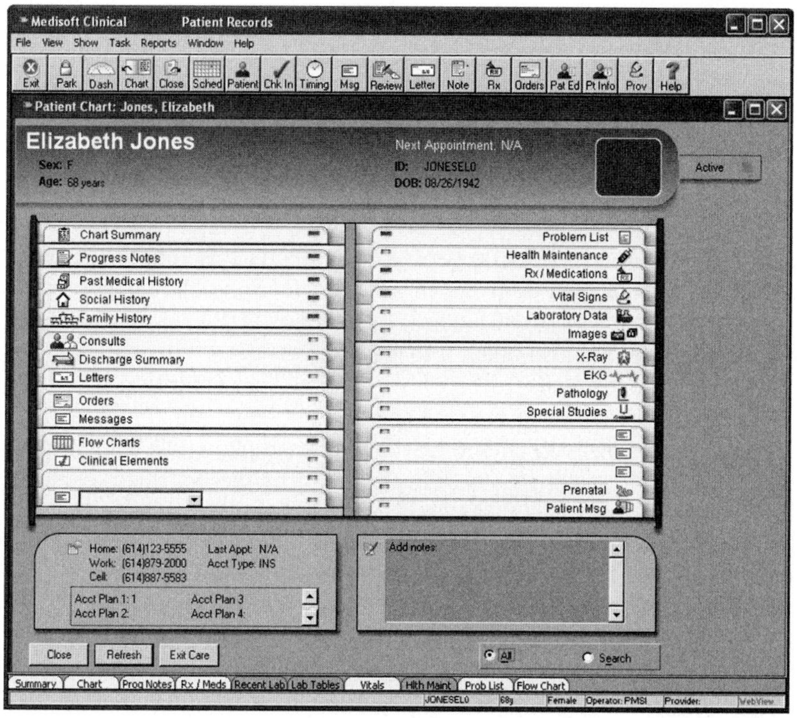

FIGURE 2.2 Screen from an Electronic Health Record Program

Statistics, 2011 survey). In electronic health records, documents may be created in a variety of ways, but they are ultimately viewed on a computer screen. See Figure 2.2 as an example.

EHRs offer both patients and providers significant advantages over paper records:

▶ Immediate access to health information: The EHR is simultaneously accessible from computers in the office and in other sites such as hospitals. Compared to sorting through papers in a paper folder, an EHR database can save time when vital patient information is needed. Once information is updated in a patient record, it is available to all who need access, whether across the hall or across town.

▶ Computerized physician order management: Physicians can enter orders for prescriptions, tests, and other services at any time. This information is then transmitted to the staff for implementation or directly to pharmacies linked to the practice.

▶ Clinical decision support: An EHR system can provide access to the latest medical research on approved medical websites to help medical decision making.

▶ Automated alerts and reminders: The system can provide medical alerts and reminders for office staff to ensure that patients are scheduled for regular screenings and other preventive practices. Alerts can also be created to identify patient safety issues, such as possible drug interactions.

▶ Electronic communication and connectivity: An EHR system can provide a means of secure and easily accessible communication between physicians and staff and in some offices between physicians and patients.

▶ Patient support: Some EHR programs allow patients to access their medical records and request appointments. These programs also offer patient education on health topics and instructions on preparing for common medical tests, such as an HDL cholesterol test.

▶ Administration and reporting: The EHR may include administrative tools, including reporting systems that enable medical practices to comply with federal and state reporting requirements.

BILLING TIP

Hybrid Record Systems

Although the majority of physician practices use EHRs, most also still have paper records too. The use of electronic along with paper records is called a *hybrid record system*.

▶ Error reduction: An EHR can decrease medical errors that result from illegible chart notes, since notes are entered electronically on a computer or a handheld device. Nevertheless, the accuracy of the information in the EHR is only as good as the accuracy of the person entering the data; it is still possible to click the wrong button or enter the wrong letter.

Record Retention

retention schedule Practice policy governing the handling and storage of patients' medical records.

Patients' medical records and financial records are retained according to the practice's policy. The practice manager or providers set the retention policy after reviewing the state regulations that apply. Any federal laws, such as HIPAA (described later in this chapter) regulations, are also taken into account.

The practice's policy about keeping records is summarized in a **retention schedule**, a list of the items from a record that are retained and for how long. The retention schedule usually also covers the method of retention. For example, a policy might state that all established patients' records are stored in the practice's files for three years and then microfilmed and removed to another storage location for another four years.

The retention schedule protects both the provider and the patient. Continuity of care is the first concern: the record must be available for anyone within or outside of the practice who is caring for the patient. Also, records must be kept in case of legal proceedings. For example, a provider might be asked to justify the level and nature of treatment when a claim is investigated or challenged, requiring access to documentation.

Although state guidelines cover medical information about patients, most do not specifically cover financial records. Financial records are generally saved according to federal business records retention requirements. Under HIPAA, covered entities must keep records of HIPAA compliance for six years. In general, the storage method chosen and the means of destroying the records when the retention period ends must strictly adhere to the same confidentiality requirements as patient medical records.

THINKING IT THROUGH 2.1

1. Consider the process of switching to EHRs from paper records in a practice having 2000 patients. What are the pros and cons of moving all past patient records to the EHR at once versus doing so gradually?

2.2 Health Care Regulations

Health is a personal and private matter. The health information that patients share with physicians could change their lives or cause them to lose jobs or friends. Nevertheless, medical information must be recorded in medical records and communicated to others in the course of treatment and payment. To protect consumers' health, both federal and state governments pass laws that affect the medical services that must be offered to patients. To protect the privacy of patients' health information, additional laws cover the way health care plans and providers exchange this information as they conduct business.

Federal and State Regulation

Centers for Medicare and Medicaid Services (CMS) Federal agency that runs Medicare, Medicaid, clinical laboratories, and other government health programs.

The main federal government agency responsible for health care is the **Centers for Medicare and Medicaid Services,** known as **CMS** (formerly the Health Care Financing Administration, or HCFA). Part of the Department of Health and Human Services (HHS), CMS administers the Medicare and Medicaid programs and implements annual federal budget acts and laws. The agency also acts to ensure the quality of health care, often recommending new rules, such as increased coverage of screening procedures for diseases, that become the model for the health care industry.

States are also major regulators of the health care industry. Operating an insurance company without a license is illegal in all states. State commissioners of insurance investigate consumer complaints about the quality and financial aspects of health care. State laws ensure the solvency of insurance companies and managed care organizations, so that they will be able to pay enrollees' claims. States may also restrict price increases on premiums and other charges to patients, require that policies include a guaranteed renewal provision, and control the situations in which an insurer can cancel a patient's coverage.

HIPAA and HITECH

The foundation legislation for the privacy of patients' health information is called the **Health Insurance Portability and Accountability Act (HIPAA) of 1996.** This law is designed to:

- ▶ Protect people's private health information.
- ▶ Ensure health insurance coverage for workers and their families when they change or lose their jobs.
- ▶ Uncover fraud and abuse.
- ▶ Create standards for electronic transmission of health care transactions.

The American Recovery and Reinvestment Act (ARRA) of 2009, also known as the Stimulus Package, contains additional provisions concerning the standards for electronic transmission of health care data. The most important rules are in the **Health Information Technology for Economic and Clinical Health (HITECH) Act,** which is Title XIII of ARRA. This law guides the use of federal stimulus money to promote the adoption and meaningful use of health information technology, mainly using electronic health records.

Covered Entities

Under HIPAA/HITECH, there are three types of **covered entities (CEs)** that must follow the regulations:

- ▶ *Health plans:* The individual or group plan that provides or pays for medical care.
- ▶ *Health care **clearinghouses:*** Companies that help providers handle such electronic transactions as submitting claims and that manage electronic medical record systems.
- ▶ *Health care providers:* People or organizations that furnish, bill, or are paid for health care in the normal course of business; most medical offices are included under HIPAA.

Business Associates

Business Associates (BAs) are organizations that work under contract for covered entities but are not themselves CEs. Examples of BAs include law firms; outside medical billers, coders, and transcriptionists; accountants; and collection agencies. BAs are also responsible for following HIPAA rules.

Electronic Data Interchange

HIPAA/HITECH encourage and promote **electronic data interchange (EDI),** the computer-to-computer exchange of routine business information using publicly available standards. As an example, medical assistants use EDI to exchange health information about their practices' patients with payers and clearinghouses. Each electronic exchange is a **transaction,** which is the electronic equivalent of a business document.

EDI transactions are not visible in the way that an exchange of paperwork, such as a letter, is. An example of a nonmedical transaction is the process of getting cash from an ATM. In an ATM transaction, the computer-to-computer exchange is made up of computer language that is sent and answered between the machines. This exchange happens behind the scenes. It is documented on the customer's end with the transaction receipt that is printed; the bank also has a record at its location.

CMS Home Page
www.cms.gov

Health Insurance Portability and Accountability Act (HIPAA) of 1996 Federal act with guidelines for standardizing the electronic data interchange of administrative and financial transactions, exposing fraud and abuse, and protecting PHI.

Health Information Technology for Economic and Clinical Health (HITECH) Act Law promoting the adoption and use of health information technology.

covered entity (CE) Health plan, clearinghouse, or provider that transmits any health information in electronic form.

clearinghouse Company that converts nonstandard transactions into standard transactions and transmits the data to health plans, and the reverse procedure.

BILLING TIP

Excepted Providers

Excepted providers are only those few who do not send any claims (or other HIPAA transactions) electronically *and* do not employ any other firm to send electronic claims for them.

business associate (BA) Person or organization that performs a function or activity for a covered entity.

electronic data interchange (EDI) System-to-system exchange of data in a standardized format.

transaction Electronic exchange of health care information.

The Affordable Care Act (ACA)

The Patient Protection and Affordable Care Act, known as the **Affordable Care Act (ACA),** which is health system reform legislation signed into law by President Obama in 2010, introduced a number of significant benefits for patients. Some benefits took effect immediately, and others are being gradually phased in. Medical assistants should stay updated on all aspects of the regulations as they emerge. Here is an overview.

Improvements that are now in effect for patients with private health insurance are:

▶ A payer can no longer drop a beneficiary from a plan because of a preexisting illness or a new condition, a practice known as *rescission.*

▶ Children ages 18 and younger cannot be denied private insurance coverage if they have a preexisting medical condition.

▶ For adults with preexisting medical conditions who cannot obtain private insurance coverage, a temporary national "high-risk pool" will be established to provide coverage, with financial subsidies to make premiums more affordable, until all insurers are required to cover people with preexisting conditions in 2014.

▶ Young adults up to age 26 can remain as a dependent on their parents' private health insurance plan.

▶ Payers cannot impose lifetime financial limits on benefits.

▶ Insurance companies must spend at least 80 cents of every dollar they collect from customers on providing health care, limiting salaries and profits. If this is not the case, health plan subscribers will get a tax-free rebate.

▶ Preventive services for women such as mammograms, and immunizations for children, must be covered by insurers, with no co-payments or deductibles required.

Future patient benefits include:

▶ Preventive services for all patients in new health plans, such as annual physicals and dozens of screening tests, must be completely covered by payers, as long as in-network providers are used.

▶ U.S. citizens and legal residents cannot be denied private health insurance coverage for any reason, beginning in 2014, and they must obtain health insurance coverage or pay a minor tax penalty (although there are some exemptions).

▶ State-based health insurance exchanges will begin operating in 2014, where people who do not have access to employer-based insurance can compare the benefits and costs of private health insurance plans. These exchanges will create insurance pools that will allow people to choose among affordable coverage options. All insurance companies in the exchange must provide at least a minimum benefit package, as well as additional coverage options beyond a basic plan.

▶ Federal subsidies through tax credits or vouchers will be provided in 2014 to people who cannot afford the full cost to help them purchase coverage through the exchanges.

For patients enrolled in Medicare or Medicaid:

▶ Preventive services recommended by the U.S. Preventive Services Task Force (USPSTF), which uses a letter grading system to determine when a service is appropriate, are now provided without deductible or coinsurance requirements. Examples include bone mass measurement, colorectal cancer screening, influenza and pneumococcal vaccines, and ultrasound abdominal aortic aneurysm screening.

▶ The cost of Medicare drug coverage is reduced.

▶ A series of pilot programs will be implemented to help find new ways to improve quality and lower the cost of care.

▶ Medicaid coverage will be expanded in 2014, in many states, to all eligible children, pregnant women, parents and childless adults under age 65 who have incomes at or below 138 percent of the federal poverty level.

CMS HIPAA Home Page
www.cms.gov/hipaageninfo

THINKING IT THROUGH 2.2

1. Do covered entities and business associates follow the same rules regarding protected health information?

2.3 HIPAA Privacy Rule

Patients' medical records—the actual progress notes, reports, and other clinical materials—are legal documents that belong to the provider who created them. But the provider cannot withhold the information in the records unless providing it would be detrimental to the patient's health. The information belongs to the patient.

Patients control the amount and type of information that is released, except for the use of the data to treat them or to conduct the normal business transactions of the practice. Only patients or their legally appointed representatives have the authority to authorize the release of information to anyone not directly involved in their care.

Medical assistants handle issues such as requests for information from patients' medical records. They need to know what information can be released about patients' conditions and treatments. What information can be legally shared with other providers and health plans? What information must the patient specifically authorize to be released? The **HIPAA Privacy Rule** provides guidance on these issues. The Privacy Rule says that covered entities must:

> **HIPAA Privacy Rule** Law promoting the adoption and use of health information technology.

- ▶ Have a set of privacy practices that are appropriate for their health care services.
- ▶ Notify patients about their privacy rights and how their information can be used or disclosed.
- ▶ Train employees so that they understand the privacy practices.
- ▶ Appoint a privacy official responsible for seeing that the privacy practices are adopted and followed.
- ▶ Safeguard patients' records.

Protected Health Information

The HIPAA Privacy Rule covers the use and disclosure of patients' **protected health information (PHI).** PHI is defined as individually identifiable health information that is transmitted or maintained by electronic media, such as over the Internet or between computers.

> **protected health information (PHI)** Individually identifiable health information transmitted or maintained by electronic media.

This information includes a person's:

- ▶ Name
- ▶ Address (including street address, city, county, ZIP code)
- ▶ Names of relatives and employers
- ▶ Birth date
- ▶ Telephone numbers
- ▶ Fax number
- ▶ E-mail address
- ▶ Social Security number
- ▶ Medical record number
- ▶ Health plan beneficiary number
- ▶ Account number
- ▶ Certificate or license number
- ▶ Serial number of any vehicle or other device
- ▶ Website address
- ▶ Fingerprints or voiceprints
- ▶ Photographic images

COMPLIANCE GUIDELINE

HIPAA Exemptions

Certain benefits are always exempt from HIPAA, including coverage only for accident, disability income coverage, liability insurance, workers' compensation, automobile medical payment and liability insurance, credit-only insurance (such as mortgage insurance), and coverage for on-site medical clinics.

Use and Disclosure for Treatment, Payment, and Health Care Operations

treatment, payment, and health care operations (TPO) Legitimate reasons for the sharing of patients' protected health information without authorization.

Patients' PHI under HIPAA can be used and disclosed by providers for treatment, payment, and health care operations. *Use of PHI* means sharing or analysis *within* the entity that holds the information. *Disclosure of PHI* means the release, transfer, provision of access to, or divulging of PHI *outside* the entity holding the information.

Both use and disclosure of PHI are necessary and permitted for patients' **treatment, payment, and health care operations (TPO).** *Treatment* means providing and coordinating the patient's medical care; *payment* refers to the exchange of information with health plans; and *health care operations* are the general business management functions.

minimum necessary standard Principle that individually identifiable health information should be disclosed only to the extent needed.

Minimum Necessary Standard   When using or disclosing protected health information, a covered entity must try to limit the information to the minimum amount of PHI necessary for the intended purpose. The **minimum necessary standard** means taking reasonable safeguards to protect PHI from incidental disclosure. Here are examples of complying with these rules:

▶ A medical assistant does not disclose a patient's history of cancer on a workers' compensation claim for a sprained ankle. Only the information the recipient needs to know is given.
▶ A physician's assistant faxes appropriate patient cardiology test results before scheduled surgery.
▶ A physician sends an e-mail message to another physician requesting a consultation on a patient's case.
▶ A patient's family member picks up medical supplies and a prescription.

designated record set (DRS) Covered entity's records that contain protected health information (PHI); for providers, the medical/financial patient record.

Designated Record Set   A covered entity must disclose individuals' PHI to them (or to their personal representatives) when they request access to, or an accounting of disclosures of, their PHI. Patients' rights apply to a **designated record set (DRS).** For a provider, the designated record set means the clinical and billing records the provider maintains. It does not include appointment and surgery schedules, requests for lab tests, and birth and death records. It also does not include mental health information, psychotherapy notes, and genetic information. For a health plan, the designated record set includes enrollment, payment, claim decisions, and medical management systems of the plan.

Within the designated record set, patients have the right to:

▶ Access, copy, and inspect their PHI.
▶ Request amendments to their health information.
▶ Obtain accounting of most disclosures of their health information.
▶ Receive communications from providers via other means, such as in Braille or in foreign languages.
▶ Complain about alleged violations of the regulations and the provider's own information policies.

Notice of Privacy Practices (NPP) Description of a covered entity's principles and procedures related to the protection of patients' health information.

Notice of Privacy Practices   Covered entities must give each patient a notice of privacy practice at the first contact or encounter. To meet this requirement, physician practices give patients their **Notice of Privacy Practices (NPP)** and ask them to sign an acknowledgment that they have received it. The notice explains how patients' PHI may be used and describes their rights.

PHI and Accounting of Disclosures   Patients have the right to an accounting of disclosures of their PHI other than for TPO. When a patient's PHI is accidentally disclosed, the disclosure should be documented in the individual's medical record, since the individual did not authorize it and it was not a permitted disclosure. An example is faxing a discharge summary to the wrong physician's office. Also, under HITECH, patients can request an accounting of all disclosures—not just those other than for TPO—for the past three years if their PHI is stored in an EHR.

Authorizations for Other Use and Disclosure

For use or disclosure other than for TPO, the covered entity must have the patient sign an **authorization** to release the information. Information about substance (alcohol and drug) abuse, sexually transmitted diseases (STDs) or human immunodeficiency virus (HIV), and behavioral/mental health services may not be released without a specific authorization from the patient. The authorization document must be in plain language and include the following:

▶ A description of the information to be used or disclosed.
▶ The name or other specific identification of the person(s) authorized to use or disclose the information.
▶ The name of the person(s) or group of people to whom the covered entity may make the use or disclosure.
▶ A description of each purpose of the requested use or disclosure.
▶ An expiration date.
▶ The signature of the individual (or authorized representative) and the date.

In addition, the rule states that a valid authorization must include:

▶ A statement of the individual's right to revoke the authorization in writing.
▶ A statement about whether the covered entity is able to base treatment, payment, enrollment, or eligibility for benefits on the authorization.
▶ A statement that information used or disclosed after the authorization may be disclosed again by the recipient and may no longer be protected by the rule.

A sample authorization form is shown in Figure 2.3 on the next page.

Uses or disclosures for which the covered entity has received specific authorization from the patient do not have to follow the minimum necessary standard. Incidental use and disclosure are also allowed. For example, the practice may use reception-area sign-in sheets.

authorization (1) document signed by a patient to permit release of medical information; (2) health plan's system of approving payment of benefits for appropriate services.

Exceptions

There are a number of exceptions to the usual rules for release:

▶ Court orders: If the patient's PHI is required as evidence by a court of law, it may be released without patient approval.
▶ Workers' compensation cases: State law may allow record release to employers, the state administration board, and the responsible insurance company in workers' compensation cases.
▶ Statutory reports: Some specific types of information are required by state law to be released to state health or social services departments. For example, physicians must make statutory reports for patients' births and deaths and for cases of abuse. Because of the danger of harm to patients or others, communicable diseases such as tuberculosis, hepatitis, and rabies must usually be reported.

   A special category of communicable disease control is applied to patients with diagnoses of human immunodeficiency virus (HIV) infection and acquired immunodeficiency syndrome (AIDS). Every state requires AIDS cases to be reported. Most states also require reporting of the HIV infection that causes the syndrome. However, state law varies concerning whether just the fact of a case is to be reported or if the patient's name must also be reported. The practice guidelines reflect the state laws and must be strictly observed, as all these regulations should be, to protect patients' privacy and to comply with the regulations.
▶ Research: PHI may be made available to researchers approved by the practice.
▶ Self-pay requests for restrictions: Under HITECH, patients can restrict the access of health plans to their medical records if they pay for the service in full at the time of the visit.

All these types of disclosures must be logged, and the release information must be available to the patient who requests it.

Patient Name: _____

Health Record Number: _____

Date of Birth: _____

1. I authorize the use or disclosure of the above named individual's health information as described below.

2. The following individual(s) or organization(s) are authorized to make the disclosure: _____

3. The type of information to be used or disclosed is as follows (check the appropriate boxes and include other information where indicated)

❑ problem list

❑ medication list

❑ list of allergies

❑ immunization records

❑ most recent history

❑ most recent discharge summary

❑ lab results (please describe the dates or types of lab tests you would like disclosed): _____

❑ x-ray and imaging reports (please describe the dates or types of x-rays or images you would like disclosed): _____

❑ consultation reports from (please supply doctors' names): _____

❑ entire record

❑ other (please describe): _____

4. I understand that the information in my health record may include information relating to sexually transmitted disease, acquired immunodeficiency syndrome (AIDS), or human immunodeficiency virus (HIV). It may also include information about behavioral or mental health services, and treatment for alcohol and drug abuse.

5. The information identified above may be used by or disclosed to the following individuals or organization(s):

Name: _____

Address: _____

Name: _____

Address: _____

6. This information for which I'm authorizing disclosure will be used for the following purpose:

❑ my personal records

❑ sharing with other health care providers as needed/other (please describe): _____

7. I understand that I have a right to revoke this authorization at any time. I understand that if I revoke this authorization, I must do so in writing and present my written revocation to the health information management department. I understand that the revocation will not apply to information that has already been released in response to this authorization. I understand that the revocation will not apply to my insurance company when the law provides my insurer with the right to contest a claim under my policy.

8. This authorization will expire (insert date or event): _____

If I fail to specify an expiration date or event, this authorization will expire six months from the date on which it was signed.

9. I understand that once the above information is disclosed, it may be redisclosed by the recipient and the information may not be protected by federal privacy laws or regulations.

10. I understand authorizing the use or disclosure of the information identified above is voluntary. I need not sign this form to ensure healthcare treatment.

Signature of patient or legal representative: _____ Date: _____

If signed by legal representative, relationship to patient

Signature of witness: _____ Date: _____

Distribution of copies: Original to provider; copy to patient; copy to accompany use or disclosure

Note: This sample form was developed by the American Health Information Management Association for discussion purposes. It should not be used without review by the issuing organization's legal counsel to ensure compliance with other federal and state laws and regulations.

What specific information can be released

To whom

For what purpose

FIGURE 2.3 Sample Authorization Form

De-Identified Health Information

There are no restrictions on the use or disclosure of *de-identified health information* that neither identifies nor provides a reasonable basis to identify an individual. For example, these identifiers must be removed (also referred to as *redacted*, meaning to cross through or otherwise make data illegible): names, medical record numbers, health plan beneficiary numbers, device identifiers (such as pacemakers), and biometric identifiers, such as fingerprints and voiceprints on documentation to categorize it as de-identified.

Psychotherapy Notes

Psychotherapy notes have special protection under HIPAA. According to the American Health Information Management Association Practice Brief on Legal Process and Electronic Health Records,

> Under the HIPAA Privacy Rule, psychotherapy notes are those recorded (in any medium) by a health care provider who is a mental health professional documenting or analyzing the content of conversation during a private counseling session or a group, joint, or family counseling session and that are separated from the rest of the individual's medical record. Notes exclude medication prescription and monitoring, counseling session start or stop times, the modalities and frequencies of treatment furnished, results of clinical tests, and any summary of diagnosis, functional status, the treatment plan, symptoms, prognosis, and progress to date. The privacy rule gives such notes extra protection as may state law. (Available online at www.ahima.org/resources/ehr.aspx.)

State Statutes

Some state statutes are more stringent than HIPAA specifications. Areas in which state statutes may differ from HIPAA include the following:

► Designated record set
► Psychotherapy notes
► Rights of inmates
► Information compiled for civil, criminal, or administrative court cases

Each practice's privacy official reviews state laws and develops policies and procedures for compliance with the HIPAA Privacy Rule. The tougher rules are implemented.

THINKING IT THROUGH 2.3

1. In each of these cases of release of PHI, was the HIPAA Privacy Rule followed? Why or why not?

   A. A laboratory communicates a patient's medical test results to a physician by phone.

   B. A physician mails a copy of a patient's medical record to a specialist who intends to treat the patient.

   C. A hospital faxes a patient's health care instructions to a nursing home to which the patient is to be transferred.

   D. A doctor discusses a patient's condition over the phone with an emergency room physician who is providing the patient with emergency care.

   E. A doctor orally discusses a patient's treatment regimen with a nurse who will be involved in the patient's care.

   F. A physician consults with another physician by e-mail about a patient's condition.

   G. A hospital shares an organ donor's medical information with another hospital treating the organ recipient.

   H. A medical assistant answers questions over the phone from a health plan about a patient's dates of service on a submitted claim.

2.4 HIPAA Security Rule and HITECH Breach Notification Rule

The **HIPAA Security Rule** requires covered entities to establish safeguards to protect PHI. The security rule specifies how to secure such protected health information on computer networks, the Internet, and storage media.

Encryption Is Required

Information security is needed when computers exchange data over the Internet. Security measures rely on **encryption,** the process of encoding information in such a way that only the person (or computer) with the key can decode it. Practice management programs (PMPs) encrypt data traveling between the office and the Internet, such as patients' Social Security numbers, so that the information is secure.

Security Measures

A number of other security measures help enforce the HIPAA Security Rule. These include:

▶ Secure Internet connections
▶ Access control, passwords, and log files to keep intruders out
▶ Backups to replace items after damage
▶ Security policies to handle violations that do occur

Internet Security

Information is exchanged over the Internet between the practice and those outside of the office in a number of ways, especially by e-mail, the most important business communications method. Additionally, practices may have their own websites and patient portals for access to the physicians and for marketing purposes; taking calls from patients' mobile phones; and sending medical records to health plans via attachments. HIPAA, HITECH, and many states have laws for data security that require the use of antivirus software programs and encrypting confidential patient data that is transmitted.

Access Controls, Passwords, and Log Files

Most practices use role-based access, meaning that only people who need information can see it. Once access rights have been assigned, each user is given a key to the designated databases. Users must enter a user ID and a **password** (the key) to see files to which they have been granted access rights.

For example, receptionists may view the names of patients coming to the office on one day, but they should not see those patients' medical records. However, the nurse or physician needs to view the patient records. Receptionists are given individual computer passwords that let them view the day's schedule but that deny entry to patient records. The physicians and nurses possess computer passwords that allow them to see all patient records.

The PMP also creates activity logs of who has accessed—or tried to access—information, and passwords prevent unauthorized users from gaining access to information on a computer or network.

Backups

Backing up is the activity of copying files to another medium so that they will be preserved in case the originals are no longer available. A successful backup plan is critical in recovering from either a minor or major security incident that jeopardizes critical data. In order to be secure, backups must also be encrypted.

Security Policy

Practices have security policies that inform employees about their responsibilities for protecting electronically stored information. Many practices include this information in handbooks distributed to all employees. These handbooks contain general information about the organizations, their structures, and their policies as well as specific information about employee responsibilities.

Breach Notification

The HITECH Act requires covered entities to notify affected individuals following the discovery of a breach of unsecured health information. A **breach** is an impermissible use or disclosure under the Privacy Rule that compromises the security or privacy of PHI and also that could pose a significant risk of financial, reputational, or other harm to the affected person. Covered entities are required to monitor their handling of PHI to be sure to discover breaches, and if a breach occurs, to follow these **breach notification** procedures:

▶ Notice to patients of breaches "without reasonable delay" within 60 days.
▶ Notice to covered entities by business associates (BAs) when BAs discover a breach.
▶ Notice to "prominent media outlets" on breaches involving more than 500 individuals.
▶ Notice to "next of kin" on breaches involving patients who are deceased.
▶ Notice to the secretary of HHS about breaches involving 500 or more individuals without reasonable delay.
▶ Annual notice to the secretary of HHS about breaches of "unsecured PHI" involving less than 500 individuals that pose a significant financial risk or other harm to the individual, such as reputation.

breach Impermissible use or disclosure of PHI that could pose significant risk to the affected person.

breach notification Document notifying an individual of a breach.

HHS Breach Notifications Website

www.hhs.gov/ocr/privacy/ hipaa/administrative/ breachnotificationrule/ breachtool.html

THINKING IT THROUGH 2.4

1. Imagine that you are employed as a medical assistant for Orchard Hill Medical Center. Based on the Tip on selecting good passwords, make up a password that you will use to keep your files secure.

2. As an employee, how would you respond to another staff member who asked to see your latest claim files in order to see how you handled a particular situation?

2.5 HIPAA Electronic Health Care Transactions and Code Sets

The **HIPAA Electronic Health Care Transactions and Code Sets (TCS)** standards are rules that make it possible for physicians and health plans to exchange electronic data using the standard format and standard codes. Under this rule, three types of standards have been set:

1. Standard transactions
2. Code sets
3. Identifiers

HIPAA Electronic Health Care Transactions and Code Sets (TCS) Rule governing the electronic exchange of health information.

Table 2.1 HIPAA Electronic Transaction Standards

Number	Name
X12 837	Health care claims or equivalent encounter information as well as coordination of benefits (COB)—an exchange of information between payers when a patient is covered by more than one medical insurance plan
X12 276/277	Health care claim status inquiry/response
X12 270/271	Eligibility for a health plan inquiry/response
X12 278	Referral authorization inquiry/response
X12 835	Health care payment and remittance advice
X12 820	Health plan premium payments
X12 834	Health plan enrollment and disenrollment

Standard Transactions

The HIPAA transactions standards apply to the electronic data that are regularly sent back and forth between providers and health plans. Examples of formats are electronic forms to verify insurance coverage and electronic claims. Each standard is labeled with both a number and a name. Either the number or the name may be used to refer to the particular electronic document format. For example, the number X12 837 stands for health care claims. The complete list of transaction standards is shown in Table 2.1.

Code Sets

code set Alphabetic and/or numeric representations for data.

Under HIPAA, a **code set** is any group of codes used for encoding data elements, such as tables of terms, medical concepts, and diagnosis and procedures. There are standard sets of codes for diseases; treatments and procedures; and supplies or other items used to perform these actions. These standards are listed in Table 2.2.

Identifiers

Identifiers are numbers of predetermined length and structure, such as a person's Social Security number. They are important for billing because the unique numbers

Table 2.2 HIPAA Standard Code Sets

Purpose	Standard
Codes for diseases, injuries, impairments, and other health-related problems	*International Classification of Diseases,* Ninth Edition, *Clinical Modification* (ICD-9-CM), Volumes 1 and 2 (until 10-01-2014) *International Classification of Diseases,* Tenth Edition, *Clinical Modification* (ICD-10-CM) (after 10-01-2014)
Codes for procedures or other actions taken to prevent, diagnose, treat, or manage diseases, injuries, and impairments	Physicians' Services: *Current Procedural Terminology* (CPT) Inpatient Hospital Services: *International Classification of Diseases,* Ninth Edition, *Clinical Modification,* Volume 3: *Procedures* (until 10-01-2014) *International Classification of Diseases,* Tenth Edition, *Procedure Coding System* (ICD-10-PCS) (after 10-01-2014)
Codes for other medical services	Healthcare Common Procedures Coding System (HCPCS)
Codes for dental services	*Current Dental Terminology* (CDT-4)

can be used in electronic transactions. Two identifiers—for employers and for providers—have been set up by the federal government, and two—for patients and for health plans—are to be established in the future.

▶ The employer identifier is used to identify the patient's employer on claims. The Employer Identification Number (EIN) issued by the Internal Revenue Service is the HIPAA standard.

▶ The **National Provider Identifier (NPI)** is the standard unique health identifier for health care providers to use in filing health care claims and other transactions. The NPI replaces other identifying numbers that had been in use, such as the UPIN for Medicare. The NPI is ten positions long, with nine numbers and a check digit. The numbers are assigned to individuals, such as physicians and nurses, and also to organizations, such as hospitals, pharmacies, and clinics. If a physician is in a group practice, both the individual doctor and the group have NPIs. CMS maintains the NPIs as they are assigned in the *National Plan and Provider Enumerator System (NPPES)*, a database of all assigned numbers. Once assigned, the NPI will not change; it remains with the provider regardless of job or location changes.

National Provider Identifier (NPI) Unique ten-digit identifier assigned to each provider.

NPPES

nppes.cms.hhs.gov/NPPES/ Welcome.do

THINKING IT THROUGH 2.5

1. Gloria Traylor, an employee of National Bank, called Marilyn Rennagel, a medical assistant who works for Dr. Judy Fisk. The bank is considering hiring one of Dr. Fisk's patients, Juan Ramirez, and Ms. Traylor would like to know if he has any known medical problems. Marilyn, in a hurry to complete the call and get back to work on this week's claims, quickly explains that she remembers that Mr. Ramirez was treated for depression some years ago, but that he has been fine since that time. She adds that she thinks he would make an excellent employee.

A. In your opinion, did Marilyn handle this call correctly?

B. What problems might result from her answers?

COMPLIANCE GUIDELINE

Using NPIs

The NPI eliminates the need for health care providers to use different identification numbers to identify themselves when conducting standard transactions with multiple health plans. Many health plans—including Medicare, Medicaid, and private health insurance issuers—and all health care clearinghouses must now accept and use NPIs in standard transactions.

2.6 Avoiding Fraud and Abuse

Fraud occurs when someone intentionally misrepresents facts to receive a benefit illegally. A person who cooperates in a fraudulent situation is also personally responsible. On the other hand, **abuse** means an action that misuses money that the government has allocated, such as Medicare funds. Abuse is illegal because taxpayers' dollars are misspent. An example of abuse is an ambulance service that billed Medicare for transporting a patient to the hospital when the patient did not need ambulance service. This abuse—billing for services that were not medically necessary—resulted in improper payment for the ambulance company. Abuse is not necessarily intentional. It may be the result of ignorance of a billing rule or of inaccurate coding.

fraud Intentional deceptive act to obtain a benefit.

abuse Actions that improperly use another's resources.

Fraud and HIPAA

HIPAA clearly defines health care fraud as a crime. The act set up the *Health Care Fraud and Abuse Control Program* to coordinate federal, state, and local law enforcement through investigations, audits, evaluations, and inspections. This program is not limited to Medicare and Medicaid. It covers any plan or program that provides health benefits, such as health insurance policies. When fraud is determined, the law permits fines of up to $10,000 per item or service for which fraudulent payment was received. Criminal penalties—fines and imprisonment—exist for

BILLING TIP

Fraud versus Abuse

To bill when the task was not done is fraud; to bill when it was not necessary is abuse. Remember the rule: If a service was not documented, in the view of the payer it was not done and cannot be billed. To bill for undocumented services is fraudulent.

knowingly planning to obtain money or property owned by the health care benefit program. The federal False Claims Act, a related law, prohibits submitting a fraudulent claim or making a false statement in connection with a claim. This law has been made even stronger by the federal Fraud Enforcement and Recovery Act (FERA) of 2009 and the 2010 Affordable Care Act. Further, many states have passed similar laws.

Knowingly is a key word in fraud cases. Most physicians maintain honest relationships with insurance carriers. Some, however, do not. For example, suppose a physician asks a staff member to code a patient's headaches as a subdural hematoma (pool of blood below the dura mater membrane of the brain) in order to justify billing an expensive procedure. An employee must never falsify medical records. Here is what can happen: The physician might receive the higher payment, but the federal government audits the records of the medical office, finds that the patient's record does not match the insurance claim, and successfully prosecutes the physician and the staff member, finding the staff member responsible.

OCR Compliance and Enforcement
www.hhs.gov/ocr/privacy/

CMS HIPAA Enforcement
www.cms.gov/Enforcement/

OCR Privacy Fact Sheets
www.hhs.gov/ocr/hipaa/

Office for Civil Rights (OCR) Government agency that enforces the HIPAA Privacy Act.

Enforcement

Enforcing HIPAA is the job of a number of governmental agencies. Which agency performs which task depends on the nature of the violation and is determined by the *HIPAA Enforcement Rule*.

▶ **Office for Civil Rights** Civil violations (those that are based on *civil law*, such as trespassing, divorce cases, and breach of contract proceedings) of the HIPAA privacy and security standards are enforced by the **Office for Civil Rights (OCR)**, an agency of HHS. OCR has the authority to receive and investigate complaints as well as to issue subpoenas for evidence in cases it is investigating. It is charged with enforcing the privacy standards because privacy and security of one's health information are considered a civil right.

▶ **Department of Justice** Criminal violations (those that involve crimes, such as kidnapping, robbery, and arson) of HIPAA privacy standards are prosecuted by the federal government's Department of Justice (DOJ). DOJ is America's "law office" and central agency for enforcement of federal laws.

Office of E-Health Standards and Services (OESS) Government agency that enforces the other HIPAA standards.

Office of the Inspector General (OIG) Government agency that investigates and prosecutes fraud.

▶ **Office of E-Health Standards and Services (OESS)** Part of CMS, the **Office of E-Health Standards and Services (OESS)** enforces the other HIPAA standards.

▶ **Office of the Inspector General** The HHS **Office of the Inspector General (OIG)** has the task of detecting health care fraud and abuse, and enforcing all laws relating to them. OIG works with the U.S. Department of Justice (DOJ), which includes the Federal Bureau of Investigation (FBI), to prosecute those suspected of medical fraud and abuse.

The Medical Assistant's Role

To the best of their ability, administrative staff strive to ensure that health care claims are accurate reflections of the work that was done and documented. It is important to avoid fraudulent or abusive billing practices, such as:

▶ *Intentionally billing for services that were not performed or documented.*

   Example: A lab bills Medicare for two tests when only one was done.

   Example: A physician asks a coder to report a physical examination that was just a telephone conversation.

▶ *Reporting services at a higher level than was carried out.*

   Example: After a visit for a flu shot, the provider bills the encounter as a comprehensive physical examination plus a vaccination.

▶ *Performing and billing for procedures that are not related to the patient's condition and therefore not medically necessary.*

> *Example:* After reading an article about Lyme disease, a patient is worried about having worked in her garden over the summer, and she requests a Lyme disease diagnostic test. Although no symptoms or signs have been reported, the physician orders and bills for the *Borrelia burgdorferi* (Lyme disease) confirmatory immunoblot test.

Also, because of their contracts with physicians, many health plans have the right to **audit** the physician's billing practices. Payers may audit selected physicians because they provide very specialized services or because fraud or other misrepresentation of services is suspected. The health plan will notify the physician before an audit is conducted, and the types of records that will be audited are specified ahead of time. The role of the medical assistant is to make sure the records are available, complete, and signed by the physician.

audit   Formal examination of a physician's records.

THINKING IT THROUGH 2.6

1. Mary Kelley, a patient of the Good Health Clinic, asked Kathleen Culpepper, the medical insurance specialist, to help her out of a tough financial spot. Her medical insurance authorized her to receive four radiation treatments for her condition, one every 35 days. Because she was out of town, she did not schedule her appointment for the last treatment until today, which is one week beyond the approved period. The insurance company will not reimburse Mary for this procedure. She asks Kathleen to change the date on the record to last Wednesday so that it will be covered, explaining that no one will be hurt by this change and, anyway, she pays the insurance company plenty.

   A. What type of action is Mary asking Kathleen to do?

   B. How should Kathleen handle Mary's request?

2.7 Compliance Plans

A wise slogan is that "the best defense is a good offense." For this reason, medical practices write and implement **compliance plans** to uncover compliance problems and correct them to avoid risking liability. A compliance plan is a process for finding, correcting, and preventing illegal medical office practices. It is a written document prepared by a compliance officer and committee that sets up the steps needed to (1) audit and monitor compliance with government regulations, especially in the area of coding and billing, (2) have policies and procedures that are consistent, (3) provide for ongoing staff training and communication, and (4) respond to and correct errors. The goals of the compliance plan are to:

compliance plan   Medical practice's written plan for complying with regulations.

▶ Prevent fraud and abuse through a formal process to identify, investigate, fix, and prevent repeat violations relating to reimbursement for health care services.
▶ Ensure compliance with applicable federal, state, and local laws, including employment and environmental laws as well as antifraud laws.
▶ Help defend the practice if it is investigated or prosecuted for fraud by substantiating the desire to behave compliantly and thus reduce any fines or criminal prosecution.

Having a compliance plan demonstrates to outside investigators that the practice has made honest, ongoing attempts to find and fix weak areas. Compliance plans cover more than just coding and billing. They also cover all areas of government regulation of medical practices, such as Equal Employment Opportunity (EEO) regulations (for example, hiring and promotion policies) and Occupational Safety and Health Administration (OSHA) regulations (for example, fire safety and handling of hazardous materials such as blood-borne pathogens).

Generally, according to OIG, plans should contain seven elements:

1. Consistent written policies and procedures
2. Appointment of a compliance officer and committee
3. Ongoing training
4. Communication
5. Disciplinary systems
6. Auditing and monitoring
7. Responding to and correcting errors

Following OIG's guidance can help in the defense against a false claims accusation. Having a plan in place shows that efforts are made to understand the rules and correct errors. This indicates to OIG that the problems may not add up to a pattern or practice of abuse, but may simply be errors.

THINKING IT THROUGH 2.7

1. As a medical assistant, why would ongoing training be important to you?

Chapter Summary

Learning Outcomes	Key Concepts/Examples

2.1 Explain the importance of accurate documentation when working with medical records. Pages 26–30	• Accurate medical records provide continuity and communication among physicians and other health care professionals that are involved in a patient's care.
	 • Medical records are created based on a variety of different types of documentation for patient encounters.
	 • Some advantages of EHRs include:
	    Immediate access to health information
	    Computerized physician order management
	    Clinical decision support
	    Automated alerts and reminders
	    Electronic communication and connectivity
	    Patient support
	    Administration and reporting
	    Error reduction

Learning Outcomes	Key Concepts/Examples
2.2 Compare the major regulations affecting patient records in medical offices. Pages 30–33	• HIPAA is a law designed to: Protect people's private health information. Ensure health insurance coverage for workers and their families when they change or lose jobs. Uncover fraud and abuse. Create standards for electronic transmission of health care transactions. • The ARRA of 2009, which includes the rules in the HITECH Act: Contains additional provisions concerning the standards for electronic transmission of health care data. Guides the use of federal stimulus money to promote the adoption and meaningful use of health information technology, mainly using EHRs.
2.3 Discuss the purpose of the HIPAA Privacy Rule. Pages 33–37	• The HIPAA Privacy Rule provides guidance on what information can be released about a patient's condition or treatment. • It regulates the use and disclosure of patients' PHI. • Both use and disclosure of PHI are necessary and permitted for patients' treatment, payment, and health care operations (TPO). • Some exceptions to the usual rules of PHI release may include court cases, workers' compensation cases, statutory reports, research, and self-pay requests for restriction.
2.4 Briefly state the purpose of the HIPAA Security Rule and the HITECH Breach Notification Rule. Pages 38–39	• The HIPAA Security Rule requires covered entities to establish administrative, physical, and technical safeguards to protect the confidentiality, integrity, and availability of health information. • Providers follow this rule through the use of encryption, access control, passwords, log files, backups to replace items after damage, and by developing security policies to handle violations when they do occur. • The HITECH Breach Notification Rule requires covered entities to notify affected individuals following the discovery of a breach of unsecured health information. • Covered entities have specific breach notification procedures that they must follow in the event of a breach.
2.5 Describe the HIPAA Electronic Health Care Transactions and Code Sets Standards. Pages 39–41	• TCS establishes standards for the exchange of financial and administrative data among covered entities. • The standards require the covered entities to use common electronic transactions methods and code sets. • Identifiers are unique numbers that can be used in electronic transactions.
2.6 Explain how to guard against potentially fraudulent situations. Pages 41–43	Avoid fraudulent or abusive billing practices such as: • Intentionally billing for services that were not performed or documented. • Reporting services at a higher level than was carried out. • Performing and billing for procedures that are not related to the patient's condition and therefore not medically necessary.
2.7 Discuss the purpose of compliance plans. Pages 43–44	The goal of a compliance plan is to: • Prevent fraud and abuse through a formal process to identify, investigate, fix, and prevent repeat violations relating to reimbursement for health care services. • Ensure compliance with applicable federal, state, and local laws, including employment and environmental laws as well as antifraud laws. • Help defend the practice if it is investigated or prosecuted for fraud by substantiating the desire to behave compliantly and thus reduce any fines or criminal prosecution.

Using Terminology

Match the key terms in the left column with the definitions in the right column.

_____ 1. [LO 2.5] Code set

_____ 2. [LO 2.3] Protected health information

_____ 3. [LO 2.3] Authorization

_____ 4. [LO 2.3] HIPAA privacy rule

_____ 5. [LO 2.3] Notice of privacy practices

_____ 6. [LO 2.2] Business associate

_____ 7. [LO 2.3] Minimum necessary standards

_____ 8. [LO 2.4] HIPAA security rule

_____ 9. [LO 2.2] Clearinghouse

_____ 10. [LO 2.2] Covered entity

A. Document signed by a patient that permits release of medical information under the specific stated conditions.

B. A person or organization that performs a function or activity for a covered entity but is not part of its workforce.

C. A company that offers providers, for a fee, the service of receiving electronic or paper claims, checking and preparing them for processing, and transmitting them in proper data format to the correct carriers.

D. A coding system used to encode elements of data.

E. Under HIPAA, a health plan, health care clearinghouse, or health care provider who transmits any health information in electronic form in connection with a HIPAA transaction.

F. Law that regulates the use and disclosure of patients' protected health information.

G. Law that requires covered entities to establish administrative, physical, and technical safeguards to protect the confidentiality of health information.

H. The principle that individually identifiable health information should be disclosed only to the extent needed to support the purpose of the disclosure.

I. A HIPAA-mandated document that presents a covered entity's principles and procedures related to the protection of patients' protected health information.

J. Individually identifiable health information that is transmitted or maintained by electronic media.

Checking Your Understanding

Write the letter of the choice that best completes the statement or answers the question.

1. [LO 2.3] Under the HIPAA Privacy Rule, physician practices must _____.
   A. Train employees about the practice's privacy policy
   B. Appoint a staff member as privacy officer
   C. Have privacy practices appropriate for its health care services
   D. All of these

2. [LO 2.3] A notice of privacy practices is given to _____.
   A. The health plans with which a practice contracts
   B. A practice's business associates
   C. A practice's patients
   D. None of these

3. [LO 2.3] A patient's PHI may be released without authorization to _____.
   A. Local newspapers
   B. Employers' workers' compensation cases
   C. Social workers
   D. Family and friends

4. [LO 2.6] Which government agency has the authority to enforce the HIPAA Privacy Rule? _____
   A. CIA
   B. OIG
   C. OCR
   D. OESS

connect plus+
Enhance your learning at mcgrawhillconnect.com!
• Practice Exercises   • Worksheets
• Activities   • Integrated eBook

5. **[LO 2.3]** Patients have the right to _____.
   A. Authorize the release of information to anyone not directly involved in their care
   B. Alter the information in their medical records
   C. Block the release of information about their communicable diseases to the state department
   D. Deny the court of law access to PHI that is required for evidence

6. **[LO 2.3]** The authorization to release information must contain _____.
   A. The number of pages to be released
   B. The Social Security number of the patient
   C. A description of the information to be disclosed
   D. The names of all physicians that have treated the patient in the past year

7. **[LO 2.3]** Health information that does not identify an individual is referred to as _____.
   A. Protected health information
   B. Authorized health release
   C. Statutory data
   D. De-identified information

8. **[LO 2.4]** Which of the following help to enforce the HIPAA security rule? _____
   A. Controlling access to protected health information
   B. Securing Internet connections
   C. Using a system to back up data
   D. All of these

9. **[LO 2.7]** A compliance plan contains _____.
   A. Consistent written policies and procedures
   B. Medical office staff names
   C. The practice's main health plans
   D. Medical office staff addresses

10. **[LO 2.1]** Complete and comprehensive documentation shows that physicians have followed _____.
    A. The minimum necessary standards
    B. The minimum service requirements
    C. The medical standards of care
    D. The retention schedule

Define the following abbreviations:

1. **[LO 2.2]** CMS _____
2. **[LO 2.2]** HIPAA _____
3. **[LO 2.2]** EDI _____
4. **[LO 2.2]** ACA _____
5. **[LO 2.3]** PHI _____

6. **[LO 2.3]** NPP _____
7. **[LO 2.5]** NPI _____
8. **[LO 2.6]** OCR _____
9. **[LO 2.6]** OIG _____
10. **[LO 2.6]** DOJ _____

Applying Your Knowledge

[LO 2.3]   Case 2.1   Applying HIPAA

Rosalyn Ramirez is a medical insurance specialist employed by Valley Associates, PC, a midsized multispecialty practice with an excellent record of complying with HIPAA rules. Rosalyn answers the telephone and hears this question: "This is Jane Mazloum, I'm a patient of Dr. Olgivy. I just listened to a phone message from your office about coming in for a checkup. My husband and I were talking about this. Since this is my first pregnancy and I am working, we really don't want anyone else to know about it yet. Has this information been given to anybody outside the clinic?" How do you recommend that she respond?

[LO 2.3]   Case 2.2   Handling Authorizations

Angelo Diaz signed the authorization form shown on the next page. When his insurance company called for an explanation of a reported procedure that Dr. Handlesman performed to treat a stomach ulcer, George Welofar, the clinic's registered nurse, released copies of his complete file. On reviewing Mr. Diaz's history of treatment for alcohol abuse, the insurance company refused to pay the claim, stating that Mr. Diaz's alcoholism had caused the condition. Mr. Diaz complained to the practice manager about the situation. Should the information have been released?

connect (plus+)
Enhance your learning at mcgrawhillconnect.com!
• Practice Exercises   • Worksheets
• Activities   • Integrated eBook

Patient Name: _Angelo Diaz_____

Health Record Number: __ADI00_____

Date of Birth: __10-12-1945_____

1. I authorize the use or disclosure of the above named individual's health information as described below.

2. The following individual(s) or organization(s) are authorized to make the disclosure: _____Dr. L. Handlesman_____

3. The type of information to be used or disclosed is as follows (check the appropriate boxes and include other information where indicated)

❏ problem list
❏ medication list
❏ list of allergies
❏ immunization records
☑ most recent history
❏ most recent discharge summary
❏ lab results (please describe the dates or types of lab tests you would like disclosed): _____
☑ x-ray and imaging reports (please describe the dates or types of x-rays or images you would like disclosed): _____
❏ consultation reports from (please supply doctors' names): _____
❏ entire record
☑ other (please describe): __Progress notes_____

4. I understand that the information in my health record may include information relating to sexually transmitted disease, acquired immunodeficiency syndrome (AIDS), or human immunodeficiency virus (HIV). It may also include information about behavioral or mental health services, and treatment for alcohol and drug abuse.

5. The information identified above may be used by or disclosed to the following individuals or organization(s):

Name: _Blue Cross & Blue Shield_____

Address: _____

Name: _____

Address: _____

6. This information for which I'm authorizing disclosure will be used for the following purpose:
❏ my personal records
❏ sharing with other health care providers as needed/other (please describe): _____

7. I understand that I have a right to revoke this authorization at any time. I understand that if I revoke this authorization, I must do so in writing and present my written revocation to the health information management department. I understand that the revocation will not apply to information that has already been released in response to this authorization. I understand that the revocation will not apply to my insurance company when the law provides my insurer with the right to contest a claim under my policy.

8. This authorization will expire (insert date or event): _____

If I fail to specify an expiration date or event, this authorization will expire six months from the date on which it was signed.

9. I understand that once the above information is disclosed, it may be redisclosed by the recipient and the information may not be protected by federal privacy laws or regulations.

10. I understand authorizing the use or disclosure of the information identified above is voluntary. I need not sign this form to ensure healthcare treatment.

Signature of patient or legal representative: _____Angelo Diaz_____ Date: 3-1-2016_____

If signed by legal representative, relationship to patient

Signature of witness: _____ Date: _____

Distribution of copies: Original to provider; copy to patient; copy to accompany use or disclosure

Note: This sample form was developed by the American Health Information Management Association for discussion purposes. It should not be used without review by the issuing organization's legal counsel to ensure compliance with other federal and state laws and regulations.

Case 2.3   Working with Medical Records

The following chart note contains typical documentation abbreviations and shortened forms for words.

> 65-yo female; hx of right breast ca seen in SurgiCenter for bx of breast mass. Frozen section reported as benign tumor. Bleeding followed the biopsy. Reopened the breast along site of previous incision with coagulation of bleeders. Wound sutured. Pt adm. for observation of post-op bleeding. Discharged with no bleeding recurrence.

> Final Dx: Benign neoplasm, left breast.

Research the meanings of the following abbreviations (see the Abbreviations list at the end of this book), and write their meanings:

A. **[LO 2.1]** yo

B. **[LO 2.1]** hx

C. **[LO 2.1]** ca

D. **[LO 2.1]** bx

E. **[LO 2.1]** Pt

F. **[LO 2.1]** adm.

G. **[LO 2.1]** op

H. **[LO 2.1]** Dx

connect (plus+)

Enhance your learning at mcgrawhillconnect.com!
- Practice Exercises
- Worksheets
- Activities
- Integrated eBook

PATIENT ENCOUNTERS AND BILLING INFORMATION

Acknowledgment of Receipt of
    Notice of Privacy Practices
assignment of benefits
birthday rule
certification number
charge capture
chart number
coordination of benefits (COB)
encounter form
established patient (EP)
gender rule
guarantor
HIPAA Coordination of Benefits
HIPAA Eligibility for a Health Plan
HIPAA Referral Certification and Authorization
insured
network
new patient (NP)
nonparticipating provider (nonPAR)
out-of-network
participating provider (PAR)
patient information form
primary insurance
prior authorization number
referral number
referral waiver
referring physician
secondary insurance
subscriber
supplemental insurance
tertiary insurance
trace number

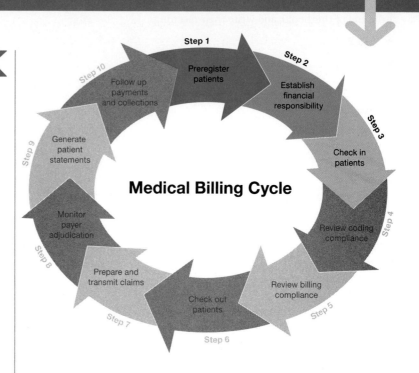

Medical Billing Cycle

Step 1 — Preregister patients
Step 2 — Establish financial responsibility
Step 3 — Check in patients
Step 4 — Review coding compliance
Step 5 — Review billing compliance
Step 6 — Check out patients
Step 7 — Prepare and transmit claims
Step 8 — Monitor payer adjudication
Step 9 — Generate patient statements
Step 10 — Follow up payments and collections

Learning Outcomes

After studying this chapter, you should be able to:

3.1 Explain the method used to classify patients as new and/or established.

3.2 List the information that is gathered from new patients.

3.3 Discuss the procedures that are followed to update established patient information.

3.4 Explain the process for verifying patients' eligibility for insurance benefits.

3.5 Discuss the importance of requesting referral or preauthorization approval.

3.6 Determine the primary insurance for patients who have more than one health plan.

3.7 Summarize the use of encounter forms.

3.8 Describe the types of communications with payers, providers, and patients that are most effective.

Processing encounters for billing purposes makes up the preclaim section of the medical billing cycle. This chapter discusses the important aspects of these steps:

▶ *Information about patients and their insurance coverage is gathered and verified.*
▶ *The encounter is documented by the provider and medical assistant.*
▶ *The primary insurance is determined.*
▶ *The patient's diagnoses and procedures are posted on an encounter form that will be used for billing and medical necessity.*

3.1 New versus Established Patients

To gather accurate information for billing and medical care, practices ask patients to supply information and then double-check key data. Patients who are new to the medical practice complete many forms before their first encounters with their providers. A **new patient (NP)** is someone who has not received any services from the provider (or another provider of the same specialty or subspecialty who is a member of the same practice) within the past three years.

A returning patient is called an **established patient (EP).** This patient has seen the provider (or another provider in the practice who has the same specialty/subspecialty) within the past three years. Established patients review and update the information that is on file about them. Figure 3.1 illustrates how to decide which category fits the patient.

new patient (NP) Patient who has not seen a provider within the past three years.

established patient (EP) Patient who has seen a provider within the past three years.

THINKING IT THROUGH 3.1

1. Carol Veras saw Dr. Alex Roderer, a gynecologist with the Alper Group, a multispecialty practice of 235 physicians, on October 24, 2014. On December 3, 2016, she made an appointment to see Dr. Judy Fisk, a gastroenterologist also with the Alper Group. Did the medical assistant handling Dr. Fisk's patients classify Carol as a new or an established patient?

3.2 Information for New Patients

When the patient is new to the practice, five types of information are important to gather:

1. Preregistration and scheduling information
2. Medical history
3. Patient/guarantor and insurance data
4. Assignment of benefits
5. Acknowledgment of Receipt of Notice of Privacy Practices

Preregistration and Scheduling Information

The collection of information begins before the patient presents at the front desk for an appointment. Most medical practices have a preregistration process to check that patients' health care requirements are appropriate for the medical practice and to schedule appointments of the correct length.

Preregistration Basics

When new patients call for appointments, basic information is usually gathered:

▶ Full name.
▶ Telephone numbers (cell, home, work).
▶ Address.
▶ Date of birth.

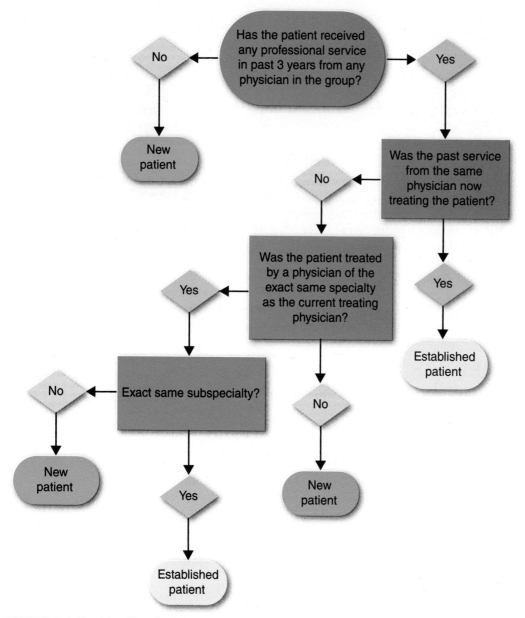

FIGURE 3.1 Decision Tree for New versus Established Patients

▶ Gender.

▶ Reason for call or nature of complaint, including information about previous treatments of problems.

▶ If insured, the name of the health plan and whether a copay or coinsurance payment at the time of service is required.

▶ If referred, the name of the **referring physician.**

referring physician Physician who transfers care of a patient to another physician.

Scheduling Appointments

Front office employees handle appointments and scheduling in most practices and may also handle prescription refill requests. Patient-appointment scheduling systems are often used; some permit online scheduling. Scheduling systems can be used to automatically send reminders to patients, to trace follow-up appointments, and to schedule recall appointments according to the provider's orders. Some offices use open-access (walk-ins) scheduling, where patients can see providers without having made advance appointments; follow-up visits are scheduled.

Provider Participation

New patients, too, may need information before deciding to make appointments. Most patients in managed care organizations such as PPOs and HMOs must use physicians in the managed care **network** to avoid paying higher charges. For this reason, patients check whether the provider is a **participating provider,** or **PAR,** in their plan. When patients see **nonparticipating,** or **nonPAR, providers,** they must pay more for these **out-of-network** visits—a higher copayment, greater coinsurance, or both—so a patient may choose not to make an appointment because of the additional expense.

Medical History

New patients complete medical history forms. Some practices give printed forms to patients when they come in. Others make the form available for completion ahead of time by posting it online or mailing it to the patient. The form asks for information about the patient's personal medical history, the family's medical history, and the social history. Social history covers lifestyle factors such as smoking, exercise, and alcohol use. Many specialists use less-detailed forms that cover the histories needed for treatment.

The physician or medical assistant reviews this information with the patient during the visit. The patient's answers and the physician's notes are documented in the medical record.

Patient/Guarantor and Insurance Data

A new patient arriving at the front desk for an appointment completes a **patient information form** (see Figure 3.2). This form is also called a patient registration form. It is used to collect the following demographic information about the patient:

▶ First name, middle initial, and last name.
▶ Gender (*F* for female or *M* for male).
▶ Marital status (*S* for single, *M* for married, *D* for divorced, *W* for widowed).
▶ Race and ethnicity.
▶ Primary language.
▶ Birth date, using four digits for the year.
▶ Home address and telephone numbers; e-mail address.
▶ Social Security number.
▶ Employer's name, address, and telephone number.
▶ A contact person for the patient in case of a medical emergency.
▶ For a married patient, the name and employer of the spouse.
▶ If the patient is a minor (under the age of majority according to state law) or has a medical power of attorney in place (such as a person who is handling the medical decisions of another person), the responsible person's name, gender, marital status, birth date, address, Social Security number, telephone number, and employer information. In most cases, the responsible person is a parent, guardian, adult child, or other person acting with legal authority to make health care decisions on behalf of the patient.
▶ The name of the patient's health plan.
▶ The health plan's policyholder's name (the policyholder may be a spouse, divorced spouse, guardian, or other relation), birth date, plan type, Social Security number, policy number or group number, telephone number, and employer.
▶ If the patient is covered by another health plan, the name and policyholder information for that plan.

BILLING TIP

Subscriber, Insured, or Guarantor?

Other terms for policyholder are **insured** and **subscriber.** This person is the holder of the insurance policy that covers the patient and is not necessarily also a patient of the practice. The **guarantor** is the person who is financially responsible for the bill.

---

network   Group of providers in a managed care organization.

participating provider (PAR)   Provider who agrees to provide medical services to a payer's policyholders according to a contract.

nonparticipating provider (nonPAR)   Provider who does not join a particular health plan.

out-of-network   Provider that does not have a participation agreement with a plan.

patient information form   Form that includes a patient's personal, employment, and insurance company data.

insured   Policyholder or subscriber to a health plan or policy.

subscriber   The insured.

guarantor   Person who is the insurance policyholder for a patient.

Patient

Last Name		First Name		MI	Sex __ M __ F	Date of Birth / /

Address	City	State	Zip

Home Ph # ( )	Cell Ph # ( )	Marital Status	Student Status

Race __ American Indian or Alaskan Native __ Asian __ Black __ Caucasian __ Other __ Pacific Islander __ Declined	Ethnicity __ Hispanic __ Non-Hispanic __ Declined	Language

SS#	Email	Allergies

Employment Status	Employer Name	Work Ph # ( )	Primary Insurance ID#

Employer Address	City	State	Zip

Referred By	Ph # of Referral ( )

Responsible Party (Complete this section if the person responsible for the bill is not the patient)

Last Name	First Name	MI	Sex __ M __ F	Date of Birth / /

Address	City	State	Zip	SS#

Relation to Patient __ Spouse __ Parent __ Other	Employer Name	Work Phone # ( )

Spouse, or Parent (if minor):	Home Phone # ( )

Insurance (If you have multiple coverage, supply information from both carriers)

Primary Carrier Name	Secondary Carrier Name
Name of the Insured (Name on ID Card)	Name of the Insured (Name on ID Card)
Patient's relationship to the insured __ Self __ Spouse __ Child	Patient's relationship to the insured __ Self __ Spouse __ Child
Insured ID #	Insured ID #
Group # or Company Name	Group # or Company Name
Insurance Address	Insurance Address

Phone #	Copay $	Phone #	Copay $
	Deductible $		Deductible $

Other Information

Is patient's condition related to: __ Employment __ Auto Accident (if yes, state in which accident occurred: ___) __ Other Accident	Reason for visit:

Date of Accident: /   /   Date of First Symptom of Illness: /   /

Financial Agreement and Authorization for Treatment

I authorize treatment and agree to pay all fees and charges for the person named above. I agree to pay all charges shown by statements, promptly upon their presentation, unless credit arrangements are agreed upon in writing.	I authorize payment directly to ORCHARD HILL MEDICAL CENTER of insurance benefits otherwise payable to me. I hereby authorize the release of any medical information necessary in order to process a claim for payment in my behalf.

Signed: _____   Date: _____

FIGURE 3.2 Patient Information Form

Insurance Cards

For an insured new patient, the front and the back of the insurance card are scanned or photocopied. All data from the card that the patient has written on the patient information form are double-checked for accuracy.

Most insurance cards have the following information (see Figure 3.3):

▶ Group identification number.
▶ Date on which the member's coverage became effective.
▶ Member name.
▶ Member identification number.
▶ The health plan's name, type of coverage, copayment/coinsurance requirements, and frequency limits or annual maximums for services; sometimes the annual deductible.
▶ Optional items, such as prescription drugs that are covered, with the payment requirements.

BILLING TIP

Matching the Patient's Name

Payers want the name of the patient on a claim to be exactly as it is shown on the insurance card. Do not use nicknames, do not skip middle initials, and do not make any other changes. Compare the patient information form carefully with the insurance card, and resolve any discrepancies before the encounter.

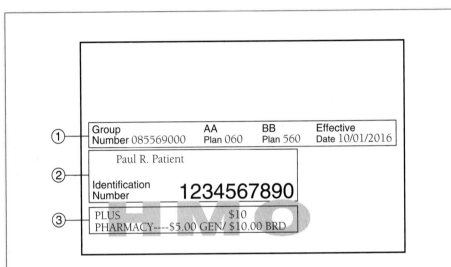

1. **Group identification number**
   The 9-digit number used to identify the member's employer.

   Plan codes
   The numbers used to identify the codes assigned to each plan: used for claims submissions when medical services are rendered out-of-state.

   Effective date
   The date on which the member's coverage became effective.

2. **Member name**
   The full name of the cardholder.

   Identification number
   The 10-digit number used to identify each plan member.

3. **Health plan**
   The name and 1-800 telephone number of the health plan and the type of coverage; usually lists any copayment amounts, frequency limits or annual maximums for home and office visits; may also list the member's annual deductible amount.

   Additional coverage
   The type(s) of riders (additional coverages) that are included in the member's benefits (DME, Visions).

   Pharmacy
   The type of prescription drug coverage; lists copayment amounts.

FIGURE 3.3 An Example of an Insurance Card

Photo Identification

Many practices also require the patient to present a photo ID card, such as a driver's license, which the practice scans or copies for the chart.

Assignment of Benefits

Physicians usually submit claims for patients and receive payments directly from the payers. This saves patients paperwork; it also benefits providers, since payments are faster. The policyholder must authorize this procedure by signing and dating an **assignment of benefits** statement. This may be a separate form, or an entry on the patient information form (see again Figure 3.2).

Acknowledgment of Receipt of Notice of Privacy Practices

Under the HIPAA Privacy Rule (see the chapter covering HIPAA), providers do not need specific authorization in order to release patients' PHI (protected health information) for treatment, payment, and health care operations (TPO) purposes. These uses are defined as:

1. *Treatment:* This purpose primarily consists of discussion of the patient's case with other providers. For example, the physician may document the role of each member of the health care team in providing care. Each team member then records actions and observations so that the ordering physician knows how the patient is responding to treatment.
2. *Payment:* Practices usually submit claims on behalf of patients; this involves sending demographic and diagnostic information.
3. *Health care operations:* This purpose includes activities such as staff training and quality improvement.

Providers must have patients' authorization to use or disclose information that is not for TPO purposes. For example, a patient who wishes a provider to disclose PHI to a life insurance company must complete an authorization form (see Chapter 2, Figure 2.3) to do so.

Under HIPAA, providers must inform each patient about their privacy practices one time. The most common method is to give the patient a copy of the medical office's privacy practices to read, and then to have the patient sign a separate form called an **Acknowledgment of Receipt of Notice of Privacy Practices** (see Figure 3.4). This form states that the patient has read the privacy practices and understands how the provider intends to protect the patient's rights to privacy under HIPAA.

The provider must make a good-faith effort to have patients sign this document. The provider must also document—in the medical record—whether the patient signed the form. The format for the acknowledgment is up to the practice. HIPAA does not require the parent or guardian of a minor to sign. If a child is accompanied by a parent or guardian who is completing other paperwork on behalf of the minor, it is reasonable to ask that adult to sign the Acknowledgment of Receipt. On the other hand, if the child or teen is unaccompanied, the minor patient may be asked to sign.

Entering New Patient Information in the Practice Management Program

The database of patients in the practice management program (PMP) must be continually kept up-to-date. For each new patient, a new file and a new **chart number** are set up. The chart number is a unique number that identifies the patient. It links all the information that is stored in the other databases—providers, insurance plans, diagnoses, procedures, and claims—to the case of the particular patient. The PMP

Acknowledgment of Receipt of Notice of Privacy Practices

I understand that the providers of Valley Associates, PC, may share my health information for treatment, billing and healthcare operations. I have been given a copy of the organization's notice of privacy practices that describes how my health information is used and shared. I understand that Valley Associates has the right to change this notice at any time. I may obtain a current copy by contacting the practice's office or by visiting the website at www.xxx.com.

My signature below constitutes my acknowledgment that I have been provided with a copy of the notice of privacy practices.

_____

Signature of Patient or Legal Representative   Date

If signed by legal representative,
relationship to patient:_____

FIGURE 3.4 Acknowledgment of Receipt of Notice of Privacy Practices

also has a database of the payers from whom the practice usually gets payments. This database contains each payer's name and the contact's name; the plan type, such as HMO, PPO, Medicare, Medicaid, or other; and telephone and fax numbers. The medical assistant selects the payer that is the patient's insurer from the insurance database. If the particular payer has not already been entered, the PMP is updated with the payer's information.

GAINING EXPERTISE IN USING A PRACTICE MANAGEMENT PROGRAM (PMP)

Options for *Insurance in the Medical Office 7e*

Completing on-the-job tasks using PMPs is an important aspect of a medical assistant's work. *Insurance in the Medical Office* offers options that your instructor may implement to help you gain experience completing these tasks.

- **Connect Plus** Connect Plus provides simulated Medisoft exercises in four modes: Demo, Practice, Test, and Assessment. The simulated exercises, offered online, cover key practice management tasks to provide experience in working with patient, insurance, procedure, diagnosis, claims, and transaction databases. If you are assigned this option, read Appendix A, *Guide to Medisoft,* as your first step, and then follow the instructions that are printed in each chapter's Connect Plus Exercises, indicated with the connect(PLUS+).

For the exercises that include the use of an insurance claim form, there is the option to complete these using Connect Plus, a paper CMS-1500 form, or the electronic CMS-1500 form provided at the book's website.

- **Paper Claim Form** If you are gaining experience by completing a paper CMS-1500 claim form, use the blank form supplied to you (from the back of *Insurance in the Medical Office* or printed out from the book's Online Learning Center, www.mhhe.com/newbycarr), and follow the instructions in the text chapter that is appropriate for the particular payer to fill in the form by hand.

- **Electronic CMS-1500 Form** If you are assigned to use the electronic CMS-1500 form, access the form at the book's Online Learning Center, www.mhhe.com/newbycarr. See Appendix B, *The Interactive Simulated CMS-1500 Form,* for further instructions.

Exercise 3.1 Creating a New Patient Account

In this scenario, a new patient, Ann Ingram, arrives at Orchard Hill Medical Center for her appointment with Dr. Clarke. Ann has been experiencing throat pain and has a fever. Dr. Clarke examines Ann and orders a throat culture. Complete the Patient/Guarantor dialog box for Ann Ingram, a new patient of Dr. Clarke.

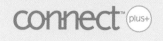

Follow the steps at www.mhhe.com/newbycarr to complete the exercise at connect.mcgraw-hill.com on your own once you have watched the demo and tried the steps with prompts in practice mode. Use the information provided in the scenario to complete the exercise.

THINKING IT THROUGH 3.2

1. Why is it important to verify a patient's insurance coverage before an office visit?

3.3 Information for Established Patients

When established patients present for appointments, the front desk staff member asks whether any pertinent personal or insurance information has changed. This update process is important because different employment, marital status, dependent status, or plans may affect patients' coverage. Patients may also phone in changes, such as new addresses or employers.

To double-check that information is current, most practices periodically ask established patients to review and sign off on their patient information forms when they come in. This review should be done at least once a year. A good time is an established patient's first appointment in a new year. The file is also checked to be sure that the patient has been given a current NPP. If the insurance of an established patient has changed, both sides of the new card are copied, and all data are checked. Many practices routinely scan or copy the card at each visit as a safeguard.

Updating Established Patient Information in the Practice Management Program

Usually, a new *case* or record for an established patient is set up in the program when the patient's chief complaint for an encounter is different than the previous chief complaint. For example, a patient might have had an initial appointment for a comprehensive physical examination. Subsequently, this patient sees the provider because of stomach pain. Each visit is set up as a separate case in the PMP.

The medical assistant also updates any changed patient demographic information that is relevant to the PMP, most importantly facts about the patient's insurance coverage and the guarantor for the bill.

Exercise 3.2 Updating an Existing Patient Account

In this scenario, an established patient of Orchard Hill Medical Center, Herbert Bell, has called to provide a new smart phone number to the office. Update his data.

Follow the steps at www.mhhe.com/newbycarr to complete the exercise at connect.mcgraw-hill.com on your own once you have watched the demo and tried the steps with prompts in practice mode. Use the information provided in the scenario to complete the exercise.

connect (plus+)

THINKING IT THROUGH 3.3

1. Review these multiple versions of the same name:

   Ralph Smith

   Ralph P. Smith

   Ralph Plane Smith

   R. Plane Smith

   R. P. Smith

   If "Ralph Plane Smith" appears on the insurance card and his mother writes "Ralph Smith" on the patient information form, which version should be used for the medical practice's records? Why?

3.4 Verifying Patient Eligibility for Insurance Benefits

To be paid for services, medical practices need to establish financial responsibility. Medical insurance specialists are vital employees in this process. For insured patients, they follow three steps to establish financial responsibility:

1. Verify patients' eligibility for insurance benefits.
2. Determine preauthorization and referral requirements.
3. Determine the primary payer if more than one insurance plan is in effect.

The first step is to verify patients' eligibility for benefits. Medical assistants abstract information about the patient's payer/plan from the patient's information form (PIF) and the insurance card. They then contact the payer to verify three points:

1. Patients' general eligibility for benefits.
2. The amount of the copayment or coinsurance required at the time of service.
3. Whether the planned encounter is for a covered service that is medically necessary under the payer's rules.

These items are checked before an encounter except in a medical emergency, where care is provided immediately and insurance is checked after the encounter.

Factors Affecting General Eligibility

General eligibility for benefits depends on a number of factors. If premiums are required, patients must have paid them on time. For government-sponsored plans where income is the criterion, like Medicaid, eligibility can change monthly. For patients with employer-sponsored health plans, employment status can be the deciding factor:

▶ Coverage may end on the last day of the month in which the employee's active full-time service ends, such as for disability, layoff, or termination.
▶ The employee may no longer qualify as a member of the group. For example, some companies do not provide benefits for part-time employees. If a full-time employee changes to part-time employment, the coverage ends.
▶ An eligible dependent's coverage may end on the last day of the month in which the dependent status ends, such as reaching the age limit stated in the policy.

If the plan is an HMO that requires a primary care provider (PCP), a general or family practice must verify that (1) the provider is a plan participant, (2) the patient is listed on the plan's enrollment master list, and (3) the patient is assigned to the PCP as of the date of service.

The medical assistant checks with the payer to confirm whether the patient is currently covered. If online access is used, Web information and e-mail messages are exchanged with provider representatives. If the payer requires the use of the telephone, the provider representative is called. Based on the patient's plan, eligibility for these specific benefits may also need checking:

▶ Office visits
▶ Lab coverage
▶ Diagnostic X-rays
▶ Maternity coverage
▶ Pap smear coverage
▶ Coverage of psychiatric visits
▶ Physical or occupational therapy
▶ Durable medical equipment (DME)
▶ Foot care

Checking Out-of-Network Benefits

If patients have insurance coverage but the practice does not participate in their plans, the medical insurance specialist checks the out-of-network benefit. When the patient has out-of-network benefits, the payer's rules concerning copayments/coinsurance and coverage are followed. If a patient does not have out-of-network benefits, as is common when the health plan is an HMO, the patient is responsible for the entire bill.

Verifying Copayment or Coinsurance Amounts

The amount of the copayment, or coinsurance, if required at the time of service, must be checked. It is sometimes the case that the insurance card is out of date, and a different amount needs to be collected.

BILLING TIP

Double-Checking Patients' Information

Review the payer's spelling of the insured's and the patient's first and last names as well as the dates of birth and identification numbers. Correct any mistakes in the PMP, so that when a health care claim is later transmitted for the encounter, it will be accepted for processing.

Determining Covered Services

The medical assistant also must attempt to determine whether the planned encounter is for a covered service. If the service will not be covered, that patient can be informed and made aware of financial responsibility in advance. The resources for covered services include knowledge of the major plans held by the practice's patients, information from the provider representative and payer websites, and the electronic benefit inquiries described below. Medical assistants are familiar with what the plans cover in general. For example, most plans cover regular office visits, but they may not cover preventive services or some therapeutic services. Unusual or unfamiliar services must be researched, and the payer must be queried.

Electronic Benefit Inquiries and Responses

An electronic transaction, a telephone call, or a fax or e-mail message may be used to communicate with the payer. Electronic transaction, the most efficient, is called the **HIPAA Eligibility for a Health Plan** transaction or the *X12 270/271*. The number 270 refers to the inquiry that is sent, and 271 to the answer returned by the payer.

When an eligibility benefits transaction is sent, the computer program assigns a unique **trace number** to the inquiry. Often, eligibility transactions are sent the day before patients arrive for appointments. If the PMP has this feature, the eligibility transaction can be sent automatically.

The health plan responds to an eligibility inquiry with this information:

▶ Trace number, as a double-check on the inquiry.
▶ Benefit information, such as whether the insurance coverage is active.
▶ Covered period—the period of dates that the coverage is active.
▶ Benefit units, such as how many physical therapy visits.
▶ Coverage level—that is, who is covered, such as spouse and family or individual.

The following information may also be transmitted:

▶ The copay amount.
▶ The yearly deductible amount.
▶ The out-of-pocket expenses.
▶ The health plan's information on the insured's/patient's first and last names, dates of birth, and identification numbers.
▶ Primary care provider.

Procedures When the Patient Is Not Covered

If an insured patient's policy does not cover a planned service, this situation is discussed with the patient before treatment. Patients should be informed that the payer does not pay for the service and that they are responsible for the charges. Some payers require the physician to use specific forms to tell the patient about uncovered services. These financial agreement forms, which patients must read and sign, prove that patients have been told about their obligation to pay the bill before the services are given. For example, the Medicare program provides a form called an advance beneficiary notice (ABN) that must be used to show patients the charges. The signed form, as explained in the chapter on Medicare, allows the practice to collect payment for a provided service or supply directly from the patient if Medicare refuses reimbursement. Figure 3.5 is

HIPAA Eligibility for a Health Plan HIPAA X12N 270/271 transaction in which a provider asks for and receives an answer about a patient's eligibility for benefits.

trace number Number assigned to a HIPAA 270 electronic transaction.

Service to be performed: _____
Estimated charge: _____
Date of planned service: _____
Reason for exclusion: _____
_____

I, _____, a patient of _____, understand the service described above is excluded from my health insurance. I am responsible for payment in full of the charges for this service.

FIGURE 3.5 Sample Financial Agreement for Patient Payment of Noncovered Services

an example of a form used to tell patients in advance of the probable cost of procedures that are not going to be covered by their plan and to secure their agreement to pay.

Exercise 3.3 Verifying Patient Eligibility

In this scenario, new patient Ann Ingram's insurance eligibility must be checked in advance of her appointment with Dr. Clarke.

Follow the steps at www.mhhe.com/newbycarr to complete the exercise at connect.mcgraw-hill.com on your own once you have watched the demo and tried the steps with prompts in practice mode. Use the information provided in the scenario to complete the exercise.

THINKING IT THROUGH 3.4

1. What is the advantage of using electronic transactions for verifying a patient's eligibility for benefits?

3.5 Determining Preauthorization and Referral Requirements

Preauthorization

prior authorization number/ certification number
Identifying code assigned when preauthorization is required.

A managed care payer often requires preauthorization before the patient sees a specialist, is admitted to the hospital, or has a particular procedure. The medical assistant may request preauthorization over the phone, by e-mail or fax, or by an electronic transaction. If the payer approves the service, it issues a **prior authorization number** that must be entered in the PMP so that it will be stored and appear later on the health care claim for the encounter. (This number may also be called a **certification number**.)

To help secure preauthorization, best practice is to:

▶ Be as specific as possible about the planned procedure when exchanging information with a payer.
▶ Collect and have available all the diagnosis information related to the procedure, including any pertinent history.
▶ Query the provider and then request preauthorization for all procedures that may potentially be used to treat the patient.

Referrals

referral number Authorization number given to the referred physician.

Often, a physician needs to send a patient to another physician for evaluation and/or treatment. For example, an internist might send a patient to a cardiologist to evaluate heart function. If a patient's plan requires it, the patient is given a **referral number** and a referral document, which is a written request for the medical service. The patient is usually responsible for bringing these items to the encounter with the specialist.

Referral Form

Label with Patient's Demographic & Insurance Information

Physician referred to ______________________________

Referred for:

□ Consult only
□ Follow-up
□ Lab
□ X-ray
□ Procedure
□ Other

Reason for visit ______________________________

Number of visits __________

Appointment requested: Please contact patient; phone: ____________

Primary care physician

Name ______________________________

Signature ______________________________

Phone ______________________________

FIGURE 3.6 Referral Form

A paper referral document (see Figure 3.6) describes the services the patient is certified to receive. This approval may instead be communicated electronically using the **HIPAA Referral Certification and Authorization** transaction, also called the *X12 278.*

HIPAA Referral Certification and Authorization HIPAA X12 278 transaction in which a provider asks a health plan for approval of a service and gets a response.

The specialist's office handling a referred patient must:

- Check that the patient has a referral number.
- Verify patient enrollment in the plan.
- Understand restrictions to services, such as regulations that require the patient to visit a specialist in a specific period of time after receiving the referral or that limit the number of times the patient can receive services from the specialist.

Two other situations arise with referrals:

1. A managed care patient may "self-refer"—that is, come for specialty care without being referred by a physician and thus without a referral number when one is required. The medical assistant then asks the patient to sign a form acknowledging responsibility for the services. A sample form is shown in Figure 3.7a.
2. A patient who is required to have a referral document does not bring one. The medical assistant then asks the patient to sign a document such as that shown in Figure 3.7b. This **referral waiver** ensures that the patient will pay for services received if in fact a referral is not documented in the time specified.

referral waiver Document a patient signs to guarantee payment when a referral authorization is pending.

Member Self-Referral Acknowledgment

I, _____, understand that I am seeking the care
of this specialty physician or health care provider, _____,
without a referral from my primary care physician. I understand that
the terms of my Plan coverage require that I obtain that referral, and
that if I fail to do so, my Plan will not cover any part of the charges,
costs or expenses related to this specialist's services to me.

Signed,

_____   _____
(member's name)   (date)

****

Specialty physician or other health care provider:

Please keep a copy of this form in your patient's file

(a)

Referral Waiver

I did not bring a referral for the medical services I will receive today.
If my primary care physician does not provide a referral within two
days, I understand that I am responsible for paying for the services I
am requesting.

Signature: _____

Date: _____

(b)

FIGURE 3.7 (a) Self-Referral Document, (b) Referral Waiver

THINKING IT THROUGH 3.5

1. What is the difference between a referral and a preauthorization
requirement?

3.6 Determining the Primary Insurance

primary insurance Health
plan that pays benefits first.

secondary insurance Second
payer on a claim.

tertiary insurance Third payer
on a claim.

supplemental insurance
Health plan that covers services
not normally covered by a
primary plan.

The medical assistant also examines the patient information form and insurance
card to see if other insurance coverage is in effect. A patient may have more than one
health plan. The assistant then decides which is the **primary insurance**—the plan
that pays first when more than one plan is in effect—and which is the **secondary
insurance**—an additional policy that provides benefits. **Tertiary insurance,** a third
payer, is possible. Some patients have **supplemental insurance,** a "fill-in-the-gap"
insurance plan that covers parts of expenses, such as coinsurance, that they must
otherwise pay under the primary plan.

As a practical matter for billing, determining the primary insurance is important
because this payer is sent the first claim for the encounter. A second claim is sent to
the secondary payer after the payment is received for the primary claim.

Deciding which payer is primary is also important because insurance policies contain a provision called **coordination of benefits (COB).** The coordination of benefits guidelines ensure that when a patient has more than one policy, maximum appropriate benefits are paid, but without duplication. Under the law, to protect the insurance companies, if the patient has signed an assignment of benefits statement, the provider is responsible for reporting any additional insurance coverage to the primary payer.

Coordination of benefits in government-sponsored programs follows specific guidelines. Primary and secondary coverage under Medicare, Medicaid, and other programs is discussed in the chapters devoted to those topics. Note that COB information can also be exchanged between provider and health plan or between a health plan and another payer, such as auto insurance. The **HIPAA Coordination of Benefits** transaction is used to send the necessary data to payers. This transaction is also called the *X12 837*—the same transaction used to send health care claims electronically—because it goes along with the claim.

coordination of benefits (COB) Explains how an insurance policy will pay if more than one policy applies.

HIPAA Coordination of Benefits HIPAA X12 837 transaction sent to a secondary or tertiary payer.

Guidelines for Determining the Primary Insurance

How do patients come to have more than one plan in effect? Possible answers are that a patient may have coverage under more than one group plan, such as a person who has both employer-sponsored insurance and a policy from union membership. A person may have primary insurance coverage from an employer but also be covered as a dependent under a spouse's insurance, making the spouse's plan the person's additional insurance. General guidelines for determining the primary insurance are shown in Table 3.1.

Guidelines for Children with More than One Insurance Plan

A child's parents may each have primary insurance. If both parents cover dependents on their plans, the child's primary insurance is usually determined by the **birthday rule.** This rule states that the parent whose day of birth is earlier in the calendar year is primary. For example, Rachel Foster's mother and father both work and have employer-sponsored insurance policies. Her father, George Foster, was born on October 7, 1971, and her mother, Myrna, was born on May 15, 1972. Since the mother's date of birth is

birthday rule Guideline that determines which parent has the primary insurance for a child.

Table 3.1 Determining Primary Coverage

- If the patient has only one policy, it is primary.
- If the patient has coverage under two group plans, the plan that has been in effect for the patient for the longest period of time is primary. However, if an active employee has a plan with the present employer and is still covered by a former employer's plan as a retiree or a laid-off employee, the current employer's plan is primary.
- If the patient has coverage under both a group and an individual plan, the group plan is primary.
- If the patient is also covered as a dependent under another insurance policy, the patient's plan is primary.
- If an employed patient has coverage under the employer's plan and additional coverage under a government-sponsored plan, the employer's plan is primary. For example, if a patient is enrolled in a PPO through employment and is also on Medicare, the PPO is primary.
- If a retired patient is covered by a spouse's employer's plan and the spouse is still employed, the spouse's plan is primary, even if the retired person has Medicare.
- If the patient is a dependent child covered by both parents' plans and the parents are not separated or divorced (or if the parents have joint custody of the child), the primary plan is determined by the *birthday rule*.
- If two or more plans cover dependent children of separated or divorced parents who do not have joint custody of their children, the children's primary plan is determined in this order:
  —The plan of the custodial parent.
  —The plan of the spouse of the custodial parent if remarried.
  —The plan of the parent without custody.
- Dependent coverage can be determined by a court decision, which overrules these guidelines.

earlier in the calendar year (although the father is older), her plan is Rachel's primary insurance. The father's plan is secondary for Rachel. Note that if a dependent child's primary insurance does not provide for the complete reimbursement of a bill, the balance may usually be submitted to the other parent's plan for consideration.

Another, much less common, way to determine a child's primary coverage is called the **gender rule.** When this rule applies, if the child is covered by two health plans, the father's plan is primary. In some states, insurance regulations require a plan that uses the gender rule to be primary to a plan that follows the birthday rule.

The insurance policy also covers which parent's plan is primary for dependent children of separated or divorced parents. If the parents have joint custody, the birthday rule usually applies. If the parents do not have joint custody of the child, unless otherwise directed by a court order, usually the primary benefits are determined in this order:

- ▶ The plan of the custodial parent.
- ▶ The plan of the spouse of the custodial parent, if the parent has remarried.
- ▶ The plan of the parent without custody.

gender rule Coordination of benefits rule for a child insured under both parents' plans.

Exercise 3.4 Entering a Patient's Insurance Information

In this scenario, Ann Ingram's insurance information that was verified in Exercise 3.3 is entered into the PMP by completing the Policy 1 tab.

Follow the steps at www.mhhe.com/newbycarr to complete the exercise at connect.mcgraw-hill.com on your own once you have watched the demo and tried the steps with prompts in practice mode. Use the information provided in the scenario to complete the exercise.

connect plus+

THINKING IT THROUGH 3.6

1. When a patient has secondary insurance, the claim for that payer is sent after the claim to the primary payer is paid. Why is that the case? What information do you think the medical assistant provides to the secondary payer?

3.7 Working with Encounter Forms

After the registration process is complete, patients are shown to rooms for their appointments with providers. Typically, a clinical medical assistant documents the patient's vital signs. Then the provider conducts and documents the examination. After the visit, the medical assistant uses the documented diagnoses and procedures to update the practice management program.

BILLING TIP

Double-Checking Billing Data

Completed encounter forms need to be double-checked for accurate **charge capture.** Correct any mistakes in the PMP when charges are entered.

charge capture Procedures that ensure billable services are recorded and reported for payment.

Encounter Forms

The diagnosis and procedure codes are recorded on an **encounter form,** also known as a superbill, charge slip, or routing slip. Traditionally, the encounter form has been a paper form. Offices that use integrated EHR and PMPs use an electronic version of the form. Whether on paper or in electronic form, encounter form codes must be recorded in the PMP, as they will be submitted to the health plan in the form of a claim.

encounter form List of the diagnoses, procedures, and charges for a patient's visit.

The encounter form is completed by a provider to summarize billing information for a patient's visit. This may be done using a device such as a laptop computer, tablet PC, or PDA (personal digital assistant), or by checking off items on a paper form. Physicians should sign and date the completed encounter forms for their patients.

Encounter forms record the services provided to a patient, as shown in the completed office encounter form in Figure 3.8. These forms list the medical

ORCHARD HILL MEDICAL PRACTICE
Ruth J. Clarke, MD - Internal Medicine

PATIENT NAME	APPT. DATE/TIME
Ingram, Ann	10/6/2016 9:30 am

PATIENT NO.	DX
INGRAAN0	1. Z00.00 Exam, Adult 2. 3. 4.

DESCRIPTION	✓	CPT	FEE	DESCRIPTION	✓	CPT	FEE
OFFICE VISITS				**PROCEDURES**			
New Patient				Diagnostic Anoscopy		46600	
LI Problem Focused		99201		ECG Complete	✓	93000	70
LII Expanded		99202		I&D, Abscess		10060	
LIII Detailed		99203		Pap Smear		88150	
LIV Comp./Mod.		99204		Removal of Cerumen		69210	
LV Comp./High		99205		Removal 1 Lesion		17000	
Established Patient				Removal 2-14 Lesions		17003	
LI Minimum		99211		Removal 15+ Lesions		17004	
LII Problem Focused		99212		Rhythm ECG w/Report		93040	
LIII Expanded		99213		Rhythm ECG w/Tracing		93041	
LIV Detailed		99214		Sigmoidoscopy, diag.		45330	
LV Comp./High		99215					
				LABORATORY			
PREVENTIVE VISIT				Bacteria Culture		87081	
New Patient				Fungal Culture		87101	
Age 12-17		99384		Glucose Finger Stick		82948	
Age 18-39		99385		Lipid Panel		80061	
Age 40-64	✓	99386	180	Specimen Handling		99000	
Age 65+		99387		Stool/Occult Blood		82270	
Established Patient				Tine Test		85008	
Age 12-17		99394		Tuberculin PPD		86580	
Age 18-39		99395		Urinalysis	✓	81000	17
Age 40-64		99396		Venipuncture		36415	
Age 65+		99397					
				INJECTION/IMMUN.			
CONSULTATION: OFFICE/OP				Immun. Admin.	✓	90471	20
Requested By:				Ea. Addl.		90472	
LI Problem Focused		99241		Hepatitis A Immun		90632	
LII Expanded		99242		Hepatitis B Immun		90746	
LIII Detailed		99243		Influenza Immun	✓	90661	68
LIV Comp./Mod.		99244		Pneumovax		90732	
LV Comp./High		99245					
				TOTAL FEES			355

FIGURE 3.8 Sample Completed Encounter Form

practice's most frequently performed procedures with their procedure codes. It also often has blanks where the diagnosis and its code(s) are filled in. (Some forms include a list of the diagnoses that are most frequently made by the practice's physicians.)

Other information is often included on the form:

▶ A checklist of managed care plans under contract and their utilization guidelines.
▶ The patient's prior balance due, if any.
▶ Check boxes to indicate the timing and need for a follow-up appointment to be scheduled for the patient during checkout.

Preprinted or Computer-Generated Forms

The paper form may be designed by the practice manager and/or physicians based on analysis of the practice's medical services. It is then printed, usually with carbonless copies available for distribution according to the practice's policy. For example, the top copy may be filed in the medical record; the second copy may be filed in the financial record; and the third copy may be given to the patient. Alternatively, the form may be printed for each patient's appointment using the practice management program. A customized encounter form lists the date of the appointment, the patient's name, and the identification number assigned by the medical practice. It can also be designed to show the patient's previous balance, the day's fees, payments made, and the amount due. Encounter forms must be updated when new codes are issued and old codes are modified or dropped.

THINKING IT THROUGH 3.7

Review the completed encounter form shown in Figure 3.8.

1. What is the age range of the patient?
2. Is this a new or an established patient?
3. What procedures were performed during the encounter?
4. What laboratory tests were ordered?

3.8 Communications Are Key
Communications with Payers

Communications with payers' representatives—whether to check on eligibility, receive referral certification, or resolve billing disputes—are frequent and are vitally important to the medical practice. Getting answers quickly means quicker payment for services. Medical assistants follow these guidelines for effective communication:

▶ Learn the name, telephone number/extension, and e-mail address of the appropriate representative at each payer. If possible, invite the representative to visit the office and meet the staff.
▶ Use a professional, courteous telephone manner or writing style to help build good relationships.
▶ Keep current with changing reimbursement policies and utilization guidelines by regularly reviewing information from payers. Usually, the medical practice receives Internet or printed bulletins or newsletters that contain up-to-date information from health plans and government-sponsored programs.

All communications with payer representatives should be documented. The representative's name, the date and time of the communication, and the outcome should be described. This information is sometimes needed later to explain or defend a charge on a patient's insurance claim.

Communications with Providers

At times, medical assistants find incorrect or conflicting data on encounter forms. It may be necessary to check the documentation and, if still problematic, to communicate with the physician to clear up the discrepancies. In such cases, it is important to remember that medical practices are extremely busy places. Providers often have crowded schedules, especially if they see many patients, and have little time to go over billing and coding issues. Questions must be kept to those that are essential.

Also, paper encounter forms (and practice management programs) list procedure codes and, often, diagnosis codes that change periodically. Medical assistants must be sure that these databases are updated when new codes are available.

Communications with Patients

Service to patients—the customers of medical practices—is as important as, if not more important than, billing information. Satisfied customers are essential to the financial health of every business, including medical practices. Medical practice staff members must be dedicated to retaining patients by providing excellent service.

The following are examples of good communication:

▶ Established and new patients who call or arrive for appointments are always given friendly greetings and are referred to by name.
▶ Patients' questions about forms they are completing and about insurance matters are answered with courtesy.
▶ When possible, patients in the reception area are told the approximate waiting time until they will see the provider.
▶ Fees for providers' procedures and services are explained to patients.
▶ The medical practice's guidelines about patients' responsibilities, such as when payments are due from patients and the need to have referrals from primary care physicians, are prominently posted in the office.
▶ Patients are called a day or two before their appointments to remind them of appointment times.

Like all businesses, even the best-managed medical practices have to deal with problems and complaints. Patients sometimes become upset over scheduling or bills or have problems understanding lab reports or instructions. Medical assistants often handle patients' questions about benefits and charges. They must become good problem solvers, willing to listen to and empathize with the patient while sorting out emotions from facts to get accurate information. Phrases such as these reduce patients' anger and frustration:

"I'm glad you brought this to our attention. I will look into it further."

"I can appreciate how you would feel this way."

"It sounds like we have caused some inconvenience, and I apologize."

"I understand that you are angry. Let me try to understand your concerns so we can address the situation."

"Thank you for taking the time to tell us about this. Because you have, we can resolve issues like the one you raised."

Medical assistants need to use the available resources and to investigate solutions to problems. Following through on promised information is also critical. An assistant who says to a patient, "I will call you by the end of next week with that information," must do exactly that. Even if the problem is not solved, the patient needs an update on the situation within the stated time frame.

COMPLIANCE GUIDELINE

Answering Machine Messages

If possible, ask patients whether staff members may leave messages on answering machines or with friends or family during their first visits. If this is not done, messages should follow the minimum necessary standard by leaving a phone number and a request for the patient to call back. For example: "This is the doctor's office with a message for Mr. Warner. Please call us at 555-123-4646."

THINKING IT THROUGH 3.8

1. Which of the following actions indicate communications that are effective and positive? Put a Y before those that seem positive, and an N before those that seem negative and ineffective to you.

_____ **A.** Mumbling

_____ **B.** Listening carefully

_____ **C.** Showing boredom during a patient's explanation of problems paying

_____ **D.** Speaking slowly and clearly

_____ **E.** Breaking in during a phone call to tell the payer's representative that you have a personal call

_____ **F.** Remaining calm in the face of an angry patient

Chapter Summary

Learning Outcomes	Key Concepts/Examples
3.1 Explain the method used to classify patients as new and/or established. Page 51	• Practices gather accurate information from patients to perform billing and medical care. • New patients are those who have not received any services from the provider within the past three years. • Established patients have seen the provider within the past three years. • Established patients review and update the information that is on file about them.
3.2 List the information that is gathered from new patients. Pages 51–58	• Basic personal preregistration and scheduling information. • The patient's detailed medical history. • Insurance data for the patient or guarantor. • A signed and dated assignment of benefits statement by the policyholder. • A signed Acknowledgement of Receipt of Notice of Privacy Practices authorizing the practice to release the patient's PHI for TPO purposes.
3.3 Discuss the procedures that are followed to update established patient information. Pages 58–59	• Patient information forms are reviewed at least once per year by established patients. • Patients are often asked to double-check their information at their encounters. • The PMP is updated to reflect any changes as needed, and the provider strives for good communication with the patient to provide the best possible service.
3.4 Explain the process for verifying patients' eligibility for insurance benefits. Pages 59–62	To verify patients' eligibility the provider • Checks the patient's information form and medical insurance card (except in medical emergency situations). • Contacts the payer to verify the patient's general eligibility for benefits, the amount of copayment or coinsurance that is due at the encounter, and to determine if the planned encounter is for a covered service that is considered medically necessary by the payer.
3.5 Discuss the importance of requesting referral or preauthorization approval. Pages 62–64	• Preauthorization is requested before a patient is given certain types of medical care. • In cases of referrals, the provider often needs to issue a referral number and a referral document in order for the patient to see a specialist under the terms of the medical insurance. • Providers must handle these situations correctly to ensure that the services are covered if possible.

Learning Outcomes	Key Concepts/Examples
3.6 Determine the primary insurance for patients who have more than one health plan. Pages 64–66	• Patient information forms and insurance cards are examined to determine if more than one health insurance policy is in effect. • If so, the provider determines which policy is the primary insurance based on coordination of benefits rules. • This information is then entered into the PMP and all necessary communications with the payers are performed.
3.7 Summarize the use of encounter forms. Pages 66–68	• Encounter forms may include a list of the medical practice's most commonly performed services, procedures, and assigned diagnoses. • The provider checks off the services and procedures a patient received, and the encounter form is then used for billing.
3.8 Describe the types of communications with payers, providers, and patients that are most effective. Pages 68–70	• All communication with payer representatives should be documented. • The representative's name, the date of the communication, and the outcome should be described. • It is important to be mindful of a provider's schedule and only query the physician when necessary. • Medical practice staff must be dedicated to retaining patients by providing excellent customer service.

Using Terminology

Match the key terms in the left column with the definitions in the right column.

_____ 1. **[LO 3.2]** Network

_____ 2. **[LO 3.2]** Assignment of benefits

_____ 3. **[LO 3.2]** Patient information form

_____ 4. **[LO 3.6]** Secondary insurance

_____ 5. **[LO 3.1]** Established patient

_____ 6. **[LO 3.2]** Guarantor

_____ 7. **[LO 3.6]** Coordination of benefits

_____ 8. **[LO 3.1]** New patient

_____ 9. **[LO 3.7]** Encounter form

_____ 10. **[LO 3.2]** Insured

A. Authorization by a policyholder that allows a payer to pay benefits directly to the provider.

B. A patient who has not received professional services from a provider, or another provider in the same practice with the same specialty, in the past three years.

C. The insurance plan that pays benefits after payment by the primary payer when a patient is covered by more than one insurance plan.

D. Form used to summarize the treatments and services patients receive during visits.

E. A patient who has received professional services from a provider, or another provider in the same practice with the same specialty, in the past three years.

F. The policyholder or subscriber to a health plan.

G. A clause in the insurance policy that explains how the policy will pay if more than one insurance policy applies to the claim.

H. Form completed by patients that summarizes their demographic and insurance information.

I. The person financially responsible for the bill.

J. A group of providers having participation agreements with a health plan.

connect plus+

Enhance your learning at mcgrawhillconnect.com!
• Practice Exercises   • Worksheets
• Activities   • Integrated eBook

Checking Your Understanding

Write the letter of the choice that best completes the statement or answers the question.

1. **[LO 3.4]** If a health plan member receives medical services from a provider who does not participate in the plan, the cost to the member is _____.
   A. Lower
   B. Higher
   C. The same
   D. Negotiable

2. **[LO 3.2]** What information does a patient information form gather? _____
   A. The patient's personal information, employment data, and insurance information
   B. The patient's history of present illness, past medical history, and examination results
   C. The patient's chief complaint
   D. The patient's insurance plan deductible and/or copayment requirements

3. **[LO 3.6]** If a husband has an insurance policy but is also eligible for benefits as a dependent under his wife's insurance policy, the wife's policy is considered _____ for him.
   A. Primary
   B. Participating
   C. Secondary
   D. Coordinated

4. **[LO 3.5]** A certificate number for a procedure is the result of which transaction? _____
   A. Claim status
   B. Health care payment and remittance advice
   C. Coordination of benefits
   D. Referral certification and authorization

5. **[LO 3.7]** A completed encounter form contains _____.
   A. Information about the patient's diagnosis
   B. Information on the procedures performed during the encounter
   C. Both information about the patient's diagnosis and information on the procedures performed during the encounter
   D. None of these

6. **[LO 3.7]** The encounter form is a source of _____ information for the medical insurance specialist.
   A. Billing
   B. Treatment plan
   C. Third-party payment
   D. Credit card

7. **[LO 3.2]** When registering new patients, the practice must make a good-faith effort to have them sign
   A. The encounter form
   B. The coordination of benefits form
   C. The referral form
   D. The Acknowledgement of Receipt of Notice of Privacy Practices

8. **[LO 3.6]** The tertiary insurance pays _____.
   A. After the first and second payers
   B. After the first payer
   C. After receipt of the claim
   D. None of these

9. **[LO 3.6]** If a patient is a dependent child covered by both parents' health insurance plans, the child's primary insurance is usually determined by _____.
   A. The policy that covered the child first
   B. The age of the parent
   C. The cost of the policy
   D. The birthday rule

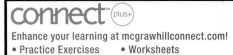
Enhance your learning at mcgrawhillconnect.com!
- Practice Exercises
- Worksheets
- Activities
- Integrated eBook

10. **[LO 3.8]** When communicating with a payer representative which of the following should be documented? _____
   - **A.** The outcome of the billing dispute
   - **B.** The date of the communication
   - **C.** The name of the representative
   - **D.** All of these

Define the following abbreviations:

1. **[LO 3.2]** nonPar _____

2. **[LO 3.6]** COB _____

3. **[LO 3.2]** PAR _____

4. **[LO 3.1]** NP _____

5. **[LO 3.1]** EP _____

Applying Your Knowledge

Case 3.1   Documenting Communications

[LO 3.8]   Harry Cornprost, a patient of Dr. Connelley, calls on October 25, 2016, to cancel his appointment for October 31 because he will be out of town. The appointment is rescheduled for December 4. How would you document this call?

Case 3.2   Coordinating Benefits

Based on the information provided, determine the primary insurance in each case.

- **A.** **[LO 3.6]**   George Rangley enrolled in the individual ACR plan in 2008 and in the New York Health group plan in 2006. What is George's primary plan?

- **B.** **[LO 3.6]**   Mary is the child of Gloria and Craig Bivilaque, who are divorced. Mary is a dependent under both Craig's and Gloria's plans. Gloria has custody of Mary. What is Mary's primary plan?

- **C.** **[LO 3.6]**   Karen Kaplan's date of birth is 10/11/1970; her husband Carl was born on 12/8/1971. Their child Ralph was born on 4/15/2000. Ralph is a dependent under both Karen's and Carl's plans. What is Ralph's primary plan?

- **D.** **[LO 3.6]**   Belle Estaphan has medical insurance from Internet Services, from which she retired last year. She is on Medicare but is also covered under her husband Bernard's plan from Orion International, where he works. What is Belle's primary plan?

- **E.** **[LO 3.6]**   Jim Larenges is covered under his spouse's plan and also has medical insurance through his employer. What is Jim's primary plan?

connect plus+

Enhance your learning at mcgrawhillconnect.com!
- Practice Exercises
- Worksheets
- Activities
- Integrated eBook

KEY TERMS

Alphabetic Index
category
chief complaint (cc)
combination code
convention
diagnostic statement
eponym
etiology
exclusion notes
external cause code
GEM
ICD-9-CM
ICD-10-CM
ICD-10-CM *Official Guidelines for Coding and Reporting*
inclusion notes
Index to External Causes
laterality
main term
manifestation
NEC (not elsewhere classified)
Neoplasm Table
nonessential modifier
NOS (not otherwise specified)
outpatient
placeholder character (x)
sequelae
seventh-character extension
subcategory
subterm
Table of Drugs and Chemicals
Tabular List
Z code

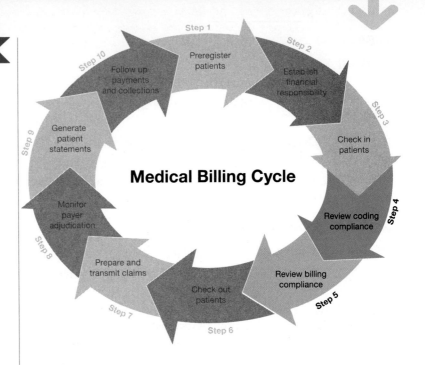

Medical Billing Cycle

Step 1 Preregister patients
Step 2 Establish financial responsibility
Step 3 Check in patients
Step 4 Review coding compliance
Step 5 Review billing compliance
Step 6 Check out patients
Step 7 Prepare and transmit claims
Step 8 Monitor payer adjudication
Step 9 Generate patient statements
Step 10 Follow up payments and collections

Learning Outcomes

After studying this chapter, you should be able to:

4.1 Discuss the purpose and organization of ICD-10-CM.

4.2 Summarize the structure, content, and key conventions of the Alphabetic Index.

4.3 Summarize the structure, content, and key conventions of the Tabular List.

4.4 Explain the use of external cause codes and Z codes.

4.5 Discuss the types of rules that are provided in the ICD-10-CM *Official Guidelines for Coding and Reporting.*

4.6 Assign correct ICD-10-CM diagnosis codes.

In place of written descriptions of the many different symptoms, conditions, and illnesses people have, standardized diagnosis codes have been developed for reporting them on claims. During the course of office encounters (visits) with patients, physicians document their evaluations of patients' conditions in their medical records. The diagnosis, often abbreviated Dx in the medical record, describes illnesses or injuries using medical terminology. After the physician determines the diagnosis, that physician, a medical coder, or other administrative staff member may assign the diagnostic codes, a vital element of information on a health care claim.

Coding affects the medical billing and payment process. Diagnosis codes give insurance carriers clearly defined diagnoses to help process claims efficiently. An error in coding conveys to an insurance carrier the wrong reason a patient received medical services. This causes confusion, a delay in processing, and possibly a reduced payment or denial of the claim. An incorrect code may also raise the question of fraudulent billing if the payer decides that, based on the diagnosis, the services provided were not medically necessary.

4.1 ICD-10-CM

Under HIPAA, the diagnosis codes that must be used in the United States starting on October 1, 2014, are based on the *International Classification of Diseases (ICD)*, Tenth Revision. The ICD-10 lists diseases and codes according to a system copyrighted by the World Health Organization of the United Nations. ICD has been revised a number of times since the coding system was first developed more than a hundred years ago.

ICD-10 has been the classification used by the federal government to categorize mortality data from death certificates since 1999. An expanded version of this tenth revision was published prior to the mandated compliance date for review by the health care community. A committee of health care professionals from various organizations and specialties prepared this version, which is called the ICD-10's *Clinical Modification*, or **ICD-10-CM.** It is used to code and classify morbidity data from patient medical records, physician offices, and surveys conducted by the National Center for Health Statistics. Codes in ICD-10-CM describe conditions and illnesses more precisely than does the World Health Organization's ICD-10 because the codes are intended to provide a more complete picture of patients' conditions.

ICD-10-CM HIPAA-mandated diagnosis code set as of October 1, 2014.

Code Makeup

An ICD-10-CM diagnosis code has between three and seven alphanumeric characters. The system is built on categories for diseases, injuries, and symptoms. A category has three characters. Most categories have subcategories of either four- or five-character codes. Valid codes themselves are either three, four, five, six, or seven characters in length, depending on the number of subcategories provided. For example, the code for the first visit for a closed and displaced fracture of the right tibial spine requires seven characters:

Example ICD-10-CM Diagnosis Code

Category S82 **Fracture of lower leg, including ankle**

Subcategory S82.1 **Fracture of upper end of tibia**

Subcategory S82.11 **Fracture of tibial spine**

Code S82.111 **Displaced fracture of right tibial spine**

Code S82.111A **Displaced fracture of tibial spine, closed fracture, initial encounter** ◄

This variable structure enables coders to assign the most specific diagnosis that is documented in the patient medical record. A sixth character is more specific than the fourth or fifth characters, and the seventh character extension can provide additional specific information about the health-related condition. When they are available for assignment in the ICD-10-CM code set, sixth and seventh characters are not optional; they must be used. For example, Centers for Medicare and Medicaid Services (CMS) rules state that a Medicare claim will be rejected when the most specific code available is not used.

Updates

The National Center for Health Statistics and CMS release ICD-10-CM updates called *addenda*. Since ICD-10-CM is new, it can be anticipated that many, many changes will be made during its first years of use. The major new, invalid, and revised codes are posted on the appropriate websites, such as the NCHS and CMS websites.

New codes must be used as of the date they go into effect, and invalid (deleted) codes must not be used. The U.S. Government Printing Office (GPO) publishes the official ICD-10-CM on the Internet and in CD-ROM format every year. Various commercial publishers include the updated codes in annual coding books that are printed soon after the updates are released. The current reference must always be in use for the date of service of the encounter being coded.

ICD-9-CM: Accessing the Previously Required Code Set

ICD-10-CM, as the name implies, is the tenth version of the diagnostic code set. The previous version is called **ICD-9-CM.** The major advantages of ICD-10-CM are many more categories for disease and other health-related conditions and much greater flexibility for adding new codes in the future. It is a larger code set, having about 69,000 versus ICD-9-CM's approximately 13,000. It also offers a higher level of specificity and additional characters and extensions for expanded detail. There are also many more codes that combine etiology and manifestations, poisoning and external cause, or diagnosis and symptoms.

Differences and Similarities between ICD-9 and ICD-10-CM

ICD-10-CM contains 21 chapters versus ICD-9-CM's 17 chapters and two supplemental classifications, V codes, and E codes, and there are differences in the order of chapters. Further, ICD-10-CM codes are alphanumeric and have five, six, or seven characters, whereas ICD-9-CM codes have three to five characters. However, there are two major similarities that exist between the code sets: The two major sections of the ICD-9-CM and the ICD-10-CM code sets are the Alphabetic Index and the Tabular List, and the same steps that will be covered in this chapter apply to researching ICD-9-CM codes.

GEMS

In some situations, coders will be called upon to research an ICD-9-CM code. Perhaps an old claim has resurfaced, or an audit forces a review of pre-2014 codes that were reported. Workers' compensation claims may also specify a non-ICD-10-CM code set, because WC is not regulated by HIPAA law and therefore is not required to use ICD-10-CM.

The federal government has prepared **GEMs,** an acronym that stands for general equivalence mappings. Although imperfect, GEMs may be helpful in these situations. Both files of equivalent codes and a conversion tool may be located via an Internet search. Particularly useful is the translator tool located on the American Association of Professional Coders (AAPC) website.

Note that confusion may result if the coder mixes up the ICD-9-CM codes that start with the capital letter E with those in ICD-10-CM that also start with E. There are a number of codes that are the same in both systems but have different meaning. Being clear on which system is in use will help the coder avoid these problems.

ICD-10-CM Updates

www.cdc.gov/nchs/icd/
icd10cm.htm

www.cms.gov/ICD10

ICD-9-CM   Previously HIPAA-mandated diagnosis code set.

**ICD-10-CM to ICD-9-CM
Conversion Tool**

www.aapc.com/icd-10/codes/
index.aspx

GEMs   Acronym for general equivalence mappings, reference tables of related ICD-10-CM and ICD-9-CM codes.

Organization of ICD-10-CM

ICD-10-CM has two major parts:

ICD-10-CM Index to Diseases and Injuries: The major section of this part, known as the **Alphabetic Index,** provides an index of the disease descriptions in the second major part, the Tabular List. Many descriptions are listed in more than one manner.

ICD-10-CM Tabular List of Diseases and Injuries: The **Tabular List** is made up of 21 chapters of disease descriptions and their codes.

ICD-10-CM's first part also has three additional sections that provide resources for researching correct codes:

ICD-10-CM Neoplasm Table: The **Neoplasm Table** provides code numbers for neoplasms by anatomical site and divided by the description of the neoplasm.

ICD-10-CM Table of Drugs and Chemicals: The **Table of Drugs and Chemicals** provides an index in table format of drugs and chemicals that are listed in the Tabular List.

ICD-10-CM Index to External Causes: The **Index to External Causes** provides an index of all the external causes of diseases and injuries that are listed in the related chapter of the Tabular List.

The process of assigning ICD-10-CM codes begins with the physician's **diagnostic statement,** which contains the medical term describing the condition for which a patient is receiving care. For each encounter, this medical documentation includes the main reason for the patient encounter. It may also provide descriptions of additional conditions or symptoms that have been treated or that are related to the patient's current illness.

In each part of ICD-10-CM, **conventions,** which are typographic techniques that provide visual guidance for understanding information, help coders understand the rules and select the right code. The primary rule is that both the Alphabetic Index and the Tabular List are used sequentially to pick a code. The coder first locates the description/code in the Alphabetic Index and then verifies the proposed code selection by turning to the Tabular List and studying its entries.

This process must be followed when assigning all codes. A code followed by a hyphen in the Alphabetic Index is a clear reminder of this rule. The hyphen means that the coder will need to drill down to select the right code. For example, the index entry for otitis media is H66.9-. The coder turns to the Tabular List and reviews these entries:

H66.90 Otitis media, unspecified, unspecified ear

H66.91 Otitis media, unspecified, right ear

H66.92 Otitis media, unspecified, left ear

H66.93 Otitis media, unspecified, bilateral

Based on the documentation, one of these must be selected for compliant coding; just H66.9 is not sufficient.

Alphabetic Index Part of ICD-CM-10 listing disease and injuries alphabetically with corresponding diagnosis codes.

Tabular List Part of ICD-10-CM listing diagnosis codes in chapters alphanumerically.

Neoplasm Table Provides code numbers for neoplasms by anatomical site and divided by the description of the neoplasm.

Table of Drugs and Chemicals Index in table format of drugs and chemicals that are listed in the Tabular List.

Index to External Causes Index of all the external causes of diseases and injuries classified in the Tabular List.

diagnostic statement Physician's description of the main reason for a patient's encounter.

convention Typographic technique that provides visual guidance for understanding information.

THINKING IT THROUGH 4.1

1. The annual updates to the ICD-10-CM code set often contain new codes for diseases that have recently been discovered. What are examples of diseases that have been diagnosed in the last two decades?

2. Why is it important to use current ICD codes?

4.2 The Alphabetic Index

The Alphabetic Index contains all the medical terms in the Tabular List classifications. For some conditions, it also lists common terms that are not found in the Tabular List. The index is organized by the *condition*, not by the body part (anatomical site) in which it occurs.

Alphabetic Index Example

The term *wrist fracture* is located by looking under *fracture* (the condition) and then, below it, *wrist* (the location), rather than under *wrist* to find *fracture*. ◄

Main Terms, Subterms, and Nonessential Modifiers

main term Word that identifies a disease or condition in the Alphabetic Index.

The assignment of the correct code begins with looking up the medical term that describes the patient's condition based on the diagnostic statement. Figure 4.1 illustrates the format of the Alphabetic Index. Each **main term** appears in boldface type and is followed by its *default code*, the one most frequently associated with it. For example, if the diagnostic statement is "the patient presents with blindness," the main term *blindness* is located in the Alphabetic Index (see Figure 4.1); the default code shown is H54.0.

subterm Word or phrase that describes a main term in the Alphabetic Index.

Below the main term, any **subterms** with their codes appear. Subterms are essential in the selection of correct codes. They may show the **etiology** of the disease—its cause or origin—or describe a particular type or body site for the main term. For example, the main term *blindness* in Figure 4.1 includes 21 subterms, each indicating a different etiology or type—such as color blindness—for that condition.

etiology Cause or origin of a disease or condition.

nonessential modifier Supplementary word or phrase that helps define a code in ICD-10-CM.

Any **nonessential modifiers** for main terms or subterms are shown in parentheses on the same line. Nonessential modifiers are supplementary terms that are not essential to the selection of the correct code. They help point to the correct term, but they do not have to appear in the physician's diagnostic statement for the coder to correctly select the code. In Figure 4.1, for example, any of the supplementary terms *acquired*, *congenital*, and *both eyes* may modify the main term in the diagnostic statement, such as "the patient presents with blindness acquired in childhood," or none of these terms may appear.

Common Terms

Many terms appear more than once in the Alphabetic Index. Often, the term in common use is listed, as well as the accepted medical terminology. For example, there is an entry for *flu*, with a cross-reference to *influenza*.

Eponyms

eponym Name or phrase formed from or based on a person's name.

An **eponym** (pronounced ĕp'-∩-nĭm) is a condition (or a procedure) named for a person, such as the physician who discovered or invented it; some are named for patients. An eponym is usually listed both under that name and under the main term *disease* or *syndrome*. For example, Hodgkin's disease appears as a subterm under *disease* and as a key term. The Alphabetic Index is the guide for coding other syndromes, such as battered child syndrome or HIV infection; if the syndrome is not identified, its manifestations are assigned codes.

Indention: Turnover Lines

If the main term or subterm is too long to fit on one line, as is often the case when many nonessential modifiers appear, turnover (or carryover) lines are used. Turnover lines are always indented farther to the right than are subterms. It is important to read carefully to distinguish a turnover line from a subterm line. For example, under the main term *blindness* (Figure 4.1) and the subterm *transient*, the information

Blind (*see also* Blindness)
    bronchus (congenital) Q32.4
    loop syndrome K90.2
        congenital Q43.8
    sac, fallopian tube (congenital) Q50.6
    spot, enlarged—*see* Defect, visual field, localized,
        scotoma, blind spot area
    tract or tube, congenital NEC—*see* Artresia, by site

Blindness (acquired) (congenital) (both eyes) H54.0
    blast S05.8x-
    color—*see* Deficiency, color vision
    concussion S05.8x-
    cortical H47.619
        left brain H47.612
        right brain H47.611
    day H53.11
    due to injury (current episode) S05.9-
        sequelae—code to injury with extension S
    eclipse (total)—*see* Retinopathy, solar
    emotional (hysterical) F44.6
    face H53.16
    hysterical F44.6
    legal (both eyes) (USA definition) H54.8
    mind R48.8
    night H53.60
        abnormal dark adaptation curve H53.61
        acquired H53.62
        congenital H53.63
        specified type NEC H53.69
        vitamin A deficiency E50.5
    one eye (other eye normal) H54.40
        left (normal vision on right) H54.42
            low vision on right H54.12
        low vision, other eye H54.10
        right (normal vision on left) H54.41
            low vision on left H54.11
    psychic R48.8
    river B73.01
    snow—*see* Photokeratitis
    sun, solar—*see* Retinopathy, solar
    transient—*see* Disturbance, vision, subjective, loss,
        transient
    traumatic (current episode) S05.9-
    word (developmental) F81.0
        acquired R48.0
        secondary to organic lesion R48.0

FIGURE 4.1 Format of the Alphabetic Index

under "*See*" is long enough to require a turnover line. Without close attention, it is possible to confuse a turnover entry with a subterm.

Cross-References

Some entries use cross-references. If the cross-reference *see* appears after a main term, the coder *must* look up the term that follows the word *see* in the index. The *see* reference means that the main term where the coder first looked is not correct; another category must be used. In Figure 4.1, for example, to code the subterm snow under *blind*, the term *Photokeratitis* must be found.

See also, another type of cross-reference, points the coder to additional, related index entries. *See also category* indicates that the coder should review the additional categories that are mentioned. For example, in Figure 4.1, the *see also* note at Blind directs the coder to check *Blindness* as well.

The Abbreviations NEC and NOS

NEC (not elsewhere classifiable) Abbreviation indicating the code to use when a disease or condition cannot be placed in any other category.

Not elsewhere classifiable, or **NEC,** appears with a term when there is no code that is specific for the condition. This abbreviation means that no code matches the exact situation. For example:

Hemorrhage, eye NEC H57.8

NOS (not otherwise specified) Indicates the code to use when no information is available for assigning the disease or condition a more specific code; unspecified.

Another abbreviation, **NOS,** or **not otherwise specified,** means *unspecified.* This term or abbreviation indicates that the code to be located in the Tabular List should be used when a condition is not completely described in the medical record. For example:

Enteritis, bacillary NOS A03.9

Multiple Codes, Connecting Words, and Combination Codes

Some conditions may require two codes, one for the etiology and a second for the **manifestation,** the disease's typical signs, symptoms, or secondary processes. This requirement is indicated when two codes, the second in brackets, appear after a term:

manifestation Characteristic sign or symptom of a disease.

Pneumonia in rheumatic fever I00 [J17]

This entry indicates that the diagnostic statement "pneumonia in rheumatic fever" requires two codes, one for the etiology (rheumatic fever, I00) and one for the manifestation (pneumonia, J17). The use of brackets in the Alphabetic Index around a code means that it cannot be the *first-listed code* in coding this diagnostic statement; these codes are listed after the codes for the etiology.

The use of connecting words, such as *due to, during, following,* and *with,* may also indicate the need for two codes or for a single code that covers both conditions. For example, the main term below is followed by a *due to* subterm:

Cramp(s), muscle, R25.2

    due to immersion T75.1

When the Alphabetic Index indicates the possible need for two codes, the Tabular List entry is used to determine whether in fact they are needed. In some cases, a **combination code** describing both the etiology and the manifestation is available instead of two codes. For example:

combination code Single code describing both the etiology and the manifestation(s) of a particular condition.

Influenza due to identified novel influenza A virus J09.X3

Combination codes may also exist that classify two diagnoses or a diagnosis with an associated complication.

THINKING IT THROUGH 4.2

1. The following entry appears in the Alphabetic Index: Pompe's disease (glycogen storage) E74.02.

    A. What type of term is "Pompe's disease"?

    B. What type of term is shown in parentheses?

2. Locate the following main terms in the Alphabetic Index. List and interpret any cross-references you find next to the entries.

    A. Stieda's disease _____

    B. Atrophia _____

    C. Branchial _____

3. Are "See" cross-references in the Alphabetic Index followed by codes? Why?

4.3 The Tabular List

The Tabular List received its name from the language of statistics; the word *tabulate* means to count, record, or list systematically. The diseases and injuries in the Tabular List are organized into chapters according to etiology, body system, or purpose. The organization of the Tabular List and the ranges of codes each part covers are shown in Table 4.1.

Categories, Subcategories, and Codes

Each Tabular List chapter is divided into categories, subcategories, and codes.

1. A **category** is a three-character alphanumeric code that covers a single disease or related condition. For example, the category LO3 covers cellulitis and acute lymphangitis.

category Three-character code for classifying a disease or condition.

Table 4.1 ICD-10-CM Chapter Structure

Chapter	Code Range	Title
1	A00-B99	Certain infectious and parasitic diseases
2	C00-D49	Neoplasms
3	D50-D89	Diseases of the blood and blood-forming organs and certain disorders involving the immune mechanism
4	E00-E89	Endocrine, nutritional and metabolic diseases
5	F01-F99	Mental and behavioral disorders
6	G00-G99	Diseases of the nervous system
7	H00-H59	Diseases of the eye and adnexa
8	H60-H95	Diseases of the ear and mastoid process
9	I00-I99	Diseases of the circulatory system
10	J00-J99	Diseases of the respiratory system
11	K00-K94	Diseases of the digestive system
12	L00-L99	Diseases of the skin and subcutaneous tissue
13	M00-M99	Diseases of the musculoskeletal system and connective tissue
14	N00-N99	Diseases of the genitourinary system
15	O00-O9A	Pregnancy, childbirth and the puerperium
16	P00-P96	Certain conditions originating in the perinatal period
17	Q00-Q99	Congenital malformations, deformations and chromosomal abnormalities
18	R00-R99	Symptoms, signs and abnormal clinical and laboratory findings, not elsewhere classified
19	S00-T88	Injury, poisoning and certain other consequences of external causes
20	V01-Y99	External causes of morbidity
21	Z00-Z99	Factors influencing health status and contact with health services

2. A **subcategory** is a four- or five-character alphanumeric subdivision of a category. It provides a further breakdown of the disease to show its etiology, site, or manifestation. For example, the L03 category has six subcategories:

L03   Cellulitis and acute lymphangitis
L03.0   Cellulitis and acute lymphangitis of finger and toe
L03.1   Cellulitis and acute lymphangitis of other parts of limb
L03.2   Cellulitis and acute lymphangitis of face and neck
L03.3   Cellulitis and acute lymphangitis of trunk
L03.8   Cellulitis and acute lymphangitis of other sites
L03.9   Cellulitis and acute lymphangitis, unspecified

3. A *code*, the smallest division, has either 3, 4, 5, 6, or 7 alphanumeric characters. For example, Figure 4.2 shows the entries under the first subcategory of the L03 category.

Note that the first character in a code is always a letter. The complete alphabet, except for the letter U, is used. The second and third characters may be either numbers or letters, although currently the second character is usually (but not always) a number. A valid code has to have at least three characters. If it has more than that, a period is placed following the third character:

L03.042   Acute lymphangitis of left toe

Each character beyond the category level provides greater specificity to the code's meaning.

Placeholder Character Requirement

ICD-10-CM uses a **placeholder character** (also known as the "dummy placeholder") designated as "x" in some codes when a fifth, sixth, or seventh digit character is required but the digit space to the left of that character is empty.

L03.0	**Cellulitis and acute lymphangitis of finger and toe**	
	Infection of nail	
	Onychia	
	Paronychia	
	Perionychia	
	L03.01	**Cellulitis of finger**
		Felon
		Whitlow
		Excludes 1 herpetic whitlow (B00.89)
		L03.011 **Cellulitis of right finger**
		L03.012 **Cellulitis of left finger**
		L03.019 **Cellulitis of unspecified finger**
	L03.02	**Acute lymphangitis of finger**
		Hangnail with lymphangitis of finger
		L03.021 **Acute lymphangitis of right finger**
		L03.022 **Acute lymphangitis of left finger**
		L03.029 **Acute lymphangitis of unspecified finger**
	L03.03	**Cellulitis of toe**
		L03.031 **Cellulitis of right toe**
		L03.032 **Cellulitis of left toe**
		L03.039 **Cellulitis of unspecified toe**
	L03.04	**Acute lymphangitis of toe**
		Hangnail with lymphangitis of toe
		L03.041 **Acute lymphangitis of right toe**
		L03.042 **Acute lymphangitis of left toe**
		L03.049 **Acute lymphangitis of unspecified toe**

FIGURE 4.2 Format of Tabular List Subcategory

For example, the subcategory T46.1 Poisoning by, adverse effect of and underdosing of calcium-channel blockers, uses the *sixth* digit to describe whether the poisoning was accidental (unintentional), intentional self-harm, caused by assault, undetermined, or related to an adverse effect or underdosing. Since there is no fifth digit assigned, an x is used to hold that fifth space.

T46.1x2   Poisoning by calcium-channel blockers, intentional self-harm

Seventh-Character Extension

ICD-10-CM requires assigning a seventh character in some categories, usually to specify the sequence of the visit (for example, the initial encounter for the problem, the subsequent encounter for the problem, or sequela—the problem results from a previous disease or injury; the plural is *sequelae*). The **seventh-character extension** requirement is contained in a note at the start of the codes it covers. The seventh character must always be in position 7 of the alphanumeric code, so if the code is not at least six characters long, the placeholder character "x" must be used to fill that empty space.

For example, category S64, Injury of nerves at wrist and hand level, leads off with this note:

The appropriate 7th character is to be added to each code from category S64.

A   initial encounter

D   subsequent encounter

S   sequela

Subcategory S64.22, Injury of radial nerve at wrist and hand level of left arm, has no sixth digit but requires the seventh, so the correct code for an initial encounter would be:

S64.22xA   Injury of radial nerve at wrist and hand level of left arm, initial encounter

Depending on the publisher of ICD-10-CM, a section mark (§) or other symbol (such as a number enclosed in a circle) appears next to a chapter, a category, a subcategory, or a code that requires a fifth, sixth, or seventh digit to be assigned. These are important reminders to assign the appropriate characters.

seventh-character extension Necessary assignment of a seventh character to a code; often for the sequence of an encounter.

Inclusion Notes

Inclusion notes are headed by the word *includes* and refine the content of the category appearing above them.

inclusion note Tabular List entry addressing the applicability of certain codes to specified conditions.

Exclusion Notes

Exclusion notes are headed by the word *excludes* and indicate conditions that are not classifiable to the code above. Two types of exclusion notes are used. *Excludes 1* is used when two conditions could not exist together, such as an acquired and a congenital condition; it means "not coded here." *Excludes 2* means "not included here," but a patient could have both conditions at the same time. An example of an exclusion note occurs in the category L03 in Figure 4.2. This *excludes* note states that the code L03.01 Cellulitis of finger does not include herpetic whitlow. The note may also give the code(s) of the excluded condition(s), as in this case.

exclusion note Tabular List entry limiting applicability of particular codes to specified conditions.

Punctuation

Colons

A colon (:) indicates an incomplete term. One or more of the entries following the colon is required to make a complete term. Unlike terms in parentheses or brackets, when the colon is used, the diagnostic statement must include one of the terms after the colon to be assigned a code from the particular category. For example, the *excludes* note after the information for chorioretinal disorders is as follows:

> H32 Chorioretinal disorders in diseases classified elsewhere
>> *Excludes 1: chororetinitis (in):*
>>> *toxoplasmosis (acquired) (B58.01)*
>>> *tuberculosis (A18.53)*

For the *excludes* note to apply to *chororetinitis,* "acquired toxoplasmosis" or "tuberculosis" must appear in the diagnostic statement.

Parentheses

Parentheses ( ) are used around descriptions that do not affect the code—that is, nonessential, supplementary terms. For example, the subcategory G24.1, Genetic torsion dystonia, is followed by the entry "Idiopathic (torsion) dystonia NOS."

Brackets

Brackets [ ] are used around synonyms, alternative wordings, or explanations. They have the same meaning as parentheses. For example, category E52 is described as "Niacin deficiency [pellagra]."

Abbreviations: NEC versus NOS

NEC and NOS are used in the Tabular List with the same meanings as in the Alphabetic Index.

Etiology/Manifestation Coding

The convention that addresses multiple codes for conditions that have both an underlying etiology and manifestations is indicated in the Tabular List by some phrases that contain instructions about the need for additional codes. The phrases point to situations in which more than one code is required. For example, a statement that a condition is "due to" or "associated with" may require an additional code.

Use Additional Code

The etiology code may be followed by the instruction *use an additional code* or a note saying the same thing. The order of the codes must be the same as shown in the Alphabetic Index: the etiology comes first, followed by the manifestation code.

Code First Underlying Disease

The instruction *code first underlying disease* (or similar wording) appears below a manifestation code that must not be used as a first-listed code. These codes are for symptoms only, never for causes. At times, a specific instruction is given, such as in this example:

> **F07   Personality and behavioral disorders due to known physiological condition**
> *Code first the underlying physiological condition*

Other "Use Additional Code" Requirements

The "use additional code" note also appears when ICD-10-CM requires assignment of codes for health factors such as tobacco use and alcohol use.

Laterality

laterality Use of ICD-10-CM classification system to capture the side of the body that is documented; the fourth, fifth, or sixth characters of a code specify the affected side(s).

The Tabular List provides a coding structure based on the concept of **laterality.** In ICD-10-CM, this is the idea that the classification system should capture the side of the body that is documented for a particular condition. The fourth, fifth, or sixth characters specify the affected side, such as right arm, left wrist, both eyes. (In general usage, laterality means a preference for one side of the body, like lefthandedness.)

When the affected side of the condition is not known, an unspecified code is assigned. If a condition is documented as bilateral but there is no appropriate code for bilaterality (that is, both), two codes for the left and right sides are assigned.

THINKING IT THROUGH 4.3

Provide the following information about codes found in the Tabular List.

1. What condition is excluded from category B58, Toxoplasmosis?

2. What is the meaning of the phrase that follows the entry J44.0?

3. What is the meaning of the note that follows category S80, Superficial injury of knee and lower leg?

4. What types of diabetes are included in category E11, Type 2 diabetes mellitus?

5. Review the instructions for category H67, Otitis media in diseases classified elsewhere. Can any of the codes be first-listed?

4.4 Using External Cause Codes and Z Codes

Codes in Chapter 20 of ICD-10-CM classify **external cause codes,** which report the cause of injuries from various environmental events, such as transportation accidents, falls, and fires. External cause codes are not used alone or as first-listed codes. They always supplement a code that identifies the injury or condition itself.

external cause code ICD-10-CM code for an external cause of a disease or injury.

Many blocks of accident and injury codes in this chapter require additional external cause codes for

▶ The encounter (A = initial, D = subsequent, or S = sequela)
▶ The place of occurrence (category Y92)
▶ The activity (category Y93)
▶ The status (category Y99)

External cause codes are located by first using the third section of the Alphabetic Index, Index to External Causes. This index is organized by main terms describing the accident, circumstance, or event that caused the injury. Codes are verified in Chapter 20 of the Tabular List.

External cause codes are often used in collecting public health information. They capture cause, intent, place, and activity. As many external cause codes as are needed to describe these factors should be reported. Note, however, that these codes are not needed if the external cause and intent are already included in a code from another chapter.

Chapter 21 contains **Z codes** that are used to report encounters for circumstances other than a disease or injury, such as factors influencing health status, and to describe the nature of a patient's contact with health services. There are two chief types:

Z code Abbreviation for ICD-10-CM codes that identify factors that influence health status and encounters that are not due to illness or injury.

▶ Reporting visits with healthy (or ill) patients who receive services other than treatments, such as annual checkups, immunizations, and normal childbirth. This use is coded by a Z code that identifies the service, such as:

Z00.01 Encounter for general adult medical examination with abnormal findings

▶ Reporting encounters in which a problem not currently affecting the patient's health status needs to be noted, such as personal and family history. For example, a person with a family history of breast cancer is at higher risk for the disease, and a Z code is assigned as an additional code for screening codes to explain the need for a test or procedure, as is shown here:

Z80.3 Family history of malignant neoplasm of breast

Table 4.2 — Terminology Associated with Z Codes

Term	Example
Contact/exposure	Z20.1 Contact with and (suspected) exposure to tuberculosis
Contraception	Z30.01 Encounter for initial prescription of contraceptive pills
Counseling	Z31.5 Encounter for genetic counseling
Examination	Z00.110 Health examination for newborn under 8 days old
Fitting of	Z46.51 Encounter for fitting and adjustment of gastric lap band
Follow-up	Z08 Encounter for follow-up examination following completed treatment for malignant neoplasm
History (of)	Z92.23 Personal history of estrogen therapy
Screening/test	Z11.51 Encounter for screening for human papillomavirus (HPV)
Status	Z67.10 Type A blood, Rh positive
Superision (of)	Z34.01 Supervision of normal first pregnancy, first trimester
Vaccination/inoculation	Z23 Encounter for immunization

BILLING TIP

Use Z Codes to Show Medical Necessity

Z codes such as family history or a patient's previous condition help demonstrate why a service was medically necessary.

A Z code can be used as either a primary code for an encounter or as an additional code. It is researched in the same way as other codes, using the Alphabetic Index to point to the term's code and the Tabular List to verify it. The terms that indicate the need for Z codes, however, are not the same as other medical terms. They usually have to do with a reason for an encounter other than a disease or its complications. When found in diagnostic statements, the words listed in Table 4.2 often point to Z codes.

THINKING IT THROUGH 4.4

1. Patient Betty Standover received an endometrial biopsy and pelvic ultrasound to monitor any changes of the endometrium that may be caused by a medication she is taking. What type of code is used to describe the medical need for the biopsy and the ultrasound?

2. Patient Frank Sherchasy fell off a ladder while on the job at Right's Painting Service. He sprained his left ankle and has a simple fracture of the right femur. What type of code is used in addition to the main codes to describe his diagnosis?

4.5 ICD-10-CM *Official Guidelines for Coding and Reporting*

ICD-10-CM *Official Guidelines for Coding and Reporting* General rules, inpatient (hospital) coding guidance, and outpatient (physician office/clinic) coding guidance from the four cooperating parties (CMS advisers and participants from the AHA, AHIMA, and NCHS).

Assigning HIPAA-mandated diagnosis codes follows both the conventions that are incorporated in the Alphabetic Index/Tabular List as well as a separate set of rules called **ICD-10-CM *Official Guidelines for Coding and Reporting.*** Known as the "*Official Guidelines,*" these rules are developed by a group known as the four cooperating parties made up of CMS advisers and participants from the American Hospital Association (AHA), the American Health Information Management Association (AHIMA), and the National Center for Health Statistics (NCHS).

The *Official Guidelines* have sections for general rules, inpatient (hospital) coding, and **outpatient** (physician office/clinic) coding:

▶ Section I, *Conventions, general coding guidelines, and chapter-specific guidelines*, first reviews the Alphabetic Index and Tabular List conventions and broad coding rules, and then discusses key topics affecting the use of codes in each of the 21 chapters.

▶ Section II, *Selection of Principal Diagnosis*, and Section III, *Reporting Additional Diagnoses*, explain the guidelines for establishing the diagnosis or diagnoses for inpatient cases.

▶ Section IV, *Diagnostic Coding and Reporting Guidelines for Outpatient Services*, explains the guidelines for establishing the diagnosis or diagnoses for all outpatient encounters. The key points from this section can be summarized as follows:

1. Code the primary diagnosis first, followed by current coexisting conditions.
2. Code to the highest level of certainty.
3. Code to the highest level of specificity.

ICD-10-CM Official Guidelines
www.cdc.gov/nchs/icd/
icd10cm.htm

Code the Primary Diagnosis First, Followed by Current Coexisting Conditions

ICD-10-CM code for the primary diagnosis is listed first.

Example

Diagnostic Statement: Patient is an elderly female complaining of back pain. For the past five days, she has had signs of pyelonephritis, including urinary urgency, urinary incontinence, and back pain. Has had a little hematuria, but no past history of urinary difficulties.
Primary Diagnosis: N12 Pyelonephritis ◀

After the first diagnosis code, additional codes may be used to describe all current documented coexisting conditions that must be actively managed because they affect patient treatment or that require treatment during the encounter. *Coexisting conditions* may be related to the primary diagnosis, or they may involve a separate illness that the physician diagnoses and treats during the encounter.

Example

Diagnostic Statement: Patient, a forty-five-year-old male, presents for complete physical examination for an insurance certification. During the examination, patient complains of occasional difficulty hearing; wax is removed from the left ear canal.
Primary Diagnosis: Z02.6 Routine physical examination for insurance certification
Coexisting Condition: H61.22 Impacted cerumen ◀

It is important to note that patients may have diseases or conditions that do not affect the encounter being coded. Some physicians add notes about previous conditions to provide an easy reference to a patient's history. Unless these conditions are directly involved with the patient's treatment, they are not considered in selecting codes. Also, conditions that were previously treated and no longer exist are not coded.

Example

Chart Note: Mrs. Mackenzie, whose previous encounter was for her regularly scheduled blood pressure check to monitor her hypertension, presents today with a new onset of psoriasis.
Primary Diagnosis: L40.9 Psoriasis, NOS ◀

Coding Acute versus Chronic Conditions

The reasons for patient encounters are often *acute* symptoms—generally, relatively sudden or severe problems. Acute conditions are coded with the specific code that is designated acute, if listed. Many patients, however, receive ongoing treatment for *chronic* conditions—those that continue over a long period of time or recur frequently. For example, a patient may need a regular injection for the management of rheumatoid arthritis. In such cases, the disease is coded and reported for as many times as the patient receives care for the condition.

In some cases, an encounter covers both an acute and a chronic condition. Some conditions do not have separate entries for both manifestations, so a single code applies. If both the acute and the chronic illnesses have codes, the acute code is listed first, for example:

Acute Renal Failure N17.9

Chronic Renal Failure N18.9

Coding Sequelae

sequelae Conditions that remain after an acute illness or injury has been treated and resolved.

A **sequela** is a condition that remains after a patient's acute illness or injury has ended. Often called residual effects or late effects, some happen soon after the disease is over, and others occur later. The diagnostic statement may say:

▶ Due to an old . . . (for example, swelling due to old contusion of knee)
▶ Late . . . (for example, nausea as a late effect of radiation sickness)
▶ Due to a previous . . . (for example, abdominal mass due to a previous spleen injury)
▶ Traumatic (if not a current injury); including scarring or nonunion of a fracture (for example, malunion of fracture, left humerus)

In general, the main term *sequela* is followed by subterms that list the causes. Two codes are usually required. First reported is the code for the specific effect (such as muscle soreness), followed by the code for the cause (such as the late effect of rickets). The code for the acute illness that led to the sequela is never used with a code for the late effect itself.

Code to the Highest Level of Certainty

Diagnoses are not always established at a first encounter. Follow-up visits over time may be required before the physician determines a primary diagnosis. During this process, although possible diagnoses may appear in the physician's documentation as diagnostic work is progressing, these inconclusive diagnoses are not used to determine the codes reported for reimbursement of service fees.

Signs and Symptoms

Instead of inconclusive diagnoses, the specific signs and symptoms are coded and reported. A *sign* is an objective indication that can be evaluated by the physician, such as weight loss. A *symptom* is a subjective statement by the patient that cannot be confirmed during an examination, such as pain.

The following case provides an example of how symptoms and signs are coded:

Example

Diagnostic Statement: Middle-aged male presents with abdominal pain and weight loss. He had to return home from vacation due to acute illness. He has not been eating well because of a vague upper- abdominal pain. He denies nausea, vomiting. He denies changes in bowel habit or blood in stool. Physical examination revealed no abdominal tenderness.
Primary Diagnosis: R10.13 Abdominal pain, epigastric region
Coexisting Condition: R63.4 Abnormal loss of weight ◀

Suspected Conditions

Similarly, possible but not confirmed diagnoses, such as those preceded by "rule out," "suspected," "probable," or "likely," are not coded in the outpatient (physician practice) setting.

Note that in the inpatient setting, however, the guidance is different. For hospital coding, the first-listed diagnosis is referred to as the *principal diagnosis* and is defined as the condition established after study to be chiefly responsible for the admission. "After study" means at the patient's discharge from the facility. If a definitive condition has not been established, then, at discharge, the inpatient coder codes the condition that matches the planned course of treatment most closely as if it were established.

Coding the Reason for Surgery

Surgery is coded according to the diagnosis that is listed as the reason for the procedure. In some cases, the postoperative diagnosis is available and is different from the physician's primary diagnosis before the surgery. If so, the postoperative diagnosis is coded because it is the highest level of certainty available. For example, if an excisional biopsy is performed to evaluate mammographic breast lesions or a lump of unknown nature, and the pathology results show a malignant neoplasm, the diagnosis code describing the site and nature of the neoplasm is used.

Code to the Highest Level of Specificity

The more characters a code has, the more specific it becomes; the additional characters add to the clinical picture of the patient. Using the most specific code possible is referred to as coding to the highest level of specificity. In the following example, the most specific code has six characters.

Category L03 **Cellulitis and acute lymphangitis** (three characters)

Subcategory L03.0 **Cellulitis and acute lymphangitis of finger and toe** (four characters)

Subcategory L03.01 **Cellulitis of finger** (five characters)

Code L03.011 **Cellulitis of right finger** (six characters)

Code L03.012 **Cellulitis of left finger** (six characters)

Code L03.019 **Cellulitis of unspecified finger** (six characters)

However, note that the last code, L03.019, is considered less specific than the other six-character codes, because it indicates that the affected finger is not known. Appropriate documentation should provide this level of detail.

Other (or Other Specified) versus Unspecified

In the Tabular List, the coder may need to choose between a code described as the core condition, *other* (or *other specified*) versus *unspecified*. For example:

L70.8   Other acne

L70.9   Acne unspecified

If the documentation mentions a type or form of the condition that is not listed, the coder chooses "other," because a type is indicated but not found. If no type is mentioned, the documentation is not complete enough to assign a more specific code, and so the least-specific choice, "unspecified," is assigned. If there is no other versus unspecified coding option, select the "other specified" which in this situation represents both "other" and "unspecified."

4.6 Assigning Diagnosis Codes

The correct procedure for assigning accurate diagnosis codes has six steps, as shown in Figure 4.3.

Step 1: Review Complete Medical Documentation

chief complaint (cc) Patient's description of the symptoms or other reasons for seeking medical care.

In outpatient settings, diagnosis coding begins with the patient's **chief complaint (CC).** The chief complaint is the medical reason that the patient presents for the particular visit, as well as the duration of the medical reason. This is documented in the patient's medical record. The physician then examines the patient and evaluates the condition or complaint, documenting the diagnosis, condition, problem, or other reason that the documentation shows as being chiefly responsible for the services that are provided. This primary diagnosis provides the main term to be coded first. Documentation will also mention any coexisting complaints that should be coded. If a patient has cancer, the disease is probably the patient's major health problem. However, if that patient sees the physician for an ear infection that is not related to the cancer, the primary diagnosis for that particular claim is the ear infection.

A patient's examination might be documented as follows:

CC: Diarrhea × 5 days with strong odor and mucus, abdominal pain and tenderness, no meds.

Dx: Ulcerative colitis.

The notes mean that the patient has had symptoms for five days and has taken no medication. The chief complaint is noted after the abbreviation *CC*. The diagnosis, listed after the abbreviation *Dx*, is ulcerative colitis.

Assume that another patient's record indicates a history of heavy smoking and includes an X-ray report and notes such as these:

CC: Hoarseness, pain during swallowing, painful breathing during exertion for a week.

Dx: Emphysema and laryngitis.

The physician listed emphysema, the major health problem, first; it is the primary diagnosis. Laryngitis is a coexisting condition that is being treated.

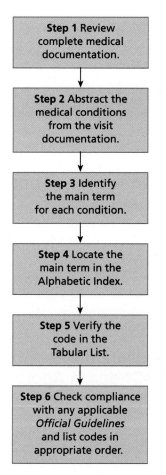

FIGURE 4.3 Diagnosis Code Assignment Flowchart

Step 2: Abstract the Medical Conditions from the Visit Documentation

The code will be assigned based on the physician's diagnosis or diagnoses. This information may be located on the encounter form or elsewhere in the patient's medical record, such as in a progress note. For example, a medical record reads:

CC: Chest and epigastric pain; feels like a burning inside for 10 days. Occasional reflux. Abdomen soft, flat without tenderness. No bowel masses or organomegaly.

Dx: Peptic ulcer.

The diagnosis is peptic ulcer.

Step 3: Identify the Main Term for Each Condition

If needed, decide which is the main term or condition of the diagnosis. For example, in the diagnosis above, the main term or condition is *ulcer.* The word *peptic* describes what type of ulcer it is. Here are other examples:

Dx: Complete paralysis.

The main term is *paralysis,* and the supplementary term is *complete.*

Dx: Heart palpitation.

The main term is *palpitation,* and the supplementary term is *heart.*

Dx: Panner's disease.

This condition can be found in either of two ways. Looking up the main term *disease,* followed by *Panner's,* or by looking up *Panner's disease.*

Step 4: Locate the Main Term in the Alphabetic Index

The main term for the patient's primary diagnosis is located in the Alphabetic Index. These guidelines should be observed in choosing the correct term:

▶ Use any supplementary terms in the diagnostic statement to help locate the main term.
▶ Read and follow any notes below the main term.
▶ Review the subterms to find the most specific match to the diagnosis.
▶ Read and follow any cross-references.
▶ Make note of a two-code (etiology and/or manifestation) indication.

Step 5: Verify the Code in the Tabular List

The code for the main term is then located in the Tabular List. These guidelines are observed to verify the selection of the correct code:

▶ Read *includes* or *excludes* notes, checking back to see if any apply to the code's category, section, or chapter.
▶ Be alert for and follow instructions for fifth-digit requirements.
▶ Follow any instructions requiring the selection of additional codes (such as "code also" or "code first underlying disease").
▶ List multiple codes in the correct order.

Step 6: Check Compliance with Any Applicable *Official Guidelines* and List Codes in Appropriate Order

The final step is to review ICD-10-CM *Official Guidelines for Coding and Reporting* to check for applicable points. Coders should be sure not to include suspected conditions (for outpatient settings) and to report the primary diagnosis code, followed by any coexisting conditions and external source codes.

Exercise 4.1 Entering a Patient's Diagnosis

Complete the Diagnosis tab for Ann Ingram.

Follow the steps at www.mhhe.com/newbycarr to complete the exercise at connect.mcgraw-hill.com on your own once you have watched the demo and tried the steps with prompts in practice mode. Use the information provided in the scenario to complete the exercise.

THINKING IT THROUGH 4.6

Place a double underline below the main terms and a single underline below any subterms in each of the following statements, and then determine the correct codes.

1. cerebral atherosclerosis _____
2. spasmodic asthma with status asthmaticus _____
3. congenital night blindness _____
4. recurrent inguinal hernia with obstruction _____
5. incomplete bundle branch heart block _____
6. acute accidental food poisoning _____
7. malnutrition following gastrointestinal surgery _____
8. frequency of urination disturbing sleep _____

Chapter Summary

Learning Outcomes	Key Concepts/Examples
4.1 Discuss the purpose and organization of ICD-10-CM. Pages 75–77	• ICD-10-CM must be used for diagnostic coding in the United States starting on October 1, 2014. • Codes are made up of between three and seven alphanumeric characters. • Addenda to codes are released regularly and must be followed as of the date they go into effect. • ICD-10-CM has two major parts that are used in medical practices: the Tabular List and the Alphabetic Index. • The Alphabetic Index has three additional sections: the Neoplasm Table, the Table of Drugs and Chemicals, and the Index to External Causes. • Conventions must be followed to select the correct code.
4.2 Summarize the structure, content, and key conventions of the Alphabetic Index. Pages 78–80	• It contains in alphabetic order the main terms that describe all diseases classified in the Tabular List. • Main terms may be followed by related subterms or supported by supplementary terms. Several conventions apply to using the Alphabetic Index correctly, including: • Turnover lines are indented farther to the right than are subterms. • *See* cross-references direct a coder to another term; *see also* cross-references point to related index entries; *see also category* cross-references indicate that additional categories should be reviewed. • Notes provide information on code selection. • The abbreviation NEC means for the code to be used when the diagnosis does not match any other available code, and the abbreviation NOS indicates the code to use when a condition is not completely described. • Multiple codes are required when two codes, the second in brackets, appear after a main term. • Brackets around a code mean that it cannot be the first-listed code.
4.3 Summarize the structure, content, and key conventions of the Tabular List. Pages 81–85	• It contains the codes, which are organized into 21 chapters according to etiology, body system, or purpose, and are listed in numerical order. • Code categories consist of three-character alphanumeric listings that cover a single disease or related condition. • Subcategories listed in a four- or five-character alphanumeric format provide further breakdown of a disease's etiology, site, or manifestation. • Codes have either 3, 4, 5, 6, or 7 alphanumeric characters. Several conventions are used in the Tabular List, including: • The first character in a code is always a letter. • Placeholder characters are designated as "x" in some codes. • The seventh-character extension requirement. • Inclusion and exclusion notes. • Colons indicate an incomplete term. • Parentheses around supplementary terms. • Brackets around synonyms, alternative wordings, or explanations. • NEC and NOS have the same meaning in the Tabular List as they do in the Alphabetic Index. • Phrases for multiple code requirements: codes that are not used as primary appear in italics and are usually followed by an instruction to *use an additional code* or *code first underlying disease*. • The concept of laterality.

Learning Outcomes	Key Concepts/Examples
4.4 Explain the use of external cause codes and Z codes. Pages 85–86	• External cause codes report the cause of injuries from various environmental events, such as transportation accidents, falls, and fires. External cause codes are not used alone or as first-listed codes. • Z codes are used to report encounters for circumstances other than a disease or injury. Many Z codes may be first listed.
4.5 Discuss the types of rules that are provided in the ICD-10-CM *Official Guidelines for Coding and Reporting.* Pages 86–90	The *Official Guidelines* have four sections containing general coding rules. Three key points are made in Section IV: • Code the primary diagnosis first, followed by current coexisting conditions. • Code to the highest level of certainty. • Code to the highest level of specificity.
4.6 Assign correct ICD-10-CM diagnosis codes. Pages 90–92	• Step 1. Review complete medical documentation. • Step 2. Abstract the medical conditions from the visit documentation. • Step 3. Identify the main term for each condition. • Step 4. Locate the main term in the Alphabetic Index. • Step 5. Verify the code in the Tabular List. • Step 6. Check compliance with any applicable *Official Guidelines* and list codes in appropriate order.

Using Terminology

Match the key terms in the left column with the definitions in the right column.

_____ **1. [LO 4.2]** Etiology

_____ **2. [LO 4.2]** Manifestation

_____ **3. [LO 4.3]** Category

_____ **4. [LO 4.4]** Z codes

_____ **5. [LO 4.1]** Convention

_____ **6. [LO 4.2]** Main term

_____ **7. [LO 4.2]** Eponym

_____ **8. [LO 4.2]** Nonessential modifier

_____ **9. [LO 4.3]** Laterality

_____ **10. [LO 4.5]** Sequelae

A. Three-character code for classifying a disease or condition.

B. Typographic technique that provides visual guidance for understanding information.

C. Name or phrase formed from or based on a person's name.

D. Cause or origin of a disease or condition.

E. Use of ICD-10-CM classification system to capture the side of the body that is documented.

F. Word that identifies a disease or condition in the Alphabetic Index.

G. Characteristic sign or symptom associated with a disease.

H. Supplementary word or phrase that helps define a code in ICD-10-CM.

I. Conditions that remain after an acute illness or injury has been treated and resolved.

J. Codes that identify factors that influence health status and encounters that are not due to illness or injury.

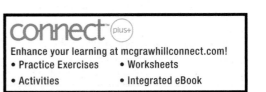

Enhance your learning at mcgrawhillconnect.com!
- Practice Exercises
- Worksheets
- Activities
- Integrated eBook

Checking Your Understanding

Write the letter of the choice that best completes the statement or answers the question.

1. **[LO 4.1]** The _____ provides an index of the disease descriptions that are found in the second major part of ICD-10-CM.
   A. Tabular List
   B. Index to External Causes
   C. Neoplasm Table
   D. Alphabetic Index

2. **[LO 4.1]** The ICD-10-CM updates released by the National Center for Health Statistics are called _____.
   A. Sequelae
   B. Addenda
   C. Eponyms
   D. Conventions

3. **[LO 4.1]** The ICD-10-CM code set contains approximately _____ codes, making it much larger than ICD-9-CM.
   A. 13,000
   B. 57,000
   C. 69,000
   D. 3,250,000

4. **[LO 4.4]** _____ are used to report encounters for circumstances other than a disease or injury in ICD-10-CM.
   A. V codes
   B. Z codes
   C. E codes
   D. A codes

5. **[LO 4.5]** A _____ is an objective indication that can be evaluated by a physician.
   A. Sign
   B. Sequela
   C. Symptom
   D. Laterality

6. **[LO 4.3]** ICD-10-CM uses _____ to indicate an incomplete term.
   A. Parentheses
   B. Brackets
   C. Colons
   D. Abbreviations

7. **[LO 4.6]** Name the final step in assigning accurate diagnosis codes. _____
   A. Locate the main term in the Alphabetic Index.
   B. Verify the code in the Tabular List.
   C. Review complete medical documentation.
   D. Check compliance with any *Official Guidelines* and list codes in appropriate order.

8. **[LO 4.1]** Typographic techniques that provide visual guidance for understanding information and help coders to understand rules and select the right code are known as _____ in ICD-10-CM.
   A. Inclusion notes
   B. Conventions
   C. Manifestations
   D. Sequelae

9. **[LO 4.2]** Tay-Sachs disease is an example of a(n) _____.
   A. Eponym
   B. Etiology
   C. Manifestation
   D. Convention

10. **[LO 4.2]** The abbreviation _____ is used with a term when there is no code that is specific for the condition.
    A. CC
    B. NOS
    C. NEC
    D. GEM

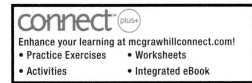

Enhance your learning at mcgrawhillconnect.com!
- Practice Exercises
- Worksheets
- Activities
- Integrated eBook

Applying Your Knowledge

Case 4.1   Coding Diagnoses

Supply the correct ICD-10-CM codes for the following diagnoses.

A. **[LO 4.6]** Brewer's infarct

B. **[LO 4.6]** Parinaud's conjunctivitis

C. **[LO 4.6]** seasonal allergic rhinitis due to pollen

D. **[LO 4.6]** cardiac arrhythmia

E. **[LO 4.6]** backache

F. **[LO 4.6]** sebaceous cyst

G. **[LO 4.6]** adenofibrosis of left breast

H. **[LO 4.6]** chronic cystitis with hematuria

I. **[LO 4.6]** normal delivery, single live birth

J. **[LO 4.6]** stage 2 pressure ulcer of right ankle

K. **[LO 4.6]** acute myocarditis due to influenza

L. **[LO 4.6]** acute otitis media, bilateral

M. **[LO 4.6]** endocarditis due to Q fever

N. **[LO 4.6]** influenza vaccination

O. **[LO 4.6]** vertigo

P. **[LO 4.6]** antineoplastic chemotherapy induced anemia

Q. **[LO 4.6]** muscle spasms, right thigh

R. **[LO 4.6]** influenza with acute respiratory infection

S. **[LO 4.6]** pneumonia due to Streptococcus, Group B

T. **[LO 4.6]** menorrhagia

Case 4.2   Auditing Code Assignment

Audit the following cases to determine whether the correct codes have been reported in the correct order. If a coding mistake has been made, state the correct code and your reason for assigning it.

A. **[LO 4.6]**

Chart note for Henry Blum, date of birth 11/4/53:

Examined patient on 12/6/2016. He was complaining of a facial rash. Examination revealed generalized pustular psoriasis and extensive seborrheic dermatitis over his upper eyebrows, nasolabial fold, and extending to the subnasal region.

The following codes were reported: L40.1, L21

B. [LO 4.6]

Physician's notes, 2/24/2016, patient George Kadar, DOB 10/11/1940:

Subjective: This 75-year-old patient complains of voiding difficulties, primarily urinary incontinence. No complaints of urinary retention.

Objective: Rectal examination: enlarged prostate. Patient catheterized for residual urine of 200 cc. Urinalysis is essentially negative.

Assessment: Prostatic hypertrophy, benign.

Plan: Refer to urologist for cystoscopy.

The following code was reported: N40.1.

C. [LO 4.6]

Patient: Gloria S. Diaz:

Subjective: This 25-year-old female patient presents with pain in her left knee both when she moves it and when it is inactive. She denies previous trauma to this area but has had right-knee pain and arthritis in the past.

Objective: Examination revealed the left knee to be warm and slightly swollen compared to the right knee. Extension is 180 degrees; flexion is 90 degrees. Some tenderness in area.

Assessment: Left-knee pain probably due to chronic arthritis.

Plan: Daypro 600 mg 2-QD 3 1 week; recheck in one week.

The following codes were reported: M25.562, M19.90.

5

PROCEDURAL CODING

Step 1
Step 2
Step 3
Step 4
Step 5
Step 6
Step 7
Step 8
Step 9
Step 10

KEY TERMS

add-on code
bundled code
Category I code
Category II code
Category III code
code linkage
consultation
Current Procedural Terminology (CPT)
E/M code
eponym
global period
Health Care Common Procedure Coding System
    (HCPCS)
key component
level of service
main number
moderate sedation
modifier
panel
place of service (POS)
primary procedure
procedure code
referral
resequenced
section guidelines
separate procedure
surgical package
unbundle
unlisted procedures

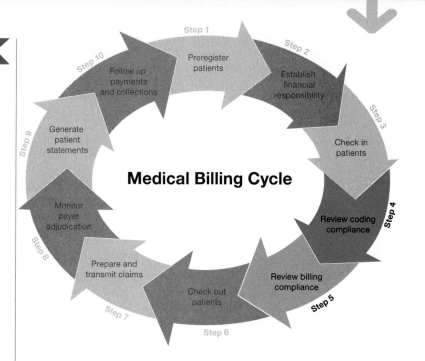

Step 10 Follow up payments and collections
Step 1 Preregister patients
Step 2 Establish financial responsibility
Step 3 Check in patients
Step 4 Review coding compliance
Step 5 Review billing compliance
Step 6 Check out patients
Step 7 Prepare and transmit claims
Step 8 Monitor payer adjudication
Step 9 Generate patient statements

Medical Billing Cycle

Learning Outcomes

After studying this chapter, you should be able to:

5.1 Discuss the use of the Current Procedural Terminology (CPT) code set.

5.2 List the six steps in the process of assigning correct CPT codes.

5.3 Explain E/M code selection and assignment.

5.4 Recognize surgical packages.

5.5 Discuss coding for laboratory panels and immunizations.

5.6 Discuss coding with the Health Care Common Procedure Coding System (HCPCS).

Procedure codes, like diagnosis codes, are an important part of the medical billing cycle. Standard procedure codes are used by physicians to report the medical, surgical, and diagnostic services they provide. These reported codes are used by payers to determine payments. Accurate procedural coding ensures that providers receive the maximum appropriate reimbursement.

5.1 Introduction to Procedure Codes in the CPT

This chapter provides a basic introduction to procedural coding that will help you work effectively with health care claims and encounter forms. When a patient sees a physician, each procedure and service performed is reported on a health care claim using a standardized **procedure code.** Procedure codes represent medical procedures, such as surgery and diagnostic tests, and medical services, such as an examination to evaluate a patient's condition.

On correct claims, each reported service is connected to a diagnosis that supports the procedure as necessary to investigate or treat the patient's condition in that health care setting. Health plans analyze this connection between the diagnostic and the procedural information, called **code linkage,** to evaluate the medical necessity of the reported charges.

Medical assistants verify procedure codes and use them to report physicians' services. The practice's physicians, medical coders, or—in some cases—medical assistants are responsible for the selection of procedure codes. To be sure that the procedure codes, as well as the diagnosis codes, are correctly linked and valid, medical assistants review the documentation to be sure it supports the codes. Often a query is communicated to the physician to resolve outstanding questions. For example, at times an additional surgical procedure is needed to remove a tumor completely, based on frozen section pathology. When this additional surgery is done controls the correct code selection. By verifying all information and following the rules of correct coding, medical assistants ensure that the provider receives the maximum appropriate reimbursement for procedures and services.

Organization of CPT

The HIPAA-required set of procedure codes is the **Current Procedural Terminology,** published by the American Medical Association (AMA) and known as the **CPT.** An updated edition of the CPT is available every year to reflect changes in medical practice. Newly developed procedures are added, some are changed, and old ones that have become obsolete are deleted. These changes are available in print and in an electronic file for medical offices that use a computer-based version of the CPT.

CPT **Category I codes**—which are most of the codes in CPT—are five-digit numbers (with no decimals). They are organized into six sections:

Section	Range of Codes
Evaluation and Management	Codes 99201–99499
Anesthesia	Codes 00100–01999
Surgery	Codes 10021–69990
Radiology	Codes 70010–79999
Pathology and Laboratory	Codes 80047–89398
Medicine	Codes 90281–99607

Table 5.1 summarizes the types of codes, organization, and guidelines of these six sections of Category I codes. With the exception of the first section, the CPT is

procedure code Code identifying medical treatment or diagnostic services.

code linkage Connection between a service and a patient's condition or illness.

Current Procedural Terminology (CPT) Contains the standardized classification system for reporting medical procedures and services.

Category I code Procedure codes found in the main body of CPT.

COMPLIANCE GUIDELINE

CPT Codes

New CPT codes are released on October 1 and must be used for services dated the following January 1 or later. The CPT codes as of the date of service—not the date of claim preparation—are required by HIPAA. Encounter forms, the PMP, and any other computer systems that store CPT codes must also be updated.

Section	Definition of Codes	Structure	Key Guidelines
Evaluation and Management	Physicians' services that are performed to determine the best course for patient care	Organized by place and/or type of service	New/established patients; other definitions Unlisted services, special reports Selecting an E/M service level
Anesthesia	Anesthesia services by or supervised by a physician; includes general, regional, and local anesthesia	Organized by body site	Time-based Services covered (bundled) in codes Unlisted services/special reports Qualifying circumstances codes
Surgery	Surgical procedures performed by physicians	Organized by body system and then body site, followed by procedural groups	Surgical package definition Follow-up care definition Add-on codes Separate procedures Subsection notes Unlisted services/special reports
Radiology	Radiology services by or supervised by a physician	Organized by type of procedure followed by body site	Unlisted services/special reports Supervision and interpretation (professional and technical components)
Pathology and Laboratory	Pathology and laboratory services by physicians or by physician-supervised technicians	Organized by type of procedure	Complete procedure Panels Unlisted services/special reports
Medicine	Evaluation, therapeutic, and diagnostic procedures by or supervised by a physician	Organized by type of service or procedure	Subsection notes Multiple procedures reported separately Add-on codes Separate procedures Unlisted services/special report

arranged in numerical order from start to end. Codes for evaluation and management, though, are listed first, out of numerical order, because they are used most often. The book as well as all sections opens with **section guidelines** that apply to its procedures. This material should be checked carefully before a procedure code is chosen.

section guidelines Usage notes at the beginnings of CPT sections.

The six primary sections of the CPT category I codes are divided into subsections. These in turn are further divided into headings according to the type of test, service, or body system. Code number ranges included on a particular page are found in the upper-right corner. This makes locating a code faster after using the index.

CPT Symbols

Symbols for Changed Codes

These three symbols have the following meanings when they appear next to CPT codes:

CPT Updates
www.ama-assn.org/go/CPT

- • A bullet (a solid circle) indicates a new procedure code. The symbol appears next to the code only the year that it is added.

▲ A triangle indicates that the code's descriptor has changed. It, too, appears in only the year the descriptor is revised.

▶ ◀ Facing triangles (two triangles that face each other) enclose new or revised text other than the code's descriptor.

Symbol for Add-On Codes

A plus sign (+) next to a code in the main text indicates an **add-on code.** Add-on codes describe *secondary procedures* that are commonly carried out in addition to a **primary procedure.** The primary procedure is the main service performed for the condition listed as the primary diagnosis. Add-on codes usually use phrases such as *each additional* or *list separately in addition to the primary procedure* to show that they are never used as stand-alone codes. For example, the add-on +15003 is used in addition to the primary procedure code for surgical preparation for a skin graft site (15002) to provide a specific percentage or dimension of body area that was involved beyond the amount covered in the primary procedure.

add-on code Procedure performed and reported in addition to a primary procedure.

primary procedure Most resource-intensive CPT procedure during an encounter.

Symbol for Moderate Sedation

In CPT, the symbol ◉ (a bullet inside a circle) next to a code means that moderate sedation is a part of the procedure that the surgeon performs. This means that for compliant coding, moderate sedation is not billed in addition to the code. **Moderate sedation** is a moderate, drug-induced depression of consciousness during which patients can respond to verbal commands. This type of sedation is typically used with procedures such as bronchoscopies.

moderate sedation Moderate, drug-induced depression of consciousness.

Symbol for FDA Approval Pending

Also used is the symbol ⚡ (a lightning bolt). This symbol is used with vaccine codes that have been submitted to the Federal Drug Administration (FDA) and are expected to be approved for use soon. The codes cannot be used until approved, at which point this symbol is removed.

Symbol for Resequenced Codes

As new procedures are developed and widely adopted, CPT has encountered situations where there are not enough numbers left in a particular numerical sequence of codes to handle all new items that need to be included. Also, at times codes need to be regrouped into related procedures for clarity. Beginning with CPT 2010, the American Medical Association (AMA) decided to change the way this situation had been accommodated. Previously, if more procedures were to be added than numbers were available, the entire list would be renumbered using *new* numbers and moved to the place in CPT where the list would be in numerical order. This approach often caused large groups of code numbers to have to be renumbered—creating confusion and requiring lots of updating of medical practice forms and databases.

The AMA decided to use the idea of *resequencing* rather than renumbering and moving codes. Resequencing is the practice of displaying the codes outside of numerical order in favor of grouping them according to the relationships among the code descriptions. This permits out-of-sequence code numbers to be inserted under the previous key procedural terms without having to renumber and move the entire list of related codes.

The codes that are **resequenced** are listed two times in CPT. First, they are listed in their original numeric position with the note that the code is now out of numerical sequence and referring the user to the code range containing the resequenced code and description.

resequenced CPT procedure codes that have been reassigned to another sequence.

46220 Code is out of numerical sequence. See 46200–46288.

Second, the resequenced symbol # is shown in front of the code and its descriptor where it appears in the group of codes to which it is related, as shown below:

46220 Excision of single external papilla or tag, anus

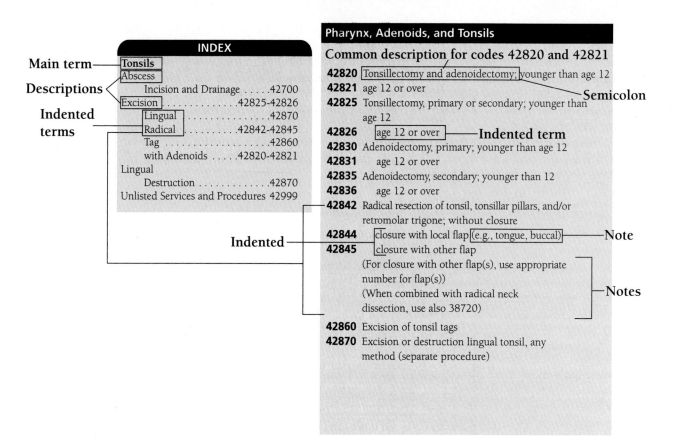

FIGURE 5.1 The CPT Format

CPT Format

The CPT uses a particular format to show codes and their descriptions. Some descriptions are indented to show that they include a common entry from above. For example, look at the descriptions for codes 42842, 42844, and 42845 in Figure 5.1. Code 42842 is the parent code in this list. Its description begins with a capital letter. Codes 42844 and 42845 are indented, and each begins with a lowercase letter. These indented codes refer to the parent code above. The words in the description of the parent code that precede the semicolon are common to all the indented codes below it. Thus, code 42844 has the full description: "Radical resection of tonsil, tonsillar pillars, and/or retromolar trigone; closure with local flap." But if the procedure is described as "closure with other flap," the correct code would be 42845.

CPT listings may also contain notes, which are explanations for categories and individual codes. Notes often appear in parentheses after a code. Many times, notes suggest other codes that should be considered before a final code is selected. For example, the note for code 42844 in Figure 5.1 is "(e.g., tongue, buccal)," meaning that either of these terms may appear in the description of the local flap.

Unlisted Procedures, Category II Codes, and Category III Codes

unlisted procedures Service not listed in CPT.

Some services or procedures occur infrequently. Others are too new to be included in the CPT. Therefore, each section provides codes to be used when a service or procedure is not listed. Codes for **unlisted procedures** are found in the guidelines at the beginning of each section, and usually under an Other Procedures subsection. Whenever a code for an unlisted procedure is used, a special report must be attached to the health care claim. It describes the procedure, its extent, and the reason it was performed. It also gives the equipment and amount of time and effort required.

Category II codes, listed at the end of the regular (Category I) CPT codes, are used to track performance measures for a medical goal, such as reducing tobacco use. Reporting these codes on health care claims is optional, and they are not paid. They help in the development of best practices and improve documentation. These codes have an alphabetic character for the fifth digit, such as 4000F for tobacco use cessation counseling.

Category III codes, also listed at the end, are temporary codes for emerging technology, services, and procedures. If a Category III code exists for a service, it, rather than an unlisted code, must be used. These codes also have an alphabetic fifth digit, such as 0184T for excision of rectal tumor, TEMS approach. A temporary code may become permanent and part of the regular codes if the service it identifies proves effective and is widely performed.

Category II code Optional CPT codes that track performance measures.

Category III code Temporary codes for emerging technology, services, and procedures.

BILLING TIP

Be Careful Using Unlisted Codes

An unlisted procedure code should not be reported until a thorough search of the CPT, especially of the Category III codes, is done using different possibilities for the proper name of the procedure. Using a code for an unlisted service requires extra time to prepare the special report and extra attention by the insurance carrier's claims department. These efforts delay or often reduce payment, particularly if the unlisted code is assigned in error.

Modifiers

One or more two-digit CPT **modifiers** may be assigned to a five-digit **main number.** Modifiers are written with a space before the two-digit number. The use of a modifier shows that some special circumstance applies to the service or procedure the physician performed. For example, in the Surgery section, the modifier 62 indicates that two surgeons worked together, each performing part of a surgical procedure, during an operation. Each physician will be paid part of the amount normally reimbursed for that procedure code. Likewise, the modifier 80 indicates that the services of a surgical assistant were used, and this person's fees are a part of the claim.

As another example, if a procedure has two parts, a technical component modifier (TC) is appended to show the work performed by a technician, such as a radiologist, and a professional component modifier (PC) is added to show the work that the physician performs, usually the interpretation and reporting of the results.

Appendix A of the CPT explains the proper use of each modifier. Some section guidelines also discuss the use of modifiers with the section's codes.

modifier Number appended to a code to report particular facts.

main number Five-digit number to which one or more two-digit CPT modifiers may be assigned.

BILLING TIP

Updating Vaccine Codes and Category III Codes

Both vaccine product codes and Category III codes are released twice a year and have a six-month period for implementation. Offices billing these services should check for updates at the CPT website.

THINKING IT THROUGH 5.1

1. After making a diagnosis, the physician determines the proper course of treatment for the patient's health situation. As in diagnostic coding, the medical assistant's role is to accurately communicate to the payer the procedures and services performed by the physician. Why is it important for the procedure codes to relate correctly to the diagnosis?

2. In CPT, what is the meaning of the symbol in front of code 93503?

3. Patient was scheduled for a total diagnostic colonoscopy, but went into respiratory distress during procedure; surgeon stopped the procedure. What modifier should be reported with the Category I CPT code?

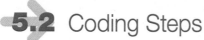

5.2 Coding Steps

The correct process for assigning accurate procedure codes has six steps, as shown in Figure 5.2.

Step 1   Review Complete Medical Documentation

The first step is to review the documentation of the patient's visit and decide which procedures and/or services were performed and where the service took place (the place of service, which may be an office, a facility, or another health care setting).

Step 2   Abstract the Medical Procedures from the Visit Documentation

Then, based on knowledge of CPT and of the payer's policies, a decision is made about which services can be charged and are to be reported.

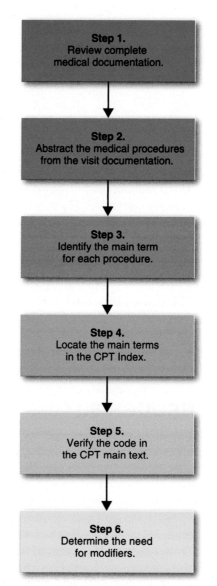

Step 1.
Review complete
medical documentation.

Step 2.
Abstract the medical procedures
from the visit documentation.

Step 3.
Identify the main term
for each procedure.

Step 4.
Locate the main terms
in the CPT Index.

Step 5.
Verify the code in
the CPT main text.

Step 6.
Determine the need
for modifiers.

FIGURE 5.2 Procedure Code Assignment Flow Chart

Step 3 Identify the Main Term for Each Procedure

The next step is to identify the main term for each procedure. Main terms may be based on the:

▶ Procedure or service (such as repair, biopsy, evaluation and management, or extraction).
▶ Organ or body part (such as chest wall, prostate, or bladder).
▶ Condition or disease being treated (such as facial nerve paralysis).
▶ Common abbreviation (such as ECG or CT) or synonym.
▶ **Eponym** (the name of a person or place for which a procedure is named, such as Cotte operation).
▶ Symptom (for example, fracture).

eponym Name or phrase formed from or based on a person's name.

Step 4 Locate the Main Terms in the CPT Index

Next, locate the procedures using the main term in the index at the back of CPT. For each term a listing of a code or a code range identifies the appropriate heading and procedure code(s) in CPT. Some entries have a *See* cross-reference or a *See also* to point to another index entry.

First, pick out a specific procedure or service, organ, or condition. Find the procedure code in the CPT's index. Remember, the number in the index is the five-digit code, not a page number. For example, to find the code for dressing change, first look alphabetically in the index for the procedure. Then, turn to the procedure code in the body of the CPT to be sure the code accurately reflects the service performed. The procedure code 15852 explains the dressing change for "other than burns" and "under anesthesia (other than local)." A dressing for a burn is listed as procedure codes 16020–16030.

In some cases, the patient's medical record shows an abbreviation, synonym, or eponym. For example, the record might state "treated for bone infection." In CPT's index, the entry for Infection, Bone, is followed by the instruction "See Osteomyelitis."

To code the excision of a vaginal cyst, one might first look under Excision. There is a listing for Cyst beneath Excision, followed by a list of organs, regions, or structures involved. Look for Vaginal to find the code. Another way to find the code is to look under Vagina and then find the listing for Cyst Excision beneath it.

Example: Code Range Index Entry

Graft

Bone and skin 20969–20970, 20972–20973

When a code range is listed, read the code descriptions for all codes within the range indicated in the index in order to select the most specific code. If the main term cannot be located in the index, review the main term selection with the physician for clarification. In some cases, there is a better or more common term that can be used. ◀

Step 5 Verify the Code in the CPT Main Text

The next step is to review the possible codes in the CPT section that the index entries point to. Check section guidelines and any notes directly under the code, within the code description, or after the code description. Items that cannot be billed separately because they are covered under another, broader code are eliminated.

The codes to be reported for each day's services are ranked in order of highest to lowest rate of reimbursement. The actual order in which they were performed on a particular day is not important. When reporting, the earliest date of service is listed first, followed by subsequent dates of service. For example:

Date	Procedure	Charge
11/17/2016	99204	$202
11/20/2016	43215	$355
11/20/2016	74235	$75

Step 6 Determine the Need for Modifiers

The circumstances involved with the procedure or service may require the use of modifiers. The patient's diagnosis may affect this determination. Check section guidelines and Appendix A to find modifiers that elaborate on details of the procedure being coded. For example, a bilateral breast reconstruction requires the modifier 50. Find the code for "breast reconstruction with free flap": 19364. To show the insurance carrier that the procedure was performed on both breasts, attach the 50 modifier: 1936450.

THINKING IT THROUGH 5.2

1. List all possible index entries for locating the service, and then assign the code. The first item is completed as an example.

Index Entry	Code
A. Excision of mucous cyst of a finger: <u>Excision, cyst, finger</u>	<u>26160</u>
B. Endoscopic biopsy of the nose: _____	
C. Arthroscopic meniscectomy of the knee joint: _____	
D. Drainage of a sublingual salivary gland cyst: _____	
E. Cystoscopy with fragmentation of ureteral calculus: _____	

5.3 Coding Evaluation and Management Services

To diagnose conditions and to plan treatments, physicians use a wide range of time, effort, and skill for different patients and circumstances. In the guidelines to the Evaluation and Management (**E/M codes**) section, CPT explains how to choose the correct codes for different levels of evaluation and management services.

New or Established Patient?

Health plans want to know whether the physician treated a new patient or an established patient. Physicians often spend more time during new patients' visits than during visits from established patients, so many E/M codes for the two types of patients are separate. Emergency patients are not classified as either new or established patients.

Place of Service

The **place of service (POS)** is also important to know, because different E/M codes apply to services performed in a physician's office, a hospital inpatient room, a hospital emergency room, a nursing facility, an extended-care facility, and a patient's home.

Referral or Consultation?

To understand the subsection of E/M codes on consultations, review the difference between a consultation and a referral in coding terminology. A **consultation** occurs when a second physician, at the request of the patient's physician, examines the patient. The second physician usually focuses on a particular issue and reports a

E/M code Covers physicians' services performed to determine the optimum course for patient care.

place of service (POS) Administrative code indicating where medical services were provided.

consultation Service in which a physician advises a requesting physician about a patient's condition and care.

written opinion to the first physician. The physician providing a consultation ("consult") may perform a service for the patient but does not independently start a full course of treatment (although the consulting physician may recommend one) or take charge of the patient's care. Consultations require use of the E/M consultation codes (the range from 99241 to 99255). Consultation requests and reports must be written documents that are stored in the medical records.

On the other hand, when the patient is *referred* to another physician, either the total care or a specific portion of care is transferred to that provider (see the chapter about patient encounters and billing information, which describes the requirement by payers for referral authorization). The patient becomes a new patient of that doctor for the referred condition and may not return to the care of the referring physician until the completion of a course of treatment. **Referrals** require use of the regular office visit E/M service codes. Although people sometimes use these terms to mean the same thing, a referral and a consultation are different. This distinction is important because the amounts that can be charged for the two types of service are different. Under a referral, the PCP or other provider is sending the patient to another physician for specialized care. If the sending provider requests a consultation, this is asking for the opinion of another physician regarding the patient's care. The patient will be returned to the care of the original provider with the specialist's written consultation report containing an evaluation of the patient's condition and/or care.

referral Transfer of patient care from one physician to another.

Level of Service

The final item to decide in assigning the right E/M code is the **level of service**—how much work, time, and decision making were involved. These **key components** documented in the patient's medical record help determine the level of service:

level of service Amount of work, time, and decision making involved in an encounter.

key component Factor documented for various levels of evaluation and management services.

1. The extent of the patient history taken.
2. The extent of the examination conducted.
3. The complexity of the medical decision making.

Eight Steps for E/M Code Assignment

To select the correct E/M code, follow these eight steps, as shown in Figure 5.3.

Step 1   Determine the Category and Subcategory of Service Based on the Place of Service and the Patient's Status

The list of E/M categories, such as office visits, hospital services, and preventive medicine services, is used to locate the appropriate place or type of service in the index. In the main text of the selected category, the subcategory—such as new or established patient—is then chosen.

> *Documentation:* initial hospital visit to established patient
>
> *Index:* Hospital Services
>
>> Inpatient Services
>>
>>> Initial Care, New or Established Patient
>
> *Code Ranges*: 99221–99223

For most types of service, such as initial hospital care for an established patient, between three to five codes are listed. To select an appropriate code from this range, three key components are considered: (1) the history the physician documented, (2) the examination that was documented, and (3) the medical decisions the physician documented. (The exception to this guideline is selecting a code for counseling or coordination of care, where the amount of time the physician spends may be the only key component in some situations.)

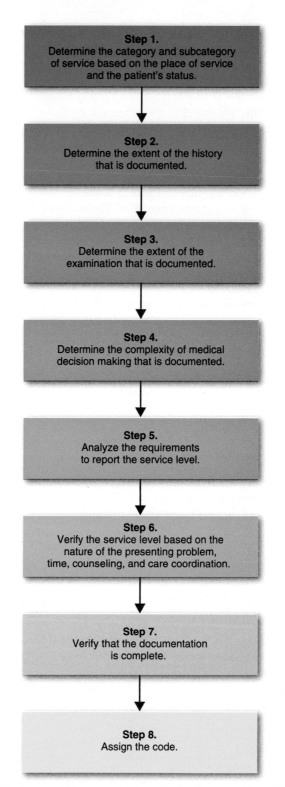

FIGURE 5.3 Evaluation and Management Code Assignment Flow Chart

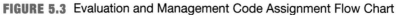

Step 2   Determine the Extent of the History That Is Documented

History is the information the physician received by questioning the patient about the chief complaint and other signs or symptoms, about all or selected body systems, and about pertinent past history, family background, and other personal factors. If the patient is incapacitated, the history may be taken from a family member.

The history is documented in the patient medical record as follows.

History of Present Illness (HPI)   The history of the illness is a description of the development of the illness from the first sign or symptom that the patient experienced to the present time. It includes everything related to the illness or condition.

These points about the illness or condition may be documented:

▶ Location *(body area of the pain/symptom)*
▶ Quality *(type of pain/symptom, such as sudden or dull)*
▶ Severity *(degree of pain/symptom)*
▶ Duration *(how long the pain/symptom lasts and when it began)*
▶ Timing *(time of day pain/symptom occurs)*
▶ Context *(any situation related to the pain/symptom, such as occurs after eating)*
▶ Modifying factors *(any factors that alter the pain/symptom)*
▶ Associated signs and symptoms *(things that also happen when the pain/symptom occurs, such as the severity, location, and timing of pain, and other signs and symptoms)*

Review of Systems (ROS)   The review of systems is an inventory of body systems. These systems are:

▶ Constitutional symptoms *(such as fever or weight loss)*
▶ Eyes
▶ Ears, nose, mouth, and throat
▶ Cardiovascular (CV)
▶ Respiratory
▶ Gastrointestinal (GI)
▶ Genitourinary (GU)
▶ Musculoskeletal
▶ Integumentary
▶ Neurological
▶ Psychiatric
▶ Endocrine
▶ Hematologic/lymphatic
▶ Allergic/immunologic

Past Medical History (PMH)   The past history of the patient's experiences with illnesses, injuries, and treatments contains data about other major illnesses and injuries, operations, and hospitalizations. It also covers current medications the patient is taking, allergies, immunization status, and diet.

Family History (FH)   The family history reviews the medical events in the patient's family. It includes the health status or cause of death of parents, brothers and sisters, and children; specific diseases that are related to the patient's chief complaint or the patient's diagnosis; and the presence of any known hereditary diseases.

Social History (SH)   The facts gathered in the social history, which depend on the patient's age, include marital status, employment, and other factors. The histories documented after the HPI are sometimes referred to as PFSH, for past, family, and social history.

The history that the physician decides to obtain is then categorized as one of four types on a scale from lesser to greater extent of amount of history obtained:

1. *Problem focused:* Determining the patient's chief complaint and obtaining a brief history of the present illness.
2. *Expanded problem focused:* Determining the patient's chief complaint and obtaining a brief history of the present illness, plus a problem-pertinent system review of the particular body system that is involved.

3. *Detailed:* Determining the chief complaint; obtaining an extended history of the present illness; reviewing both the problem-pertinent system and additional systems; and taking pertinent past, family, and/or social history.
4. *Comprehensive:* Determining the chief complaint and taking an extended history of the present illness, a complete review of systems, and a complete past, family, and social history.

Step 3   Determine the Extent of the Examination That Is Documented

The physician may examine a particular body area or organ system or may conduct a multisystem examination. The body areas are divided into the head and face; chest, including breasts and axilla; abdomen; genitalia, groin and buttocks; back; and each extremity.

The organ systems that may be examined are the eyes; the ears, nose, mouth, and throat; cardiovascular; respiratory; gastrointestinal; genitourinary; musculoskeletal; skin; neurologic; psychiatric; and hematologic/lymphatic/immunologic.

The examination that the physician documents is categorized as one of four types on a scale from lesser to greater extent:

1. *Problem focused:* A limited examination of the affected body area or system.
2. *Expanded problem focused:* A limited examination of the affected body area or system and other related areas.
3. *Detailed:* An extended examination of the affected body area or system and other related areas.
4. *Comprehensive:* A general multisystem examination or a complete examination of a single organ system.

Step 4   Determine the Complexity of Medical Decision Making That Is Documented

The complexity of the medical decisions that the physician makes involves how many possible diagnoses or treatment options were considered; how much data information (such as test results or previous records) was considered in analyzing the patient's problem; and how serious the illness is, meaning how much risk there is for significant complications, advanced illness, or death.

The decision-making process that the physician documents is categorized as one of four types on a scale from lesser to greater complexity:

1. *Straightforward:* Minimal diagnoses options, a minimal amount of data, and minimum risk.
2. *Low complexity:* Limited diagnoses options, a low amount of data, and low risk.
3. *Moderate complexity:* Multiple diagnoses options, a moderate amount of data, and moderate risk.
4. *High complexity:* Extensive diagnoses options, an extensive amount of data, and high risk.

BILLING TIP

Three Key Components

This means that to select code 99203, the medical record must show that a detailed history and examination were taken, and medical decision making was at least at the level of low complexity.

Step 5   Analyze the Requirements to Report the Service Level

The descriptor for each E/M code explains the standards for its selection. For office visits and most other services to new patients, and for initial care visits, all three of the key components must be documented. This is stated in CPT as follows:

99203   Office or other outpatient visit for the evaluation and management of a new patient, which require these three key components:
▶ **a detailed history**
▶ **a detailed examination**
▶ **medical decision making of low complexity**

For most services for established patients, and for subsequent care visits, two out of three of the key components requirements must be met. For example:

99213 Office or other outpatient visit, for the evaluation and management of an established patient, which requires at least two of these three key components:
- ▶ **an expanded problem focused history**
- ▶ **an expanded problem focused examination**
- ▶ **medical decision making of low complexity**

BILLING TIP

Two of Three Key Components

This means that to select code 99213, the medical record must show that two out of the three factors are documented.

Step 6 Verify the Service Level Based on the Nature of the Presenting Problem, Time, Counseling, and Care Coordination

Many descriptors mention two additional components: (1) how severe the patient's condition is, referred to as the *nature of the presenting problem*, and (2) how much time the physician typically spends directly treating the patient. These factors, while not the key components, help in selecting the correct E/M service level. For example, this wording statement appears in CPT after the 99214 code (office visit for the evaluation and management of an established patient):

Usually, the presenting problem(s) are of moderate to high severity. Physicians typically spend 25 minutes face-to-face with the patient and/or family.

Counseling is a discussion with a patient regarding areas such as diagnostic results, instructions for follow-up treatment, and patient education. It is mentioned as a typical part of each E/M service in the descriptor, but it is not required to be documented as a key component.

Coordination of care with other providers or agencies is also mentioned. When coordination of care is provided but the patient is not present, codes from the case management and care plan oversight services subsections' codes are reported.

BILLING TIP

The Time Factor

If a patient's visit is mainly about counseling and/or coordination of care regarding symptoms or illness, the length of time the physician spends is the controlling factor. If over 50 percent of the visit is spent counseling or coordinating care, time is the *main* factor. If an established patient's visit is thirty minutes, for example, and twenty minutes of it are spent counseling, then the E/M code is 99214.

Step 7 Verify that the Documentation is Complete

Meeting the requirements means that the documentation must contain the record of the physician's work. When an E/M code is assigned, the patient's medical record must contain the clinical details to support it. The history, examination, and medical decision making must be adequately documented, so that the medical necessity and appropriateness of the service can be understood.

Step 8 Assign the Code

After the procedure code is verified, it is assigned. If the patient has more than one diagnosis for a single claim, the primary diagnosis is listed first (see the chapter on diagnostic coding). Likewise, the corresponding primary procedure is listed first.

The physician may perform additional procedures at the same time or in the same session as the primary procedure. If additional procedures are performed, match up each procedure with its corresponding diagnosis. If this is not done, the procedures will not be considered medically necessary, and the claim will be denied.

For example, Ms. Silvers, who saw Dr. Ramirez for chest pain and shortness of breath, also has asthma. While the patient is in the office, Dr. Ramirez renews her prescription for asthma medication along with performing the ECG. If the ECG is mistakenly shown as a procedure for asthma, the claim will be denied, because that procedure is not medically necessary for that diagnosis.

The need for any modifiers, based on the documentation of special circumstances, is also reviewed.

Reporting E/M Codes on Claims

Documentation Guidelines for Evaluation and Management

Two sets of guidelines for documenting evaluation and management codes have been published by CMS and the AMA: the *1995 Documentation Guidelines for Evaluation and Management Services* and a 1997 version. CMS and most payers permit providers to use either the 1995 or the 1997 E/M guidelines. The medical practice should be clear about which set of guidelines, the 1995 or 1997, it generally follows for E/M coding and reporting.

Office and Hospital Services

Office and other outpatient services are the most often reported E/M services.

▶ When a patient is evaluated and then admitted to a health care facility, the service is reported using the codes for initial hospital care (the range 99221–99223).

▶ The admitting physician uses the initial hospital care services codes. Only one provider can report these services; other physicians involved in the patient's care, such as a surgeon or radiologist, use other E/M service codes or other codes from appropriate sections.

▶ Codes for initial hospital observation care (99218–99220), initial hospital care (99221–99223), and initial inpatient consultations (99251–99255) should be reported by a physician only once for a patient admission.

Emergency Department Services

An emergency department is hospital based and is available to patients twenty-four hours a day. When emergency services are reported, whether the patient is new or established is not applicable. Time is not a factor in selecting the E/M service code. The code ranges are 99281 to 99288.

Preventive Medicine Services

Preventive medicine services are used to report routine physical examinations in the absence of a patient complaint. These codes, in the range 99381 to 99397, are divided according to the age of the patient. Counseling is coded from code range 99401 to 99429. Immunizations and other services, such as lab tests that are normal parts of an annual physical, are reported using the appropriate codes from the Medicine and the Pathology and Laboratory sections of CPT.

THINKING IT THROUGH 5.3

1. Using the office visit E/M codes, which code would you select for Case A and Case B?

A. CASE A

Chart note for established patient:

> **S: Patient returns for removal of stitches I placed about seven days ago. Reports normal itching around the wound area, but no pain or swelling.**
>
> **O: Wound at lateral aspect of the left eye looks well healed. Decision made to remove the 5-0 nylon sutures, which was done without difficulty.**
>
> **A: Laceration, healed.**
>
> **P: Patient advised to use vitamin E for scar prophylaxis**

B. CASE B

Initial office evaluation by oncologist of a sixty-five-year-old female with sudden unexplained twenty-pound weight loss. Comprehensive history and examination performed with medical decision making of high complexity.

5.4 Coding Surgical Procedures

Codes in the Surgery section represent groups of procedures that include all routine elements. This combination of services is called a **surgical package.** According to the Surgery section guidelines in the CPT, the procedure codes for surgical procedures include the following:

▶ After the decision for surgery, one related E/M encounter on the date immediately before or on the date of the procedure.
▶ The operation: preparing the patient for surgery, including injection of anesthesia by the surgeon (local infiltration, metacarpal/metatarsal/digital block or topical anesthesia), and performing the operation, including normal additional procedures, such as debridement.
▶ Immediate postoperative care, including dictating operative notes, talking with the family and other physicians.
▶ Writing orders.
▶ Evaluating the patient in the postanesthesia recovery area.
▶ Typical postoperative follow-up care.

A complete procedure includes the operation, the use of a local anesthetic, and postoperative care, all covered under a single code.

Example

Procedural Statement: Procedure conducted 8 days ago in office to correct hallux valgus (bunions) on both feet; local nerve block administered, correction by simple exostectomy. The global period for this procedure is 10 days. Saw patient in office today for routine follow-up; complete healing.

Code: 28290 50 Bunion correction on both feet ◀

Bundled Codes and Global Periods

The procedure code for a surgical package covers a group of services that should not be listed individually. This package is called a **bundled code.** Payers assign a fee that reimburses all the services provided under a bundled code. When such services are billed, physicians must report the bundled code and not each of the other codes separately. Reporting anything that is included in the bundled code is considered **unbundling,** or fragmented billing. Doing so causes denied claims and may result in an audit.

The period of time that is covered for follow-up care is referred to as the **global period.** For example, the global period for repairing a tendon might be set at ten days. The global period for major surgery such as an appendectomy might be set at ninety days. After the global period ends, additional services that are provided can be reported separately for additional payment.

Two types of services are not included in surgical package codes. These services are reported separately and reimbursed in addition to the surgical package fee:

▶ Complications or recurrences that arise after therapeutic surgical procedures.
▶ Care for the condition for which a diagnostic surgical procedure is performed. Routine follow-up care included in the code refers only to care related to recovery from the diagnostic procedure itself, not the condition.

When health plans pay for more than one surgical procedure performed on the same day for the same patient, they pay the full amount of the first listed surgical procedure, but they often pay less than the full amount for the other procedures. For maximum payment when multiple procedures are reported, the

bundled code Procedure code for a surgical package that covers a group of services that should not be listed individually.

unbundle Incorrect billing practice of breaking a panel or package of services/procedures into component parts.

global period Days surrounding a surgical procedure when all services relating to the procedure are considered part of the surgical package.

most complex or highest-level code—the procedure with the highest reimbursement value—should be listed first. The other procedures are listed with the modifier 51 or the modifier 59. Modifier 51 is used for multiple procedures at the same body site or system. Modifier 59 indicates distinct procedures, each fully reimbursed, rather than multiple procedures. It is usually used when the surgeon performs procedures on two different body sites or organ systems, such as the excision of a lesion on the chest as well as the incision and drainage (I & D) of an abscess on the leg.

Separate Procedures

separate procedure Descriptor used for a procedure that is usually part of a surgical package but may also be performed separately.

Some procedural code descriptors in the Surgery section are followed by the words *separate procedure* in parentheses. **Separate procedure** means that the procedure is usually done as an integral part of a surgical package—usually a larger procedure—but that in some situations it is not. If a separate procedure is performed alone or along with other procedures but for a separate purpose, it may be reported separately. For example:

42870 Excision or destruction lingual tonsil, any method (separate procedure)

Lingual tonsil excision is a separate procedure. It is usually a part of a routine tonsillectomy and so cannot be reported separately when a tonsillectomy is performed. When it is done independently, however, this code can be reported.

THINKING IT THROUGH 5.4

1. Review CPT code 44180 and determine if it is correct to report a diagnostic laparoscopy (CPT code 49320) with a surgical laparoscopy.

5.5 Coding Laboratory Procedures and Immunizations

Laboratory Tests

panel Single code grouping laboratory tests frequently done together.

Organ or disease-oriented **panels** listed in the Pathology and Laboratory section of the CPT include tests frequently ordered together (see Figure 5.4). A comprehensive metabolic panel, for example, includes tests for albumin, bilirubin, calcium, carbon dioxide, chloride, glucose, and other factors. Each element of the panel has its own procedure code in the Pathology and Laboratory section. However, when the tests are performed together, the code for the panel must be used, rather than listing each test separately.

ORGAN/DISEASE PANEL	
Basic Metabolic Panel (Calcium, ionized)	80047
Basic Metabolic Panel (Calcium, total)	80048
General Health Panel	80050
Electrolyte Panel	80051
Comprehensive Metabolic Panel	80053
Obstetric Panel	80055
Lipid Panel	80061
Renal Function Panel	80069
Acute Hepatitis Panel	80074
Hepatic Function Panel	80076

FIGURE 5.4 Examples of Panels in the CPT

Coding Immunizations

Injections and infusions of immune globulins, vaccines, toxoids, and other substances require two codes, one for giving the injection and one for the particular vaccine or toxoid that is given. These codes are selected from the Medicine section of CPT. For example, for an influenza shot, the administration code 90471 is used for the injection along with one of the codes for the specific vaccine, such as 90655, 90657, 90658, or 90660.

THINKING IT THROUGH 5.5

1. If a test for ferritin and a comprehensive metabolic panel are both performed, can both be reported?

2. Is it correct to report a comprehensive metabolic panel and an electrolyte panel for the same patient on the same day?

BILLING TIP

An E/M code is not used along with the codes for immunization unless a significant separate evaluation and management service is also done.

5.6 HCPCS Codes

The **Health Care Common Procedure Coding System,** commonly referred to as **HCPCS,** was developed by the Centers for Medicare and Medicaid Services (CMS) for use in coding services for Medicare patients. The HCPCS (pronounced hic-picks) coding system has two levels:

▶ Level I codes duplicate those from the CPT.
▶ Level II codes are issued by CMS in the *Medicare Carriers Manual.* They are called national codes and cover many supplies, such as sterile trays, drugs, and DME (durable medical equipment). Level II codes also cover services and procedures not included in the CPT. The Level II HCPCS codes have five characters.

HCPCS modifiers, either two letters or a letter with a number, are also available for use. These modifiers are different from the CPT modifiers. For example, HCPCS modifiers may indicate social worker services or equipment rentals.

Examples of Level II codes are:

Code Number	Description
A0210	Nonemergency transportation: ancillary: meals, escort
J0120	Injection, tetracycline, up to 250 mg
K0001	Standard wheelchair

Health Care Common Procedure Coding System (HCPCS) Procedure codes for Medicare claims.

GO TO CODING WORKBOOK PART 2

Your successful completion of this chapter is the basis of gaining additional coding experience. If assigned by your instructor, complete Part 2, pages 79–143, of the Medical Coding Workbook for Physician Practices and Facilities, ICD-10 Edition, by Cynthia Newby, CPC, CPC-P, to reinforce and expand your knowledge and skill in CPT and HCPCS coding.

Exercise 5.1   Entering a Patient's Procedure and Charge

Enter the charge transaction for Ann Ingram's visit with Dr. Clarke.

Follow the steps at www.mhhe.com/newbycarr to complete the exercise at connect.mcgraw-hill.com on your own once you have watched the demo and tried the steps with prompts in practice mode. Use the information provided in the scenario to complete the exercise.

connect plus+

THINKING IT THROUGH 5.6

1. Using HCPCS Level II, assign the appropriate codes.

    A. Ambulance service, basic life support, nonemergency transport.

    B. Breast pump, manual, any type.

    C. Zidovudine 10 mg.

    D. Laboratory certification, wet mounts, including vaginal specimen.

    E. Hospital bed with mattress and side rails, totally electric.

Learning Outcomes	Key Concepts/Examples
5.1 Discuss the use of the Current Procedural Terminology (CPT) code set. Pages 99–103	• Current CPT codes are required by HIPAA for use in reporting medical procedures and services. • Category I codes are used to report the services performed by the provider. • Category II codes are used to track performance measures. • Category III codes are temporary codes used for emerging technology, services, and procedures.
5.2 List the six steps in the process of assigning correct CPT codes. Pages 104–106	Six steps are followed to correctly assign CPT codes. • Step 1 Review complete medical documentation. • Step 2 Abstract the medical procedures from the visit documentation. • Step 3 Identify the main term for each procedure. • Step 4 Locate the main terms in the CPT index. • Step 5 Verify the code in the CPT main text. • Step 6 Determine the need for modifiers.
5.3 Explain E/M code selection and assignment. Pages 106–112	Key components for selecting Evaluation and Management codes are • The extent of the patient history taken. • The extent of the examination conducted. • The complexity of the medical decision making. The eight steps for correct E/M code assignment are • Determine the category and subcategory of service based on the place of service and the patient's status. • Determine the extent of the history that is documented. • Determine the extent of the examination that is documented. • Determine the complexity of medical decision making that is documented. • Analyze the requirements to report the service level. • Verify the service level based on the nature of presenting problem, time, counseling, and care coordination. • Verify that the documentation is complete. • Assign the code.
5.4 Recognize surgical packages. Pages 113–114	• Codes in the Surgery section include all routine elements that occur in addition to the operation and this combination of services is called the surgical package. • Some procedure code descriptors in the Surgery section state *separate procedure*. • Separate procedures are usually done as part of a larger procedure but in some cases can be performed alone.
5.5 Discuss coding for laboratory panels and immunizations. Pages 114–115	• Laboratory panels listed in the Pathology and Laboratory section of CPT are single codes that include tests frequently ordered together. • Immunizations are coded using two codes, one for giving the injection and one for the particular vaccine that is given.
5.6 Discuss coding with the Health Care Common Procedure Coding System (HCPCS). Page 115	• The Health Care Common Procedure Coding System (HCPCS) was developed by the Centers for Medicare and Medicaid Services (CMS). • Level I codes are the Category I CPT codes. • Level II codes, known as national codes, cover supplies, durable medical equipment, services, and procedures not listed in CPT.

CPT 2013 only © 2012 American Medical Association. All rights reserved.

Using Terminology

Match the key terms in the left column with the definitions in the right column.

_____ 1. **[LO 5.1]** Add-on code

_____ 2. **[LO 5.1]** Unlisted procedures

_____ 3. **[LO 5.4]** Global period

_____ 4. **[LO 5.4]** Surgical package

_____ 5. **[LO 5.3]** Key component

_____ 6. **[LO 5.1]** Category III code

_____ 7. **[LO 5.4]** Separate procedure

_____ 8. **[LO 5.1]** Category II code

_____ 9. **[LO 5.5]** Panel

_____ 10. **[LO 5.1]** Modifier

A. A secondary procedure that is performed with a primary procedure and that is indicated in CPT by a plus sign (+) next to the code.

B. CPT codes that are used to track performance measures.

C. Temporary codes for emerging technology, services, and procedures.

D. The inclusion of follow-up care for a specified period of time in the charges for a surgical procedure.

E. Documentation in the medical record used to determine the level of service provided.

F. A two-digit number indicating that special circumstances were involved with the procedure.

G. In CPT a single code that groups laboratory tests that are frequently done together.

H. A procedure performed in addition to a primary procedure.

I. Combination of services included in one surgical code.

J. A service that is not listed in CPT and requires a special report.

Checking Your Understanding

Write the letter of the choice that best completes the statement or answers the question.

1. **[LO 5.3]** The three key factors in selecting an Evaluation and Management code are _____.
   A. Time, severity of presenting problem, and history
   B. History, examination, and time
   C. Past history, history of present illness, and chief complaint
   D. History, examination, and medical decision making

2. **[LO 5.1]** Which groups of codes are listed first in CPT? _____
   A. Anesthesia codes 00100-01999
   B. Medicine codes 90281-99607
   C. Evaluation and Management codes 99201-99499
   D. Surgery codes 10021-69990

3. **[LO 5.1]** A plus sign next to a code indicates that _____.
   A. A preventative medical service is included
   B. It cannot be reported as a standalone code
   C. Preoperative evaluation and planning are billed separately
   D. The service can be billed separately

connect (plus+)

Enhance your learning at mcgrawhillconnect.com!
• Practice Exercises   • Worksheets
• Activities   • Integrated eBook

4. **[LO 5.3]** When a patient is seen by a physician, at the request of the patient's primary care physician, to provide a medical opinion on the patient's condition, it is considered a(n) _____.
   A. Office visit
   B. Referral
   C. Consultation
   D. Follow-up service

5. **[LO 5.2]** What is the final step in the process of assigning accurate procedure codes? _____
   A. Verify the code in the CPT main text
   B. Identify the main term for each procedure
   C. Review complete medical documentation
   D. Determine the need for modifiers

6. **[LO 5.5]** When a panel code from the Pathology and Laboratory section is reported, _____.
   A. All the tests in the panel must be performed together
   B. 90 percent of the tests in the panel must be performed on the same day
   C. The lab charges additional fees
   D. Only one of the listed tests in the panel has to be completed

7. **[LO 5.6]** HCPCS level II codes are issued by _____.
   A. AMA   C. CPT
   B. CMS   D. WHO

8. **[LO 5.6]** HCPCS modifiers differ from CPT modifiers in that they contain _____.
   A. Two numbers
   B. A letter and two numbers
   C. Symbols
   D. Numbers, letters, or a combination of both

9. **[LO 5.1]** CPT stands for _____.
   A. Complete procedural terminology
   B. Current procedural text
   C. Complete procedural technology
   D. Current procedural terminology

10. **[LO 5.1]** CPT is published by _____.
    A. AMA   C. WHO
    B. CMS   D. BCBS

Applying Your Knowledge

[LO 5.2] Case 5.1   Using the Index

Find the following codes in the index of CPT. Underline the key term you used to find the code.

1. Intracapsular lens extraction

2. Coombs test

3. X-ray of duodenum

4. Unlisted procedure, maxillofacial prosthetics

5. DTaP immunization

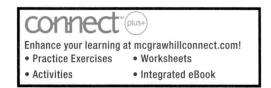

connect plus+
Enhance your learning at mcgrawhillconnect.com!
• Practice Exercises   • Worksheets
• Activities   • Integrated eBook

[LO 5.1] Case 5.2 CPT Symbols

1. Identify the symbol used to indicate a new procedure code, and list five new codes that appear in CPT.

2. Identify the symbol used to indicate a procedure that is usually done in addition to a primary procedure. Locate code 92979, and describe the unit of measure that is involved with this add-on code.

3. Identify the symbol that indicates that the code's description has been changed, and list five examples of codes with new or revised descriptors that appear in CPT.

4. Identify the symbols that enclose new or revised text other than the code's descriptor, and list five examples of codes with new or revised text that appear in CPT.

5. Identify the symbol next to a code that means that conscious sedation is a part of the procedure that the surgeon performs, and list five examples from CPT.

6. Identify the symbol next to a code that means that FDA approval is pending, and list one example from CPT's vaccines and toxoids code section (codes 90476–90749).

7. Identify the symbol next to resequenced code, and list one example from CPT 2010 or later.

[LO 5.2] Case 5.3 Procedure Codes

Find the correct procedure codes for the following:

1. Insertion, LeVeen shunt.

2. Ms. Silvers is referred to Dr. Valentine for chest pain. The patient's encounter form on her second appointment shows a cardiovascular stress test using submaximal treadmill, with continuous electrocardiographic monitoring, with physician supervision, interpretation, and report. Find the procedure code for the procedure cardiovascular stress test. (Hint: Look under the heading "Cardiology.")

3. Patient Amy Wan had surgery for ingrown toenails on the great toe of each foot. Find the procedure code for the service, including any applicable modifier.

4. Patient Judi Goldfarb had a partial mastectomy of the left breast.

5. Patient Tonisha Williams had a total abdominal hysterectomy and removal of tubes and ovaries for submucous leiomyoma of the uterus and severe polycystic disease of the ovaries.

6. Established patient: Randy Kane. Visit to Ashworth Dermatology Clinic for recurrence of forearm rash. He is a previous patient who presented with this condition twenty days ago. I saw him for a ten-minute follow-up examination because of the flare-up. Has 4 X 6 cm rash over mid-forearm with scaly, erythematous, raised papules.

7. Dr. LaFarge is called to the home of the BeGeorgs family. She is the family physician and has taken care of the patient, Ralph, since birth. He is now thirteen years old and is recovering well from a recent broken leg. She decided to visit this established patient at home to check on possible swelling or soreness due to the cast.

8. Juanita Escobar, age two, has an intramuscular injection for immunization with diphtheria and tetanus toxoids (DT). (Hint: Check the possible codes for patients' ages.)

[LO 5.3] Case 5.4 E/M

Using the most recent CPT code book available to you, find the following Evaluation and Management codes.

1. Follow-up visit, eight-year-old boy, nurse removes sutures from leg wound.

2. Office visit, twenty-nine-year-old female, established patient, follow-up on severe wrist sprain.

3. Initial office visit to evaluate gradual hearing loss, sixty-year-old female, history and physical examination, complete audiogram.

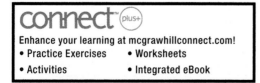

connect™ (plus+)

Enhance your learning at mcgrawhillconnect.com!
- Practice Exercises
- Worksheets
- Activities
- Integrated eBook

4. Initial office visit to evaluate forty-five-year-old male with complaint of shortness of breath and chest pain during exercise. Severe cardiovascular damage is suspected. Comprehensive history and examination performed; the decision making was moderately complex. Physician spent about forty-five minutes with the patient.

5. Annual physical examination of established patient, male, age forty-two.

6. Emergency department visit for a new patient with rash over entire trunk after exposure to poison ivy.

7. Initial intensive care for E/M of critically ill baby, fifteen days old.

8. Home visit for E/M of established patient with congestive heart failure (CHF); caregiver phoned report of sudden difficulty breathing and profuse sweating.

9. Medical conference of physician and psychiatrist to discuss patient's care; approximately thirty minutes.

10. Patient, age twenty-eight, office visit for basic evaluation for life insurance.

[LO 5.2] Case 5.5 Procedure Codes

Using the most recent CPT code book available to you, find the following procedure codes.

1. Repair of nail bed.

2. Removal of twenty skin tags.

3. Radiologic examination, chest, two views, frontal and lateral.

4. Anesthesia for vaginal delivery.

5. Electrocardiogram, routine ECG, twelve leads, interpretation and report.

6. Glucose tolerance test (GTT), three specimens (includes glucose).

7. Modifier for unusual services beyond those usually required for the procedure.

8. Modifier for laboratory procedures performed by someone other than the treating or reporting physician.

9. Unlisted surgical procedure, nervous system.

10. Modifier for repeat radiology procedure performed by the same physician.

[LO 5.6] Case 5.6 HCPCS

Using the most recent HCPCS code book available to you, supply the correct HCPCS codes for the following.

1. Administration of hepatitis B vaccine.

2. Contact layer, sterile, 16 square inches or less, each dressing.

3. Shoe lift, elevation, heel, tapered to metatarsals, per inch.

4. Screening Papanicolaou smear, cervical or vaginal, up to 3 smears by technician under physician supervision.

5. Electric heat pad, standard.

6. Half-length bedside rails.

7. Injection of bevacizumab, 10 mg.

8. Brachytherapy source, nonstranded, nonhigh dose rate iridium-192, per source.

9. Enteral nutrition infusion pump, with alarm.

10. Infusion of 1000 cc of normal saline solution.

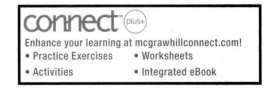

connect™ (plus+)

Enhance your learning at mcgrawhillconnect.com!
- Practice Exercises   • Worksheets
- Activities   • Integrated eBook

PAYMENT METHODS AND CHECKOUT PROCEDURES

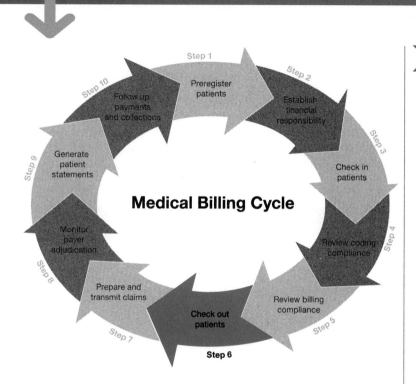

Medical Billing Cycle

- Step 1 — Preregister patients
- Step 2 — Establish financial responsibility
- Step 3 — Check in patients
- Step 4 — Review coding compliance
- Step 5 — Review billing compliance
- Step 6 — Check out patients
- Step 7 — Prepare and transmit claims
- Step 8 — Monitor payer adjudication
- Step 9 — Generate patient statements
- Step 10 — Follow up payments and collections

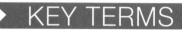

KEY TERMS

accept assignment
adjustment
allowed charge
balance billing
bundled payment
cap rate
capitation
consumer-driven health plan (CDHP)
conversion factor
discounted fee-for-service
fee schedule
financial policy
flexible savings account (FSA)
health maintenance organization (HMO)
health reimbursement account (HRA)
health savings account (HSA)
high-deductible health plan (HDHP)
independent practice association (IPA)
meaningful use
Medicare Physician Fee Schedule (MPFS)
partial payment
per member per month (PMPM)
point-of-service (POS) plan
preferred provider organization (PPO)
primary care physician (PCP)
resource-based relative value scale (RBRVS)
real-time claims adjudication (RTCA)
self-pay patient
UCR (usual, customary, reasonable)
walkout receipt
write off

Learning Outcomes

After studying this chapter, you should be able to:

6.1 Contrast provider payment under PPOs, capitated HMOs, indemnity plans, and CDHPs.

6.2 Calculate an RBRVS payment.

6.3 Discuss the influence of third-party rules on patients' charges from participating versus nonparticipating providers.

6.4 Define the eight types of time-of-service charges.

6.5 Calculate time-of-service payments.

6.6 Explain the patient checkout procedure.

Patients often have questions like "How much will my insurance pay?" "How much will I owe?" "Why are these fees different from my previous doctor's fees?" Medical assistants handle these questions based on their knowledge of the provider's current fees and their estimates of what patients' insurance plans will pay. Both to prepare compliant health claims and to estimate what patients will owe, medical assistants must be prepared to answer these key questions:

▶ *What services are covered under the plan?*
▶ *Which services are not covered and therefore cannot be billed to the plan, but rather should be billed to the patient?*
▶ *What are the billing rules, fee schedules, and payment methods of the plan?*
▶ *In addition to noncovered services, what is the patient responsible for paying?*

6.1 Types of Health Plans

Preferred provider organizations (PPOs) are the most popular type of private plan, followed by health maintenance organizations (HMOs). Few employees choose indemnity plans because they would have to pay more. Consumer-driven health plans (CDHPs) that combine a high-deductible health plan with a funding option of some type are rapidly growing in popularity among both employers and employees. Table 6.1 summarizes health plan options.

Table 6.1 Comparison of Health Plan Options

Plan Type	Provider Options	Cost-Containment Methods	Features
Indemnity Plan	Any provider	• Little or none • Preauthorization required for some procedures	• Higher costs • Deductibles • Coinsurance • Preventive care not usually covered
Health Maintenance Organization (HMO)	Only HMO network providers	• Primary care physician manages care; referral required • No payment for out-of-network nonemergency services • Preauthorization required	• Low copayment • Limited provider network • Covers preventive care
Point-of-Service (POS)	Network providers or out-of-network providers	• Within network, primary care physician manages care	• Lower copayments for network providers • Higher costs for out-of-network providers • Covers preventive care
Preferred Provider Organization (PPO)	Network providers or out-of-network providers	• Referral not required for specialists • Fees are discounted • Preauthorization for some procedures	• Higher cost for out-of-network providers • Preventive care coverage varies
Consumer-Driven Health Plan	Usually similar to PPO	• Increases patient awareness of health care costs • Patient pays directly until high deductible is met	• High deductible/low premium • Savings account

Preferred Provider Organizations

A **preferred provider organization (PPO)** is a type of managed care organization. PPOs create a network of physicians, hospitals, and other providers with whom they have negotiated discounts from the usual fees, a payment method called **discounted fee-for-service**. For example, a PPO might sign a contract with a practice stating that the fee for a brief appointment will be $60, although the practice's physicians usually charge $80. In exchange for accepting lower fees, providers—in theory, at least—see more patients, thus making up the revenue that is lost through the reduced fees.

PPOs are the most popular type of plan. An annual premium is due, benefits are usually subject to a deductible, and often a copayment must be paid for visits. A PPO plan may offer either a low deductible with a higher premium or a high deductible with a lower premium. Insured members pay a copayment at the time of each medical service. Coinsurance is often charged for in-network providers. A patient may see an out-of-network doctor without a referral or preauthorization, but the deductible for out-of-network services may be higher and the coinsurance percentage the plan will pay may be lower. Coverage for preventive care varies.

preferred provider organization (PPO) Managed care organization where a network of providers supply discounted treatment for plan members.

discounted fee-for-service Payment schedule for services based on a reduced percentage of usual charges.

Example

A PPO member using an in-network provider pays a $20 copayment at the time of service (the visit), and the PPO pays the full balance of the visit charge. A member who sees an out-of-network provider pays a $40 copayment and is also responsible for part of the visit charge. ◀

Health Maintenance Organizations

A **health maintenance organization (HMO)** combines coverage of medical costs and delivery of health care for a prepaid premium. In most states, HMOs are licensed by a state insurance authority and are legally required to provide certain services to members and their dependents, including preventive services such as immunizations and well-baby checkups for infants and screening mammograms for women.

The HMO creates a network of physicians, hospitals, and other providers by directly employing them or by negotiating contracts with them. The HMO then enrolls members in a health plan under which they use the services of those network providers. After enrolling in an HMO, members must receive services from the network. Visits to out-of-network providers are not covered, except for emergency care or urgent health problems that arise when the member is temporarily away from the geographical service area.

HMOs often require preauthorization before the patient receives many types of services. The HMO may require a second opinion—the judgment of another physician that a planned procedure is necessary—before authorizing the service. Services that are not preauthorized are not covered. Preauthorization is almost always needed for nonemergency hospital admission, and it is usually required within a certain number of days after an emergency admission.

health maintenance organization (HMO) Managed health care system in which providers offer health care to members for fixed periodic payments.

Capitation in HMOs

Capitation (from capit, Latin for head) is a fixed prepayment to a medical provider for all necessary contracted services provided to each patient who is a plan member. The capitated rate is a prospective payment—it is paid before the patient visit. It covers a specific period of time. The health plan makes the payment whether the patient receives many or no medical services during that specified period.

capitation A prepayment covering provider's services for a plan member for a specified period.

In capitation, the physician agrees to share the risk that an insured person will use more services than the fee covers. The physician also shares in the prospect that an insured person will use fewer services. In fee-for-service, the more patients the provider sees, the more charges the health plan reimburses. In capitation, the payment remains the same, and the provider risks receiving lower per-visit revenue.

Example

A family physician has a contract for a capitated payment of $30 a month for each of a hundred patients in a plan. This $3,000 monthly fee ($30 × 100 patients = $3,000) covers all office visits for all the patients. If half of the patients see the physician once during a given month, the provider in effect receives $60 for each visit ($3,000 divided by 50 visits). If, however, half of the patients see the physician four times in a month, the monthly fee is $3,000 divided by 200 visits, or $15 for each visit. ◀

A patient is enrolled in a capitated health plan for a specific time period, such as a month, a quarter, or a year. The capitated rate, usually called the **cap rate**, calculated as **per member per month (PMPM)**, is usually based on the health-related characteristics of the enrollees, such as age and gender. The health plan analyzes these factors and sets a rate based on its prediction of the amount of health care each person will need. The capitated rate of prepayment covers only services listed on the schedule of benefits for the plan. Noncovered services can be billed to patients using the provider's usual rate. Plans often require the provider to notify the patient in advance that a service is not covered and to state the fee for which the patient will be responsible.

cap rate Periodic prepayment to a provider for specified services to each plan member.

per member per month (PMPM) Periodic capitated prospective payment to a provider that covers only services listed on the schedule of benefits.

HMO Business Models

An HMO is organized around a business model. The model is based on how the terms of the agreement connect the provider and the plan. In all, however, enrollees must see HMO providers in order to be covered.

Staff Model In a staff HMO, physicians are employed by the organization. All the premiums and other revenues come to the HMO, which in turn pays the physicians' salaries. For medical care, patients visit clinics and health centers owned by the HMO.

Group (Network) Model A group (network) HMO contracts with more than one physician group. In some plans, HMO members receive medical services in HMO-owned facilities from providers who work only for that HMO. In others, members visit the providers' facilities, and the providers can also treat nonmember patients.

independent practice association (IPA) HMO in which physicians are self-employed and provide services to members and nonmembers.

Independent Practice Association Model An **independent (or individual) practice association (IPA)** type of HMO is an association formed by physicians with separately owned practices who contract together to provide care for HMO members. An HMO pays negotiated fees for medical services to the IPA. The IPA in turn pays its physician members, either by a capitated rate or a fee. Providers may join more than one IPA and usually also see nonmember patients.

primary care physician (PCP) Physician in a health maintenance organization who directs all aspects of a patient's care.

Gatekeeper Plans versus Point-of-Service Plans One cost-control method that was initially a major feature of initial HMOs required a patient to select a **primary care physician (PCP)** —also called a "gatekeeper"—from the HMO's list of general or family practitioners, internists, and pediatricians. A PCP coordinates patients' overall care to ensure that all services are, in the PCP's judgment, necessary. In gatekeeper plans, an HMO member needs a medical referral from the PCP before seeing a specialist or a consultant and for hospital admission. Members who visit providers without a referral are directly responsible for the total cost of the service. Due to this high degree of restriction, both physicians and patients became dissatisfied with the policies, and other types of plans, especially the point-of-service plan, have become more popular.

A **point-of-service (POS) plan** is a hybrid of HMO and PPO networks. Members may choose from a primary or secondary network. The primary network is HMO-like, and the secondary network is often a PPO network. Like HMOs, POS plans charge an annual premium and a copayment for office visits. Monthly premiums are slightly higher than for HMOs but offer the benefit of some coverage for visits to nonnetwork physicians for specialty care. A POS may be structured as a tiered plan, for example, with different rates for specially designated providers, regular participating providers, and out-of-network providers.

Consumer-Driven Health Plans

Consumer-driven health plans (CDHPs) combine two elements: (1) a high-deductible health plan; and (2) one or more tax-advantaged savings accounts that the patient (the "consumer") directs. The two plans work together: The high-deductible health plan covers catastrophic losses, while the savings account pays out-of-pocket or noncovered expenses. *Note:* Some payers refer to CDHPs as simply *high-deductible health plans;* the meaning is the same.

The High-Deductible Health Plan

The first part of a CDHP is a **high-deductible health plan (HDHP)**, usually a PPO. The annual deductible is over $1,000. Many of the plan's covered preventive care services, as well as coverage for accidents, disability, dental care, vision care, and long-term care, are not subject to this deductible.

The Funding Options

Three types of CDHP funding options (see Table 6.2) may be combined with high-deductible health plans to form consumer-driven health plans.

▶ A **health reimbursement account (HRA)** is a medical reimbursement plan set up and funded by an employer. HRAs are usually offered to employees with health plans that have high deductibles. Employees may submit claims to the HRA to be paid back for out-of-pocket medical expenses.

▶ The most popular type of account is the **health savings account (HSA),** which is a savings account created by an individual. Employers that wish to encourage employees to set up HSAs offer a qualified high-deductible health plan to go with it.

Table 6.2 Comparisons of CDHP Funding Options		
Health Reimbursement Account	**Health Savings Account**	**Flexible Savings (Spending) Account**
Contributions from employer	Contributions from individual (regardless of employment status), employer, or both	Contributions from employer and/or employee
Rollovers allowed within employer-set limits	Unused funds roll over indefinitely	Unused funds revert to employer
Portability allowed under employer's rules	Funds are portable (job change; retirement)	No portability
Tax-deductible deposits	Tax-deductible deposits	Tax-advantaged deposits
Tax-free withdrawals for qualified expenses	Tax-free withdrawals for qualified expenses	Tax-free withdrawals for qualified expenses
	Tax-free interest can be earned	

Both employee and employer can contribute to the HSA. The maximum amount that can be saved each year is set by the IRS.

▶ Some companies offer **flexible savings (spending) accounts (FSAs)** that augment employees' other health insurance coverage. Employees have the option of putting pretax dollars from their salaries in the FSA; they can then use the fund to pay for certain medical and dependent care expenses.

Billing under Consumer-Driven Health Plans

Consumer-driven health plans reduce providers' cash flow because visit copayments are being replaced by high deductibles that may not be collected until after claims are paid. As more employer-sponsored plan members are covered under CDHPs, physician reimbursement up to the amount of the deductible will come from the patient's funding option and, if there is not enough money there, out of pocket. CDHP payment works as follows:

▶ The group health plan establishes a funding option (HRA, HSA, FSA, or some combination) designed to help pay out-of-pocket medical expenses.
▶ The patient uses the money in the account to pay for qualified medical services.
▶ The total deductible must be met before any benefits are paid by the HDHP.
▶ Once the deductible is met, the HDHP covers a portion of the benefits according to the policy. The funding option can also be used to pay the uncovered portion.

Following is an example of payments under a CDHP with an HSA fund of $1,000 and a deductible of $1,000. The HDHP has an 80-20 coinsurance. The plan pays the visit charges as billed.

Office visits for the patient:

First visit charge	$150	$150 paid from HSA (leaving a balance in the fund of $850)
Second visit charge	$450	$450 paid from HSA (leaving a balance in the fund of $400)
Third visit charge	$600	$400 paid from HSA (emptying the fund)
		$160 paid by the HDHP (the balance of $200 on the charge × 80%)
		$40 coinsurance to be paid by the patient (the balance of $200 × 20%)

For medical practices, the best situation is an integrated CDHP in which the same plan runs both the HDHP and the funding options. This approach helps reduce paperwork and speed payment. For example, if an HSA is run by the same payer as the HDHP, a claim for charges is sent to the payer. The payer's RA/EOB states what the plan and the patient are each responsible for paying. If payment is due from the patient's HSA, that amount is withdrawn and paid to the provider. If the patient's deductible has been met, the plan pays its obligation.

Another popular payment method is a credit or a debit card provided by the plan. The patient can use it to pay for health-related expenses up to the amount in the fund. The cards may be preloaded with the member's coverage and copayment data.

Educating patients about their financial responsibility before they leave encounters, extending credit wisely, and improving collections are all key to avoiding uncollectible accounts under CDHPs.

Indemnity Plans

Indemnity plans require premium, deductible, and coinsurance payments. They typically cover 70 to 80 percent of costs for covered benefits after deductibles are

Table 6.3 Types of Payments under Health Plans

Plan Type	Participating Provider Payment Method
Preferred Provider Organization (PPO)	Discounted Fee-for-Service
Health Maintenance Organization (HMO), Capitated	Per Member Per Month
Indemnity	Fee-for-Service
Consumer-Driven Health Plan	Up to deductible: Payment by Patient
	After Deductible: Discounted Fee-for-Service

met. Some plans are structured with high deductibles, such as $5,000 to $10,000, in order to offer policyholders a relatively less expensive premium. Many have some managed care features, as payers compete for employers' contracts and try to control costs.

Provider Payments

Medical assistants become familiar with the payment approaches of the health plans patients have, so they can calculate charges due at time of service, anticipate payments after claims are processed, and explain insurance payment calculations to patients who need to know their own financial responsibilities. Table 6.3 reviews physician payments under the major types of managed care and indemnity plans.

THINKING IT THROUGH 6.1

1. A patient's total surgery charges are $1,278. The patient must pay the annual deductible of $1,000, and the policy states an 80-20 coinsurance. What does the patient owe?

2. A patient has a high-deductible consumer-driven health plan. The annual deductible is $2,500, of which $300 has been paid. After a surgical procedure costing $1,890, what does the patient owe? Can any amount be collected from a payer? Why?

3. A patient with a high-deductible consumer-driven health plan has met half of the $1,000 annual deductible before requiring surgery to repair a broken ankle while visiting a neighboring state. The out-of-network physician's bill is $4,500. The PPO that takes effect after the deductible has been met is an 80-20 in-network plan and a 60-40 out-of-network plan. How much does the patient owe? How much should the PPO be billed?

6.2 Methods for Setting Fees

Physicians establish a list of their usual fees for the procedures and services they frequently perform. Usual fees are defined as those that they charge to most of their patients most of the time under typical conditions. These fees are compiled in the physician's **fee schedule.**

Payers, too, must establish the rates they pay providers. There are two main methods: charge-based and resource-based. *Charge-based fee structures* are based on

fee schedule List of the usual fees a physician charges.

the fees that providers of similar training and experience have charged for similar services. *Resource-based fee structures* are built by comparing three factors: (1) how difficult it is for the provider to do the procedure, (2) how much office overhead the procedure involves, and (3) the relative risk that the procedure presents to the patient and to the provider.

UCR and RVS

UCR (usual, customary, reasonable)   Setting fees by comparing usual fees, customary fees, and reasonable fees.

Payers that use a charge-based fee structure create a schedule of **UCR (usual, customary, and reasonable)** fees. These UCR fees, for the most part, accurately reflect prevailing charges. However, fees may not be available for new or rare procedures. Lacking better information, a payer may set too high or low a fee for such procedures.

Another payment structure is called a relative value scale (RVS). In an RVS, each procedure in a group of related procedures is assigned a *relative value* in relation to a *base unit*. For example, if the base unit is 1 and these numbers are assigned—limited visual field examination 0.66; intermediate visual field examination 0.91; and extended visual field examination 1.33—the first two procedures are less difficult than the unit to which they are compared. The third procedure is more difficult. The relative value that is assigned is called the *relative value unit, or RVU*. To calculate the price of each service, the relative value is multiplied by a **conversion factor**, which is a dollar amount that is assigned to the base unit. The conversion factor is increased or decreased each year so that it reflects changes in the cost of living index.

conversion factor   Amount used to multiply a relative value unit to arrive at a charge.

Resource-Based Relative Value Scale (RBRVS)

resource-based relative value scale (RBRVS)   Relative value scale for establishing Medicare charges.

The payment system used by Medicare is called the **resource-based relative value scale (RBRVS).** The RBRVS establishes relative value units for services. It replaces providers' consensus on fees—the historical charges—with a relative value that is based on resources—what each service really costs to provide.

There are three parts to an RBRVS fee:

1. *The nationally uniform RVU:* The relative value is based on three cost elements—the physician's work, the practice cost (overhead), and the cost of malpractice insurance. Another way of stating this is that every $1.00 of charge is made up of *x* cents for the physician's work, *x* cents for office expenses, and *x* cents for malpractice insurance. For example, the relative value for a simple office visit, such as to receive a flu shot, is much lower than the relative value for a complicated encounter such as the evaluation and management of uncontrolled diabetes in a patient.
2. *A geographic adjustment factor:* A geographic adjustment factor called the *geographic practice cost index (GPCI)* is a number that is used to multiply each relative value element so that it better reflects a geographic area's relative costs.
3. *A nationally uniform conversion factor:* A uniform conversion factor is a dollar amount used to multiply the relative values to produce the full Medicare allowable rate for a given service. Annual changes to the conversion factor are recommended by CMS but enacted by Congress.

BILLING TIP

Medicare Outpatient versus Inpatient Payments

Medicare pays hospitals under the diagnosis-related group (DRG) method with fees based on the Medicare Inpatient Prospective Payment System (IPPS). This topic is covered later in this text.

BILLING TIP

RBRVS versus UCR Fees

When RBRVS fees are used, payments are considerably lower than when UCR fees are used. On average, according to a study done by the Medicare Payment Advisory Commission, a nonpartisan federal advisory panel, private health plans' fees are about 15 percent higher than Medicare fees.

Calculating RBRVS Payments

Each part of the RBRVS—the relative values, the GPCI, and the conversion factor—is updated each year by CMS. The year's **Medicare Physician Fee Schedule (MPFS)** is published by CMS in the *Federal Register* and is available on the CMS website.

Figure 6.1 shows the formula for calculating a Medicare payment and a worked-out example. These steps are followed to apply the formula:

1. Determine the procedure code for the service.
2. Use the Medicare Fee Schedule to find the three RVUs—work, practice expense, and malpractice—for the procedure.
3. Use the Medicare GPCI list to find the three geographic practice cost indices (also for work, practice expense, and malpractice).
4. Multiply each RVU by its GPCI to calculate the adjusted value.
5. Add the three adjusted totals, and multiply the sum by the conversion factor to determine the payment.

Work RVU x Work GPCI = W
Practice-Expense RVU x Practice-Expense GPCI = PE
Malpractice RVU x Malpractice GPCI = M
Conversion Factor = CF

$(W + PE + M)$ x CF = Payment

Example:

Work RVU = 6.39
Work GPCI = 0.998
6.39 x 0.998 = W = 6.37

Practice-Expense RVU = 5.87
Practice-Expense GPCI = 0.45
5.87 x 0.45 = PE = 2.64

Malpractice RVU = 1.20
Malpractice GPCI = 0.721
1.20 x 0.721 = M = 0.86

Conversion Factor = 34.54

(6.37 + 2.64 + 0.86) x 34.54 = $340.90 Payment

FIGURE 6.1 Medicare Physician Fee Schedule Formula

Medicare Physician Fee Schedule (MPFS) The RBRVS-based allowed fees.

THINKING IT THROUGH 6.2

1. Below are sample relative value units and geographic practice cost indices from a Medicare Physician Fee Schedule. The conversion factor for this particular year is $34.7315.

Sample RVUs

CPT/HCPCS	Description	Work RVU	Practice Expense RVU	Malpractice Expense RVU
33500	Repair heart vessel fistula	25.55	30.51	4.07
33502	Coronary artery correction	21.04	15.35	1.96
33503	Coronary artery graft	21.78	26	4.07
99203	OV new detailed	1.34	0.64	0.05
99204	OV new comprehensive	2.00	0.96	0.06

Sample GPCIs

Locality	Work GPCI	Practice Expense GPCI	Malpractice Expense GPCI
San Francisco, CA	1.067	1.299	0.667
Manhattan, NY	1.093	1.353	1.654
Columbus, Ohio	0.990	0.939	1.074
Galveston, TX	0.988	0.970	1.386

Calculate the expected payments for:

A. Office visit, new patient, detailed history/examination, low-complexity decision making, in Manhattan, NY _____

B. Coronary artery graft in San Francisco, CA _____

C. Repair heart vessel fistula in Columbus, OH _____

D. Coronary artery correction in Galveston, TX _____

6.3 Third-Party Contracts and Guidelines

Providers, like employers and employees, must evaluate participation in health plans. They judge which plans to participate in based primarily on the financial arrangements that are offered. Because managed care is the predominant type of health care, most medical practices have a number of PPO and other types of contracts with plans in their area. Practices also very often participate in Medicare, which is a fee-for-service indemnity plan with many, many guidelines and cost-containment rules in place.

Participation contracts contain important billing and compliance information, such as whether referrals and preauthorizations are required, fees, billing requirements, claim filing deadlines, patients' financial responsibilities, and other billing rules. The rules for collecting patients' payments are described, as are how to coordinate benefits when another plan is primary. The contract should also state how far back in time a plan is permitted to go for refunds of overpayments or incorrect payments.

Other than capitation, which is a small percentage of payments to providers, payers use two main methods, allowed charges and contracted fee schedules. New reimbursement models are also being introduced, such as bundled payments and incentives for particular programs.

Allowed Charges

allowed charge Maximum charge a plan pays for a service or procedure.

Many payers set an **allowed charge** for each procedure or service. This amount is the most the payer will pay any provider for that CPT code. Whether a provider actually receives the allowed charge depends on three things:

1. *The provider's usual charge for the procedure or service:* The usual charge on the physician's fee schedule may be higher than, equal to, or lower than the allowed charge.
2. *The provider's status in the particular plan or program:* The provider is either participating or nonparticipating (see the chapter on patient encounters and billing information). Participating (PAR) providers agree to accept allowed charges that are lower than their usual fees. In return, they are eligible for incentives, such as quicker payments of their claims and more patients.
3. *The payer's billing rules:* These rules govern whether the provider can bill a patient for the part of the charge that the payer does not cover.

When a payer has an allowed charge method, it never pays more than the allowed charge to a provider. If a provider's usual fee is higher, only the allowed charge is paid. If a provider's usual fee is lower, the payer reimburses that lower amount. The payer's payment is always the lower of the provider's charge or the allowed charge.

Example

The payer's allowed charge for a new patient's evaluation and management (E/M) service (CPT 99204) is $160.

Provider A Usual Charge = $180	Payment = $160
Provider B Usual Charge = $140	Payment = $140 ◄

balance billing Collecting the difference between a provider's usual fee and a payer's lower allowed charge.

write off To deduct an amount from a patient's account.

Whether a participating provider can bill the patient for the difference between a higher physician fee and a lower allowed charge—called **balance billing**—depends on the terms of the contract with the payer. Payers' rules may prohibit participating providers from balance billing the patient. Instead, the provider must **write off** the difference, meaning to subtract that amount from the patient's bill as an adjustment and never collect it.

For example, under the largest Medicare plan, called the Original Medicare Plan, Medicare-participating providers may not receive an amount greater than the Medicare allowed charge from the Medicare Physician Fee Schedule. Medicare is responsible for paying 80 percent of this allowed charge (after patients have met their annual deductibles). Patients are responsible for the other 20 percent.

Example

A Medicare PAR provider has a usual charge of $200 for a diagnostic flexible sigmoidoscopy (CPT 45330), and the Medicare allowed charge is $84. The provider must write off the difference between the two amounts. The patient is responsible for 20 percent of the allowed charge, not of the provider's usual charge:

Provider's usual fee	$200.00
Medicare allowed charge	$84.00
Medicare pays 80%	$67.20
Patient pays 20%	$16.80

The total the provider can collect is $84. The provider must deduct the $116. ◄

A provider who does not participate in a private plan can usually balance bill patients. In this situation, if the provider's usual charge is higher than the allowed charge, the patient must pay the difference. However, Medicare and other government-sponsored programs have different rules for nonparticipating providers, as explained later in this text.

Example Payer Policy

There is an allowed charge for each procedure. The plan provides a benefit of 100 percent of the provider's usual charges up to this maximum fee. Provider A is a participating provider; Provider B does not participate and can balance bill. Both Provider A and Provider B perform abdominal hysterectomies (CPT 58150). The policy's allowed charge for this procedure is $2,880.

Provider A (PAR)

Provider's usual charge	$3,100.00
Policy pays its allowed charge	$2,880.00
Provider writes off the difference between the usual charge and the allowed charge:	$220.00

Provider B (nonPAR)

Provider's usual charge	$3,000.00
Policy pays its allowed charge	$2,880.00
Provider bills patient for the $120.00 difference between the usual charge and the allowed charge; there is no write-off:	($3,000.00 − $2,880.00) ◄

Coinsurance provisions in many private plans provide for patient cost-sharing. Rather than paying the provider the full allowed charge, for example, a plan may require the patient to pay 25 percent, while the plan pays 75 percent. In this case, if a provider's usual charges are higher than the plan's allowed charge, the patient owes more for a service from a nonparticipating provider than from a participating provider. The calculations are explained below.

Example Payer Policy

A policy provides a benefit of 75 percent of the provider's usual charges, and there is a maximum allowed charge for each procedure. The patient is responsible for 25 percent of the maximum allowed charge. Balance billing is not permitted for plan participants. Provider A is a participating provider, and Provider B is a nonparticipant in the plan. Provider A and Provider B both perform total abdominal hysterectomies (CPT 58150). The policy's allowed charge for this procedure is $2,880.00.

Provider A (PAR)

Usual charge	$3,100.00
Policy pays 75% of its allowed charge	$2,160.00
	(75% of $2,880.00)
Patient pays 25% of the allowed charge	$720.00
	(25% of $2,880.00)
Provider writes off the difference between the usual charge and the allowed charge:	$220.00

Provider B (nonPAR)

Usual charge	$3,000.00
Policy pays 75% of its allowed charge	$2,160.00
	(75% of $2,880.00)
Patient pays for:	
(1) 25% of the allowed charge +	$720.00
	(25% of $2,880.00)
(2) the difference between the usual charge and the allowed charge:	$120.00
	($3,000.00 − $2,880.00)

Patient pays $840.00 ($720.00 + $120.00).

The provider has no write-off. ◄

Contracted Fee Schedule

Some payers, particularly those that contract directly with providers, establish fixed fee schedules with participating providers. They first decide what they will pay in particular geographical areas and then offer participation contracts with those fees to physician practices. If the practice chooses to join, it agrees by contract to accept the plan's fees for its member patients. The plan's contract states the percentage of the charges, if any, its patients owe, and the percentage the payer covers. Participating providers can typically bill patients their usual charges for services not covered by the plan.

Emerging Reimbursement Methods: Bundled Payments and Meaningful Use Incentives

bundled payment Single predetermined payment for an entire episode of care.

BILLING TIP

Bundled *Payment,* Not *Code*

As explained in the chapter on procedural coding, some surgical CPT codes are *bundled*—they cover a range of specific procedures from a physician. This is different from a *bundled payment,* which applies to all the providers for an episode of care.

In a traditional fee-for-service payment system, doctors and hospitals are paid more when they give patients more tests and do more procedures. Another approach that is being explored asks providers to "share" payment for services. Rather than paying all providers involved in a patient's care separately for their services, Medicare is experimenting with paying a predetermined single payment "bundle" for the entire *episode of care,* known as a **bundled payment.**

For example, Medicare would make a single payment for an episode of care, such as a knee replacement. The payment would cover physician visits, X rays, surgeon's fees, anesthesiologist's fees, inpatient care, rehabilitation services, physical therapy, and so on. The bundled amount would be lower than what Medicare would pay if it reimbursed each provider separately for the services. If the providers managed to treat the entire episode of care at a lower cost than the predetermined bundled amount, they would keep the difference. If the cost was higher than the bundled amount, the providers would not be reimbursed for the additional cost. This approach encourages doctors, hospitals, and other health care providers to better coordinate care for patients both in the hospital and after they are discharged.

Many payers, Medicare and private, also use *incentives*—extra financial rewards—to encourage providers to adopt programs that they think will both reduce costs and improve care. One approach, *pay-for-performance*, provides incentive payments for certain types of preventive care and monitoring. A part of the HITECH Act is essentially such an incentive: Under the HITECH Act, physicians who adopt and use EHRs are eligible for annual payments of up to $44,000 from Medicare and Medicaid. Physicians who derive at least 30 percent or more of their income from Medicaid are eligible for up to $64,000, and doctors who practice in underserved areas are eligible for an extra 10 percent from Medicare. To be eligible for the financial incentives, providers must do more than simply purchase EHRs; they must demonstrate meaningful use of the technology. **Meaningful use** is the utilization of certified EHR technology to improve quality, efficiency, and patient safety in the health care system. As examples, the EHR must be used to check for and prevent drug-allergy and drug-to-drug interactions, and the program must be set up to generate and transmit permissible prescriptions electronically.

meaningful use Utilization of certified EHR technology to improve quality, efficiency, and patient safety in the health care system.

THINKING IT THROUGH 6.3

1. A Medicare-participating surgeon in Galveston, TX, reports a normal charge of $6,282.00 to repair a heart vessel fistula. Using the Medicare Physician Fee Schedule RVUs and GPCIs shown on page 129, calculate the following:

   A. The allowed charge _____.

   B. The provider's expected write-off _____.

6.4 Time-of-Service (TOS) Payments

Up-front collection—money collected before the patient leaves the office—is an important part of cash flow. Practices routinely collect the following charges at the time of service:

1. Previous balances
2. Copayments
3. Coinsurance
4. Noncovered or overlimit fees
5. Charges of nonparticipating providers
6. Charges for self-pay patients
7. Deductibles for patients with consumer-driven health plans (CDHPs)
8. Charges for supplies and copies of medical records

Previous Balances

Practices routinely check their patient financial records and, if a balance is due, collect it at the time of service.

Copayments

Copayments are always collected at the time of service. In some practices, they are collected before the encounter; in others, right after the encounter. The copayment amount depends on the type of service and on whether the provider is in the patient's network. Copays for out-of-network providers are usually higher than for in-network providers. Specific copay amounts may be required for office visits to PCPs versus specialists and for lab work, radiology services such as X-rays, and surgery.

BILLING TIP

Collecting TOS Payments

- Many offices tell patients when they schedule visits what copays they will owe at the time of service.
- Keep change to make it easier for cash patients to make time-of-service payments.
- Ask for payment. "We verified your insurance coverage, and there is a copay that is your responsibility. Would you like to pay by cash, check, or credit or debit card?"

COMPLIANCE GUIDELINE

Billing for Medical Record Copies

Under HIPAA, it is permissible to bill patients a reasonable charge for supplying copies of their medical records. Costs include labor, supplies, postage, and time to prepare record summaries. Practices must check state laws, however, to see if there is a per-page charge limit.

When a patient receives more than one covered service in a single day, the health plan may permit multiple copayments. For example, copays for both an annual physical exam and for lab tests may be due from the patient. Review the terms of the policy to determine whether multiple copays should be collected on the same day of service.

Coinsurance

As health care costs have risen, employers have to pay more for their employees' medical benefit plans. As a result, employers are becoming less generous to employees, demanding that employees pay a larger share of those costs. Annual health insurance premiums are higher, deductibles are higher, and in a major trend—a shift from copayments to coinsurance—many employers have dropped the small, fixed-amount copayment requirements and replaced them with a coinsurance payment that is often due at the time of service.

Charges for Noncovered or Overlimit Services

Insurance policies require patients to pay for noncovered (excluded) services, and payers do not control what the providers charge for noncovered services. Likewise, if the plan has a limit on the usage of certain covered services, patients are responsible for paying for visits beyond the allowed number. For example, if five physical therapy encounters are permitted annually, the patient must pay for any additional visits. Practices usually collect these charges from patients at the time of service.

Charges of Nonparticipating Providers

accept assignment Participating physician's agreement to accept allowed charge as full payment.

As noted earlier in this chapter, when patients have encounters with a provider who participates in the plan under which they have coverage—such as a Medicare-participating provider—that provider has agreed to **accept assignment** for the patients—that is, to accept the allowed charge as full payment. Nonparticipating physicians usually do not accept assignment and require full payment from patients at the time of service. They also do not file claims on their behalf.

Charges for Self-Pay Patients

self-pay patient Patient with no insurance.

Patients who do not have insurance coverage are called **self-pay patients.** Since many millions of Americans do not have insurance, self-pay patients present for office visits daily. Medical insurance specialists follow the practice's procedures for informing patients of their responsibility for paying their bills. Practices may require self-pay patients to pay bills or agree to payment plans at the time of service.

Deductibles for Patients with CDHPs

Patients who have consumer-driven health plans (CDHPs) must meet large deductibles before the health plan makes a payment. Practices are responsible for determining and collecting those deductibles at the time of service.

Billing for Supplies and Other Services

Many practices bill for supplies and for other services, such as making copies of medical records, at the time of service.

Other TOS Collection Considerations

In the typical medical billing process, after the routine up-front collections are handled, for insured patients a claim is created and sent. The practice then waits to receive insurance payments, post the amount of payment to the patient's account in the PMP, and bill the patient for the balance. This process is followed because until the claim is paid by the payer, the patient's actual amount due is not known, and often the results are a change to the amount due initially calculated. Of course, how much of an annual deductible the patient has paid affects that amount. Differences in participation contracts with various payers also may reduce the physician's fee for a particular service.

However, following this process creates a problem for the practice in that it delays receipt of funds, reducing cash flow. For this reason, many practices are changing their billing process to increase time-of-service collections. For example, a practice may decide to collect patients' unmet deductibles or to adopt the policy of estimating the amount the patient will owe and collecting a **partial payment** during the checkout process. For example, if the patient is expected to owe $600 and practice policy is to collect 50 percent, the patient is asked to pay $300 today and to expect to be billed $300 after the claim is processed.

COMPLIANCE GUIDELINE

Collecting Charges

Some payers (especially government programs) do not permit providers to collect any charges except copayments from patients until insurance claims are paid. Be sure to comply with the payer's rules.

partial payment   Payment made during checkout based on an estimate.

Exercise 6.1   Entering a Patient's Copayment in the PMP

Enter the copayment that Ann Ingram made at the end of her visit with Dr. Clarke.

Follow the steps at www.mhhe.com/newbycarr to complete the exercise at connect.mcgraw-hill.com on your own once you have watched the demo and tried the steps with prompts in practice mode. Use the information provided in the scenario to complete the exercise.

connect™ (plus+)

Exercise 6.2   Billing for Supplies

Ann Ingram received a supply item during her visit that will not be covered by her insurance. Enter the amount that Ann Ingram paid for this supply at the end of her visit with Dr. Clarke.

Follow the steps at www.mhhe.com/newbycarr to complete the exercise at connect.mcgraw-hill.com on your own once you have watched the demo and tried the steps with prompts in practice mode. Use the information provided in the scenario to complete the exercise.

connect™ (plus+)

THINKING IT THROUGH 6.4

1. Why is it important to collect balances from patients at the time of service?

6.5   Calculating TOS Payments

What patients owe at the time of service for the medical procedures and services they received depends on the practice's financial policy and on the provisions of their health plans.

We sincerely wish to provide the best possible medical care. This involves mutual understanding between the patients, doctors, and staff. We encourage, you, our patient, to discuss any questions you may have regarding this payment policy.

Payment is expected at the time of your visit for services not covered by your insurance plan. We accept cash, check, MasterCard, and Visa.

Credit will be extended as necessary.

Credit Policy
Requirements for maintaining your account in good standing are as follows:

1. All charges are due and payable within 30 days of the first billing.
2. For services not covered by your health plan, payment at the time of service is necessary.
3. If other circumstances warrant an extended payment plan, our credit counselor will assist you in these special circumstances at your request.

We welcome early discussion of financial problems. A credit counselor will assist you.

An itemized statement of all medical services will be mailed to you every 30 days. We will prepare and file your claim forms to the health plan. If further information is needed, we will provide an additional report.

Insufficient Funds Payment Policy
We may charge an insufficient funds processing fee for all returned checks and bankcard chargebacks. If your payment is dishonored, we may electronically debit your account for the payment, plus an insufficient funds processing up to the amount allowed by law. If your bank account is not debited, the returned check amount (plus fee) must be replaced by cash, cashier's check, or money order.

Insurance
Unless we have a contract directly with your health plan, we cannot accept the responsibility of negotiating claims. You, the patient, are responsible for payment of medical care regardless of the status of the medical claim. In situations where a claim is pending or when treatment will be over an extended period of time, we will recommend that a payment plan be initiated. Your health plan is a contract between you and your insurance company. We cannot guarantee the payment of your claim. If your insurance company pays only a portion of the bill or denies the claim, any contact or explanation should be made to you, the policyholder. Reduction or rejection of your claim by your insurance company does not relieve the financial obligation you have incurred.

FIGURE 6.2 Example of a Financial Policy

Financial Policy and Health Plan Provisions

Patients should always be informed of their financial obligations according to practice credit and collections policy. This **financial policy** on payment for services is usually either displayed on the wall of the reception area or included in a new patient information packet. A sample of a financial policy is shown in Figure 6.2.

financial policy Practice's rules governing payment from patients.

The policy should explain what is required of the patient and when payment is due. For example, the policy may state the following:

For unassigned claims: Payment for the physician's services is expected at the end of your appointment unless you have made other arrangements with our practice manager.

For assigned claims: After your insurance claim is processed by your insurance company, you will be billed for any amount you owe. You are responsible for any part of the charges that is denied or not paid by the carrier. All patient accounts are due within thirty days of the date of the statement.

Copayments: Copayments must be paid before patients leave the office.

However, a health plan may have a contract with the practice that prohibits physicians from obtaining anything except a copayment until after the claim is paid. Medicare has such a rule; the provider is not permitted to collect the deductible or any other payment until receiving data on how the claim is going to be paid. In this case, the health plan protects patients from having to overpay the deductible amount, which could occur if multiple providers collected the deductible within a short period of visits.

Estimating What the Patient Will Owe

Many times, patients want to know what their bills will be. For practices that collect patient accounts at the time of service and for high-deductible insurance plans, the physician practice also wants to know what a patient owes. To estimate these charges, the medical assistant verifies:

▶ The patient's deductible amount and whether it has been paid in full, the covered benefits, and coinsurance or other patient financial obligations.

▶ The payer's allowed charges for the planned or provided services to the patient.

There are other tools that can be used to estimate charges. Some payers have a swipe-card reader (like a credit card processing device) that can be installed in the reception area and used by patients to learn what the insurer will pay and what the patient owes. Most practice management programs have a feature that permits estimating the patient's bill, as shown below:

	Est. Resp.		
Policy 1: Aetna Choice (EMC)	$116.00	Charges:	$116.00
Policy 2: Medicare Nationwide	$0.00	Adjustments:	$0.00
Policy 3:	$0.00	Subtotal:	$116.00
Guarantor: Williams, Vereen	-$15.00	Payment:	-$15.00
Adjustment:	$0.00	Balance:	$101.00
Policy Copay: 15.00 OA:			
Annual Deductible: 0.00 YTD: $0.00		Account Total:	$101.00

Real-time Claims Adjudication

The ideal tool for calculating charges due at the time of service is the transaction called **real-time claims adjudication (RTCA).** Offered to practices by many health plans, RTCA allows the practice to view, at the time of service, what the health plan will pay for the visit and what the patient will owe.

The process is to (1) create the claim while the patient is being checked out, (2) transmit the claim electronically to the payer, and (3) receive an immediate ("real-time") response from the payer. This response

▶ Informs the practice if there are any errors in the claim, so these can be fixed and the claim immediately resent for adjudication.

▶ States whether the patient has met the plan's deductible.

real-time claims adjudication (RTCA) Process used to generate the amount owed by a patient.

- Provides the patient's financial responsibility.
- Supplies an explanation of benefits for this patient, so that any questions the patient has about denial of coverage or payment history can be immediately answered.

Note that the RTCA does not generate a "real-time" payment—the payment follows shortly. While the waiting period varies from payer to payer, it is always an improvement over the time it normally takes payers to send payments.

BILLING TIP

Payment Plans

If patients have large bills that they must pay over time, a financial arrangement for a series of payments may be made. The payments may begin with a prepayment followed by monthly amounts. Such arrangements usually require the approval of the practice manager. They may also be governed by state laws. Payment plans are covered in greater depth later in this text.

THINKING IT THROUGH 6.5

1. Read the financial policy shown in Figure 6.2 on page 136. If a patient presents for noncovered services, when is payment expected? Does the provider accept assignment for plans in which it is nonPAR?

6.6 Checking Out Patients

The goal of an effective patient checkout procedure is that patients leave the encounter with a clear understanding of their financial responsibilities and the next steps in the billing cycle: filing of claims, insurance payments, and paying of bills they receive for balances they owe.

Patient Billing Procedures

Based on encounter form information, after the patient's visit, the medical assistant *posts* (that is, enters in the PMP) the patient's case information and diagnosis. Then the day's procedures are posted, and the program calculates the charges. Any payments from the patient are entered, and the account is brought up-to-date. These financial transactions thus may result from patients' visits:

- Charges—the amounts that providers bill for services performed.
- Payments—monies the practice receive from health plans and patients.
- **Adjustments**—changes, positive or negative, to correct patients' accounts, such as returned check fees.

adjustment Change to a patient's account.

Payment Methods

The medical assistant handles patients' payments as follows:

- *Cash:* If payment is made by cash, a receipt is issued.
- *Check:* If payment is made with a check, the amount of the payment and the check number are entered on the encounter form, and a receipt is offered.
- *Credit or debit card:* If the bill is paid with a credit or debit card, the card slip is filled out, and the card is passed through the card reader. A transaction authorization number is received from the card issuer, and the approved card slip is signed by the person paying the bill. The patient is usually offered a receipt in addition to the copy of the credit card sales slip. Telephone approval may be needed if the amount is over a specified limit.

Provider's name:_____

Provider's tax ID no.: _____

I assign my insurance benefits to the provider listed above. This credit
card authorization form is valid for one year unless I cancel the
authorization through written notice to the provider.

_____	_____
Patient name	Cardholder name
_____	
Billing address	
_____	_____ _____
City	State ZIP
_____	_____
Credit card account number	Expiration date
_____	_____
Cardholder signature	Date

I authorize _____ (provider) to keep my
signature/account number on file and to charge my American Express/
Discover/Visa/MasterCard/Other credit card account number listed above
for the balance of charges not paid by insurance within 90 days and not
to exceed $_____.

FIGURE 6.3 Preauthorized Credit Card Payment Form

Some practices ask patients who want to use a credit or debit card to complete a preauthorization form (see Figure 6.3). The patient can authorize charging copays, deductibles, and balances for all visits during a year. The authorization should be renewed according to practice policy.

If the practice accepts credit and debit cards, Payment Card Industry Data Security Standards (PCI DSS) must be followed. Similar to the rules for security under HIPAA, PCI DSS set requirements to safeguard payment card numbers, expiration dates, verification codes, and other personal data.

Walkout Receipts

If the patient makes a payment at the time of an office visit, the amount is entered into the PMP and a walkout receipt is generated. The **walkout receipt** summarizes the services and charges for that day as well as any payment the patient made (see Figure 6.4).

If the provider has not accepted assignment and is not going to file a claim for a patient, the walkout receipt is the document the patient will use to do so. Practices generally handle unassigned claims in one of two ways:

walkout receipt Report that lists the diagnoses, services provided, fees, and payments received and due after an encounter.

1. The payment is collected from the patient at the time of service (at the end of the encounter). The patient then uses the walkout receipt to report the charges and payments to the insurance company. The insurance company repays the patient (or insured) according to the terms of the plan.
2. The practice collects payment from the patient at the time of service and then sends a claim to the plan on behalf of the patient. The insurance company sends a refund check to the patient with an explanation of benefits.

Orchard Hill Medical Center

Page: 1   10/11/2016

Patient:	Walter Williams		Instructions:
	17 Mill Rd		Complete the patient information portion of your insurance
	Brooklyn, OH 44144-4567		claim form. Attach this bill, signed and dated, and all other
			bills pertaining to the claim. If you have a deductible policy,
Chart #:	WILLIWA0		hold your claim forms until you have met your deductible.
Case #:	8		Mail directly to your insurance carrier.

Date	Description	Procedure	Modify	Dx 1	Dx 2	Dx 3	Dx 4	Units	Charge
10/11/2016	EP LII Problem Focused	99212		I10	R53.1			1	46.00
10/11/2016	ECG Complete	93000		I10	R53.1			1	70.00
10/11/2016	Aetna Copayment	AETCPAY						1	-15.00

Provider Information

Provider Name:	Christopher Connolly MD
License:	37C4629
Insurance PIN:	
SSN or EIN:	161234567

Total Charges:	$ 116.00
Total Payments:	-$ 15.00
Total Adjustments:	$ 0.00
Total Due This Visit:	**$ 101.00**
Total Account Balance:	$ 101.00

Assign and Release: I hereby authorize payment of medical benefits to this physician for the services described
above. I also authorize the release of any information necessary to process this claim.

Patient Signature: _____   Date: _____

FIGURE 6.4 Walkout Receipt

Exercise 6.3 Creating a Walkout Receipt

Generate a walkout receipt for the copayment and supply payment that Ann Ingram has made at the end of her visit with Dr. Clarke.

Follow the steps at www.mhhe.com/newbycarr to complete the exercise at connect.mcgraw-hill.com on your own once you have watched the demo and tried the steps with prompts in practice mode. Use the information provided in the scenario to complete the exercise.

THINKING IT THROUGH 6.6

1. Why are up-front collections important to the practice?

Chapter Summary

Learning Outcomes	Key Concepts/Examples
6.1 Contrast provider payment under PPOs, capitated HMOs, indemnity plans, and CDHPs. Pages 122–127	• Under preferred provider organizations (PPOs), providers are paid using a discounted fee-for-service structure. • In health maintenance organizations (HMOs) capitated plans pay the provider fixed prepayments based on a per member per month (PMPM) rate. • Indemnity plans basically pay from the physician's fee schedule. • Three types of funding options are used to pay for services in a consumer-driven health plan (CDHP). • A health reimbursement account (HRA) is set up by an employer to reimburse an employee for their medical expenses. • Health savings accounts (HSAs) can be funded by an employee and employer. • Flexible savings (spending) accounts contain pretax dollars that can be used to pay for medical expenses.
6.2 Calculate an RBRVS payment. Pages 127–129	The following steps are used to calculate the resource-based relative value scale (RBRVS) payment under the Medicare Physician Fee Schedule (MPFS): • Determine the procedure code for the service. • Use the MPFS to find the three RVUs—work, practice expense, and malpractice—for the procedure. • Use the Medicare GPCI list to find the three geographic practice cost indices. • Multiply each RVU by its GPCI to calculate the adjusted value. • Add the three adjusted totals, and multiply the sum by the conversion factor to determine the payment.
6.3 Discuss the influence of third-party rules on patients' charges from participating versus nonparticipating providers. Pages 130–133	• When a maximum allowed charge is set by a payer for a service, a provider does not receive the difference from the payer if the provider's usual fee is greater. • If a provider participates in a plan the difference is written off; if the provider does not participate, the plan's rules on balance billing determine whether the patient is responsible for the amount. • Under a contracted fee schedule, the allowed charge for each service is all that the payer or the patient pays; no additional charges can be collected.

6.4 Define the eight types of time-of-service charges. Pages 133–135	• Practices routinely collect up-front money from patients at the time of their office visit as an important source of cash flow.
	• Eight different types of charges may be collected from patients at the time of service.
	    Payment owed on previous balances
	    Copayments
	    Coinsurance
	    Noncovered or overlimit fees
	    Charges of nonparticipating providers
	    Charges for self-pay patients
	    Deductibles for patients with CDHPs
	    Charges for supplies and copies of medical records

Learning Outcomes	Key Concepts/Examples
6.5 Calculate time-of-service payments. Pages 135–138	• Real-time claim adjudication tools, offered by many health plans, are used to calculate charges due at the time of service. • These tools allow the practice to view what the health plan will pay for the visit and what the patient owes.
6.6 Explain the patient checkout procedure. Pages 138–141	After the patient's visit: • The practice posts the patient's case information and diagnosis in the PMP based on the encounter form information. • The program calculates the charges. • Payments from the patient are entered at this time and the account is brought up-to-date. • Upon leaving the patient is given a walkout receipt summarizing the services and the charges for that day as well as any payment the patient made.

Using Terminology

Match the key terms in the left column with the definitions in the right column.

_____ 1. **[LO 6.1]** Health maintenance organization

_____ 2. **[LO 6.4]** Accept assignment

_____ 3. **[LO 6.2]** Resource based relative value scale

_____ 4. **[LO 6.5]** Real-time claims adjudication

_____ 5. **[LO 6.1]** Capitation

_____ 6. **[LO 6.1]** Preferred provider organization

_____ 7. **[LO 6.3]** Allowed charge

_____ 8. **[LO 6.2]** Fee schedule

_____ 9. **[LO 6.1]** Point-of-service plan

_____ 10. **[LO 6.6]** Walkout receipt

A. A participating physician's agreement to accept the allowed charge as payment in full.

B. The maximum amount that a health plan pays for a specific procedure or service.

C. A payment method in which a fixed prepayment covers the provider's services to a plan member for a specified period of time.

D. List of charges for services performed.

E. Process used to generate the amount owed by a patient.

F. Report that lists the diagnoses, services provided, fees, and payments received and due after an encounter.

G. A plan with a primary and secondary network that allows patients to receive medical services from nonnetwork providers in exchange for higher monthly premiums.

H. A managed care organization that contains a network of health care providers that agree to perform services for plan members at discounted fees.

I. Payment system used by Medicare.

J. A health plan that requires members to receive services from the contracted network of providers.

connect plus+

Enhance your learning at mcgrawhillconnect.com!
• Practice Exercises   • Worksheets
• Activities   • Integrated eBook

Checking Your Understanding

Write the letter of the choice that best completes the statement or answers the question.

1. **[LO 6.1]** Providers who participate in a PPO are paid _____.
   - **A.** A capitated rate
   - **B.** A discounted fee-for-service
   - **C.** An episode-of-care payment
   - **D.** According to their usual physician fee schedule

2. **[LO 6.1]** Consumer-driven health plans have what effect on a practice's cash flow? _____
   - **A.** There is no effect on cash flow.
   - **B.** Cash flow is increased because CDHP deductibles are higher.
   - **C.** Cash flow is increased because the health plan payment arrives faster than under other health plans.
   - **D.** Cash flow is reduced because a high deductible payment from the patient takes longer to collect than a copayment.

3. **[LO 6.3]** If a nonparticipating provider's usual fee is $200, the allowed amount is $175, and balance billing is permitted, what amount is written off? _____
   - **A.** $25
   - **B.** $50
   - **C.** Zero
   - **D.** $15

4. **[LO 6.3]** What percentage of the allowed charge does Medicare typically pay? _____
   - **A.** 50 percent
   - **B.** 60 percent
   - **C.** 70 percent
   - **D.** 80 percent

5. **[LO 6.1]** Which of the following methods of payment belong to a prospective payment system? _____
   - **A.** Discounted fee-for-service
   - **B.** Capitation
   - **C.** Fee-for-service
   - **D.** Fee schedule

6. **[LO 6.3]** If a participating provider's usual fee is $600, and the allowed amount is $450, what amount is written off? _____
   - **A.** Zero
   - **B.** $150
   - **C.** $50
   - **D.** $100

7. **[LO 6.4]** Which type of payment is always collected at the time of service? _____
   - **A.** Coinsurance
   - **B.** Copayment
   - **C.** Deductible
   - **D.** Premium

8. **[LO 6.4]** What does a provider agree to do when assignment is accepted? _____
   - **A.** To care for all patients enrolled in a health plan
   - **B.** To write off charges for services over the plan limits
   - **C.** To accept the charge allowed by the health plan as full payment
   - **D.** To write off charges for excluded services

9. **[LO 6.2]** In calculations of RBRVS fees, the three relative value units are multiplied by _____.
   - **A.** Their respective geographic practice cost indices
   - **B.** The neutral budget factor
   - **C.** The national conversion factor
   - **D.** The UCR factor

10. **[LO 6.4]** The usual fees for noncovered services are _____.
    - **A.** Written off
    - **B.** Subject to balance billing rules
    - **C.** Subtracted from the annual deductible
    - **D.** Collected at the time of service

connect™ plus+

Enhance your learning at mcgrawhillconnect.com!
- Practice Exercises
- Worksheets
- Activities
- Integrated eBook

Applying Your Knowledge

Case 6.1   Using Insurance Terms

Read the following information from a medical insurance policy.

Policy Number 054351278

Insured Jane Hellman Brandeis

Premium Due Quarterly $1,414.98

AMOUNT PAYABLE

Maximum Benefit Limit, per *covered person* $2,000,000

Stated Deductible per *covered person*, per *calendar year* $2,500

EMERGENCY ROOM DEDUCTIBLE (for each visit for illness to an emergency room when not directly admitted to the *hospital*) $50

Note: After satisfaction of the emergency room deductible, *covered expenses* are subject to any applicable *deductible amounts* and coinsurance provisions.

PREFERRED PROVIDER COINSURANCE PERCENTAGE, per *calendar year*

For *covered expenses* in excess of the applicable stated deductible, payer pays 100%

A. [LO 6.1] What type of health plan is described: HMO, PPO, or indemnity?

B. [LO 6.1] What is the annual premium?

C. [LO 6.1] What is the annual deductible?

D. [LO 6.1] What percentage of preferred provider charges does the patient owe after meeting the deductible each year?

E. [LO 6.1] If the insured incurs a $6,000 in-network medical bill after the annual deductible has been paid, how much will the health plan pay?

Case 6.2   Calculating Insurance Math

A. [LO 6.1, 6.4, 6.5] A patient's insurance policy states:

Annual deductible: $300.00

Coinsurance: 70-30

This year the patient has made payments totaling $533 to all providers. Today the patient has an office visit (fee: $80). The patient presents a credit card for payment of today's bill. What is the amount that the patient should pay?

B. [LO 6.1, 6.4, 6.5] A patient is a member of a health plan with a 15 percent discount from the provider's usual fees and a $10 copay. The day's charges are $480. What are the amounts that the HMO and the patient each pay?

C. [LO 6.1, 6.4, 6.5] A patient is a member of a health plan that has a 20 percent discount from the provider and a 15 percent copay. If the day's charges are $210, what are the amounts that the HMO and the patient each pay?

Case 6.3   Calculating Expected charges

Using the sample relative value units and GPCIs shown on page 129 and a conversion factor of $24.6712, calculate the expected charge for the following services:

A. [LO 6.2] CPT 33500 in Manhattan, NY

B. [LO 6.2] CPT 99203 in San Francisco, CA

C. [LO 6.2] CPT 33503 in Galveston, TX

connect plus+

Enhance your learning at mcgrawhillconnect.com!
- Practice Exercises   • Worksheets
- Activities   • Integrated eBook

HEALTH CARE CLAIM PREPARATION AND TRANSMISSION

7

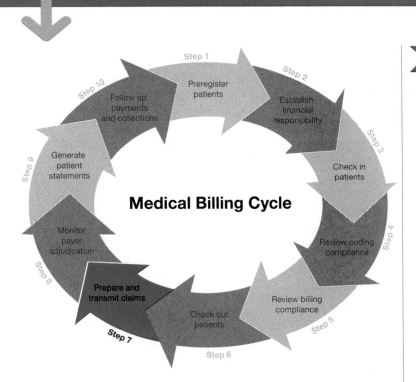

Medical Billing Cycle

Step 1 — Preregister patients
Step 2 — Establish financial responsibility
Step 3 — Check in patients
Step 4 — Review coding compliance
Step 5 — Review billing compliance
Step 6 — Check out patients
Step 7 — Prepare and transmit claims
Step 8 — Monitor payer adjudication
Step 9 — Generate patient statements
Step 10 — Follow up payments and collections

Learning Outcomes

After studying this chapter, you should be able to:

7.1 Outline the benefits of using practice management programs to prepare health care claims.

7.2 Distinguish between the electronic and paper-based claim transactions.

7.3 Complete a CMS-1500 form.

7.4 Discuss the data elements entered in the five sections of the HIPAA 837 claim transaction.

7.5 State the three major methods of electronic claim transmission.

7.6 Explain the process for billing secondary payers.

KEY TERMS

5010 format
837P claim
administrative code set
billing provider
carrier block
claim attachment
claim control number
claim filing indicator code
claim frequency code (claim submission reason code)
clean claim
CMS-1500 claim
CMS-1500 (02/12)
condition code
database
data element
destination payer
HIPAA claim
individual relationship code
line item control number
National Uniform Claim Committee (NUCC)
outside laboratory
pay-to provider
place of service (POS) code
qualifier
rendering provider
secondary claim
service line information
subscriber
taxonomy code
tertiary claim

Health care claims communicate critical data between providers and payers on behalf of patients. Understanding the internal and EDI procedures used by the practice to prepare and transmit claims is important for success. Claim processing is a major task, and the numbers can be huge. Technology makes it possible to create, send, and track a large volume of claims efficiently and effectively to ensure prompt payment.

7.1 Preparing Claims Using Practice Management Programs

database Collection of related facts.

Practice management programs (PMPs) and integrated PM/EHRs increase efficiency because repeatedly used data are stored in **databases**—collections of related facts—and quickly accessed. For example, the office's frequently used diagnosis and procedure codes, as well as fee schedules, are entered once and then stored. A medical assistant who is posting (that is, entering) the information from the encounter into the PMP does not have to enter a complete code and its description. That information has already been stored, so the correct code can be chosen from a list on the computer screen.

The major databases in PMPs are:

▶ *Provider*—The provider database has information about the licensed medical professional staff members who work in the medical office, such as names, office addresses, and NPIs.

▶ *Patient/Guarantor*—The data from each patient information form are stored in the patient/guarantor database. These data include items such as the patient's unique account number and personal information: name, address, phone number, birth date, Social Security number, gender, marital status, employer, and guarantor.

▶ *Insurance Carriers*—The payer database contains the names, addresses, plan types, and other data about the major health plans the practice has participation contracts with.

▶ *Diagnosis Codes*—The diagnosis code database contains the ICD-10-CM codes that indicate the reasons services are provided. The codes stored are those most frequently used by the office. Additional codes can easily be entered and updates made annually.

▶ *Procedure Codes*—The procedure code database contains the data needed to create charges. The CPT codes most often used by the office are selected for this database. Like the ICD codes, additional CPT codes are easy to enter or update if needed.

▶ *Transactions*—Transactions are all the financial aspects of visits—charges, payments, and adjustments. The transaction database stores information about each patient's visit charges and the related diagnoses and procedures, as well as received and outstanding payments.

When preparing claims, medical assistants work with PMPs, following these steps:

▶ Record patients' insurance and demographic information.
▶ Record diagnoses, procedures, charges, and payments for patients' encounters.
▶ Create and transmit claims to payers.

Recording Patients' Information

The first step in preparing claims is recording patients' information from new or updated patient information forms and patients' insurance cards. A new record must be created for a new patient, and facts about established patients may need to be updated.

Recording Diagnoses, Procedures, Charges, and Payments for Patients' Encounters

After the patient's visit with the medical professional staff, the diagnosis codes and the procedure codes are recorded in the PMP. (If the practice uses an integrated PM/EHR, this information crosses over from the EHR updated after the encounter.) The provider the patient saw is selected from the PMP's list of the practice's physicians and other staff members. The appropriate transactions for the visit are also entered. The source of the codes, charges, and payment information is the encounter documentation. The patient's appropriate insurance coverage for this visit is also selected. Usually, it is the patient's main (primary, if the patient has more than one plan) health plan, but if the case is for a workers' compensation claim, that insurance is selected.

Creating and Transmitting Claims to Payers

When all required data have been entered and checked, the medical assistant instructs the PMP to create a claim for the appropriate payer. Following its programmed instructions, the program draws the needed facts from the stored information and organizes these data elements into a claim file. Claims generated by PMPs can be transmitted as electronic claims to payers, or the claims can be printed and mailed to the payers. Most health care claims are submitted electronically, not on paper.

Clean Claims

Although health care claims require many data elements and are complex, it is often the simple errors that keep practices from generating **clean claims**—that is, claims that are accepted for processing by payers.

clean claim Claim accepted by a health plan for adjudication.

Data Entry Tips

Although PMPs increase efficiency and reduce errors, they are not more accurate than the individual who is entering the data. If people make mistakes while entering data, the information the computer produces will be incorrect. Many human errors occur during data entry, such as pressing the wrong key on the keyboard. Other errors are a result of a lack of computer literacy—not knowing how to use a program to accomplish tasks. For this reason, having proper training in data-entry techniques, so that errors are caught, and knowing how to use computer programs are both essential for medical assistants. Follow these tips for accurate data entry when entering data in PMPs:

▶ Do not use prefixes for people's names, such as Mr., Ms., or Dr.
▶ Unless required by a particular insurance carrier, do not use special characters such as hyphens, commas, or apostrophes.
▶ Use only valid data in all fields.
▶ Enter the required number of characters for each data element, such as four numbers for the year, but do not worry about the format. Most PMPs or claim transmission programs automatically reformat data such as dates correctly.

Common Errors to Avoid

Following are common data errors:

▶ Missing or incomplete service facility name, address, and identification for services rendered outside the office or home. This includes invalid Zip codes or state abbreviations.
▶ Missing Medicare assignment indicator or benefits assignment indicator.
▶ Invalid provider identifier (when present) for rendering provider, referring provider, or others.

- ▶ Missing part of the name or the identifier of the referring provider.
- ▶ Missing or invalid patient birth date or patient name.
- ▶ Missing payer name and/or payer identifier, required for both primary and secondary payers.
- ▶ Incomplete other payer information. This is required on all secondary claims and all primary claims that will involve a secondary payer.
- ▶ Invalid procedure codes.

THINKING IT THROUGH 7.1

1. Given that health information technology plays such an important role in claim creation, how important do you think proofreading and accuracy checking skills are? Are they more or less critical than when claims were prepared manually?

COMPLIANCE GUIDELINE

P versus I

The *P* in 837P stands for professional. For hospital billing, the mandated claim is the 837I, where I stands for institutional.

7.2 Health Care Claims

The HIPAA-mandated electronic transaction for claims (formally named the HIPAA X12 837 Health Care Claim or Equivalent Encounter Information) is often called the **HIPAA claim** or the **837P claim**. The electronic HIPAA claim is based on the **CMS-1500 claim**, formerly the HCFA-1500, which is a paper claim form. The information on the paper claim and on the electronic transaction is essentially the same.

This book covers the way to fill out the paper claim before explaining the HIPAA claim, because this is a good way to understand the data that claims generally require. Of course, the CMS-1500 is not usually filled out by transferring information directly from other office forms, like the patient information and encounter forms. Instead, claims are created using the PMP, which makes it easy to update, correct, and manage the claim process.

HIPAA claim HIPAA-mandated electronic transaction for claims.

837P claim HIPAA-mandated electronic transaction for claims.

CMS-1500 claim Paper claim for physician services.

BILLING TIP

Memorization Needed?

Medical assistants become familiar with the information most often required on claims so that they can efficiently research missing information and respond to payers' questions. Memorization is not required, but good thinking and organizational skills are.

Claim Background

The CMS-1500 was for many years the universal health claim, meaning that it was accepted by most payers. The familiar red-and-black printed form was typed or computer-generated and mailed to payers. The method of sending claims changed with the increased use of health information technology (HIT) in physician practices. HIPAA, with its emphasis on electronic transactions, has essentially made the use of IT mandatory. HIPAA requires electronic transmission of claims except from very small practices and those that never send any kind of electronic health care transactions. Only these providers can still mail or fax paper claims. Electronic transmission of the HIPAA claim is mandated for all other physician practices.

HIPAA has changed the way things work on the payer side, too. Payers may not require providers to make changes or additions to the content of the HIPAA claim. Further, they cannot refuse to accept the standard transaction or delay payment of any proper HIPAA transaction, claims included.

BILLING TIP

Staying Up-to-Date with the CMS-1500

Check the NUCC website for updated instructions.

Claim Content

The **National Uniform Claim Committee (NUCC),** led by the American Medical Association, determines the content of both HIPAA and CMS-1500 claims. The NUCC modified its instructions for the CMS-1500 in 2012, and recommended excluding selected data items that are not on the HIPAA 837P. Their goal has been to bring the CMS-1500 more in accord with a new format for the electronic claim, called the **5010 format,** without having to change the overall layout. The NUCC

National Uniform Claim Committee (NUCC) Organization responsible for claim content.

5010 format Format for electronic claims.

also made modifications to the area of the form where diagnosis codes are reported, allowing more room so the ICD-10-CM code format can be handled. In this chapter, we explain the **CMS-1500 (02/12)** version. On the job, medical assistants verify payer requirements for the paper claim in the rare instances where it is completed. Note that there may be variations in the version of the claim used by PMPs when a claim is "dropped to paper." Not all PMP vendors will update their paper forms, because most of their customers use electronic claims, which they keep current.

CMS-1500 (02/12) NUCC-revised paper claim with modified instructions.

THINKING IT THROUGH 7.2

1. What advantages can you identify for transmitting electronic claims? Are there any potential disadvantages as well?

NUCC Home Page

www.nucc.org

7.3 Completing the CMS-1500 02/12 Claim

The CMS-1500 02/12 claim contains thirty-three item numbers (INs), or information boxes, as shown in Figure 7.1 on the next page. Item numbers 1 through 13 refer to the patient and the patient's insurance coverage. This information is entered based on the patient information form and the patient insurance card. Item numbers 14 through 33 contain information about the provider and the patient's condition, including diagnoses, procedures, and charges.

COMPLIANCE GUIDELINE

CMS-1500 (02/12) Implementation

The 02/12 form is required as of October 1, 2014.

Carrier Block

The **carrier block** is located in the upper right of the CMS-1500. At the left is a Quick Response (QR) code symbol. This block allows for a four-line address for the payer. If the payer's address requires just three lines, leave a blank line in the third position, like this:

ABC Insurance Company

567 Willow Lane

Franklin IL 60605

Note that commas, periods, and other punctuation are not used in the address. However, when entering a 9-digit Zip code, the hyphen is included (for example, 60609-4563).

carrier block Data entry area in the upper right of the CMS-1500.

COMPLIANCE GUIDELINE

5010 Format: Zip Codes

9-digit Zip codes are required for all provider-related addresses.

Patient Information

The items in this part of the CMS-1500 claim form identify the patient and the insured, the health plan, and assignment of benefits/release information.

Item Number 1: Type of Insurance Item number 1 is used to indicate the patient's type of insurance coverage. Five specific government programs are listed (Medicare, Medicaid, TRICARE, CHAMPVA, FECA Black Lung), as well as Group Health Plan and Other. If the patient has group contract insurance, Group Health Plan is selected. The Other box indicates health insurance including individual health plans, HMOs, commercial insurance, automobile accident, liability, and workers' compensation. If a patient can be identified by a unique Member Identification Number, that patient is the "insured" and is reported in the insured fields rather than the patient fields.

1. MEDICARE	MEDICAID	TRICARE	CHAMPVA	GROUP HEALTH PLAN	FECA BLK LUNG	OTHER
(Medicare#)	(Medicaid#)	(ID#/DoD#)	(Member ID#)	(ID#)	(ID#)	(ID#)

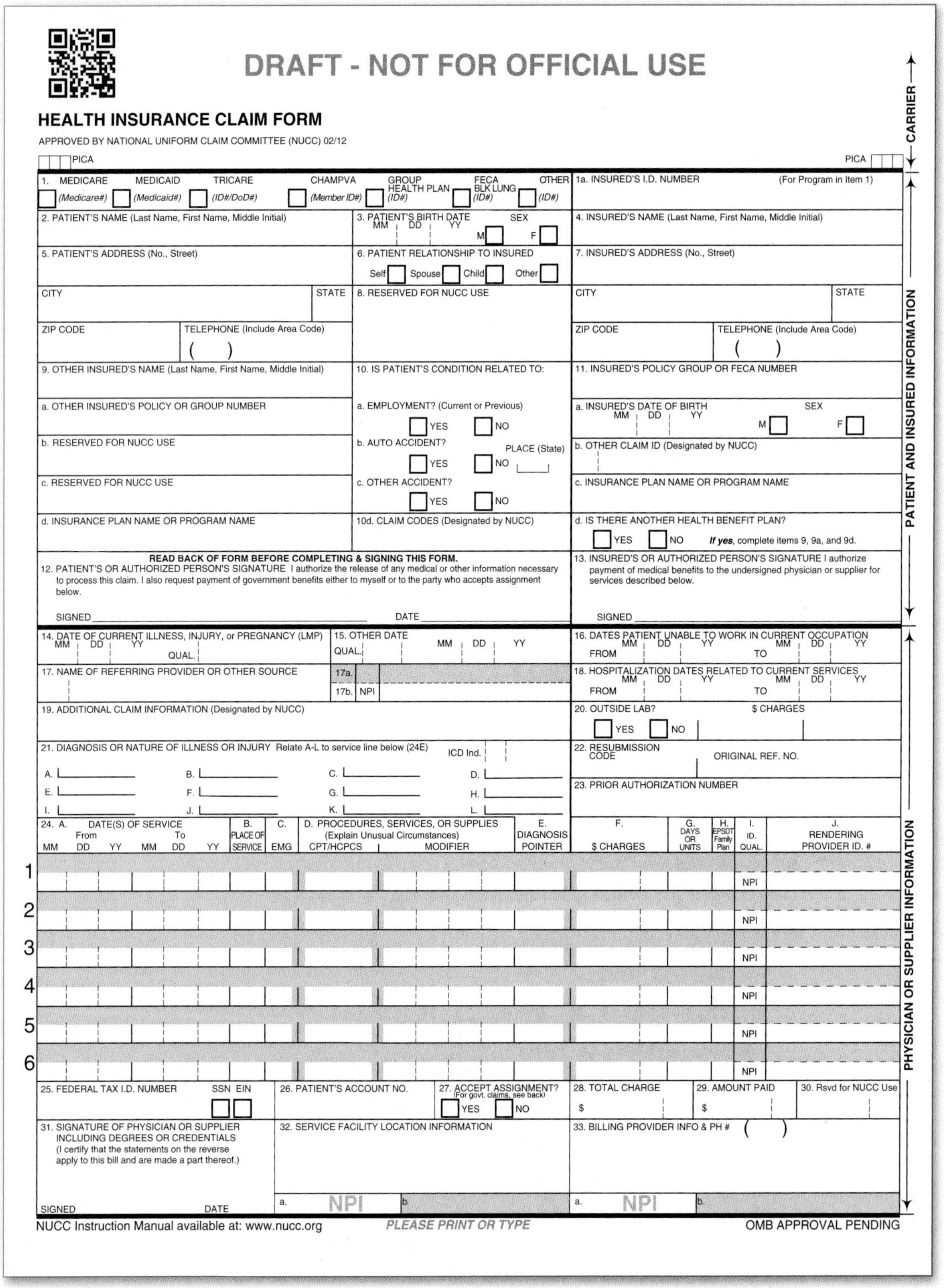

HEALTH INSURANCE CLAIM FORM

APPROVED BY NATIONAL UNIFORM CLAIM COMMITTEE (NUCC) 02/12

PICA

CARRIER

1. MEDICARE (Medicare#) | MEDICAID (Medicaid#) | TRICARE (ID#/DoD#) | CHAMPVA (Member ID#) | GROUP HEALTH PLAN (ID#) | FECA BLK LUNG (ID#) | OTHER (ID#) | 1a. INSURED'S I.D. NUMBER (For Program in Item 1)

2. PATIENT'S NAME (Last Name, First Name, Middle Initial)

3. PATIENT'S BIRTH DATE MM DD YY SEX M F

4. INSURED'S NAME (Last Name, First Name, Middle Initial)

5. PATIENT'S ADDRESS (No., Street)

6. PATIENT RELATIONSHIP TO INSURED Self Spouse Child Other

7. INSURED'S ADDRESS (No., Street)

CITY STATE

8. RESERVED FOR NUCC USE

CITY STATE

ZIP CODE TELEPHONE (Include Area Code) ( )

ZIP CODE TELEPHONE (Include Area Code) ( )

9. OTHER INSURED'S NAME (Last Name, First Name, Middle Initial)

10. IS PATIENT'S CONDITION RELATED TO:

11. INSURED'S POLICY GROUP OR FECA NUMBER

a. OTHER INSURED'S POLICY OR GROUP NUMBER

a. EMPLOYMENT? (Current or Previous) YES NO

a. INSURED'S DATE OF BIRTH MM DD YY SEX M F

b. RESERVED FOR NUCC USE

b. AUTO ACCIDENT? YES NO PLACE (State)

b. OTHER CLAIM ID (Designated by NUCC)

c. RESERVED FOR NUCC USE

c. OTHER ACCIDENT? YES NO

c. INSURANCE PLAN NAME OR PROGRAM NAME

d. INSURANCE PLAN NAME OR PROGRAM NAME

10d. CLAIM CODES (Designated by NUCC)

d. IS THERE ANOTHER HEALTH BENEFIT PLAN? YES NO If yes, complete items 9, 9a, and 9d.

READ BACK OF FORM BEFORE COMPLETING & SIGNING THIS FORM.

PATIENT AND INSURED INFORMATION

12. PATIENT'S OR AUTHORIZED PERSON'S SIGNATURE I authorize the release of any medical or other information necessary to process this claim. I also request payment of government benefits either to myself or to the party who accepts assignment below.

SIGNED _____ DATE _____

13. INSURED'S OR AUTHORIZED PERSON'S SIGNATURE I authorize payment of medical benefits to the undersigned physician or supplier for services described below.

SIGNED _____

14. DATE OF CURRENT ILLNESS, INJURY, or PREGNANCY (LMP) MM DD YY QUAL.

15. OTHER DATE QUAL. MM DD YY

16. DATES PATIENT UNABLE TO WORK IN CURRENT OCCUPATION FROM MM DD YY TO MM DD YY

17. NAME OF REFERRING PROVIDER OR OTHER SOURCE

17a. | 17b. NPI

18. HOSPITALIZATION DATES RELATED TO CURRENT SERVICES FROM MM DD YY TO MM DD YY

19. ADDITIONAL CLAIM INFORMATION (Designated by NUCC)

20. OUTSIDE LAB? YES NO $ CHARGES

21. DIAGNOSIS OR NATURE OF ILLNESS OR INJURY Relate A-L to service line below (24E) ICD Ind.

A. B. C. D.
E. F. G. H.
I. J. K. L.

22. RESUBMISSION CODE ORIGINAL REF. NO.

23. PRIOR AUTHORIZATION NUMBER

24. A. DATE(S) OF SERVICE From MM DD YY To MM DD YY | B. PLACE OF SERVICE | C. EMG | D. PROCEDURES, SERVICES, OR SUPPLIES (Explain Unusual Circumstances) CPT/HCPCS MODIFIER | E. DIAGNOSIS POINTER | F. $ CHARGES | G. DAYS OR UNITS | H. EPSDT Family Plan | I. ID. QUAL. | J. RENDERING PROVIDER ID. #

1 | | | | | | | | NPI
2 | | | | | | | | NPI
3 | | | | | | | | NPI
4 | | | | | | | | NPI
5 | | | | | | | | NPI
6 | | | | | | | | NPI

PHYSICIAN OR SUPPLIER INFORMATION

25. FEDERAL TAX I.D. NUMBER SSN EIN

26. PATIENT'S ACCOUNT NO.

27. ACCEPT ASSIGNMENT? (For govt. claims, see back) YES NO

28. TOTAL CHARGE $

29. AMOUNT PAID $

30. Rsvd for NUCC Use

31. SIGNATURE OF PHYSICIAN OR SUPPLIER INCLUDING DEGREES OR CREDENTIALS (I certify that the statements on the reverse apply to this bill and are made a part thereof.)

SIGNED _____ DATE _____

32. SERVICE FACILITY LOCATION INFORMATION a. NPI b.

33. BILLING PROVIDER INFO & PH # ( ) a. NPI b.

NUCC Instruction Manual available at: www.nucc.org

PLEASE PRINT OR TYPE

OMB APPROVAL PENDING

FIGURE 7.1 CMS-1500 02/12 Claim

1a. INSURED'S I.D. NUMBER (For Program in Item 1)

Item Number 1a: Insured's ID Number The insured's ID number is the identification number of the person who holds the policy or the dependent patient if this person has been issued a unique identifier by the payer. Item number 1a records the insurance identification number that appears on the insurance card of the person who holds the policy, who may or may not be the patient.

Item Number 2: Patient's Name The patient's name is the name of the person who received the treatment or supplies, listed exactly as it appears on the insurance card. Do not change the spelling, even if the card is incorrect. Only report the patient's information if it is different from the insured's information. The order in which the name should appear is last name, first name, and middle initial. Use commas to separate the last name, first name, and middle initial.

2. PATIENT'S NAME (Last Name, First Name, Middle Initial)

BILLING TIP

Names

When entering names with a last name suffix (e.g., Jr. or Sr.), enter the suffix after the last name and before the first name such as Jones, Jr., Edward, T.

Item Number 3: Patient's Birth Date/Sex The patient's birth date and sex (gender) helps identify the patient; this information distinguishes persons with similar names. Enter the patient's date of birth in eight-digit format (MM/DD/CCYY). Note that all four digits for the year are entered, even though the printed form indicates only two characters (YY). Use zeros before single digits. Enter an X in the correct box to indicate the sex of the patient. Leave this box blank if the patient's gender is unknown. Only report the patient's information if it is different from the insured's information.

3. PATIENT'S BIRTH DATE	SEX	
MM | DD | YY	M ☐	F ☐

Item Number 4: Insured's Name In IN 4, enter the full name of the person who holds the insurance policy (the insured). If the patient is a dependent, the insured may be a spouse, parent, or other person. Use commas to separate the last name, first name, and middle initial.

4. INSURED'S NAME (Last Name, First Name, Middle Initial)

Item Number 5: Patient's Address Item number 5 is used to report the patient's address, which includes the number and street, city, state, and ZIP code. The first line is for the street address, the second line for the city and state, and the third line for the ZIP code. Use a two-digit state abbreviation and a nine-digit ZIP code if it is available. If the patient's address is the same as the insured's address, then it is not necessary to report it here. Only report the patient's information if it is different from the insured's information. Do not report the patient's telephone number, per the NUCC.

Note that the patient's address refers to the patient's permanent residence. A temporary address or school address should not be used.

5. PATIENT'S ADDRESS (No., Street)	
CITY	STATE
ZIP CODE	TELEPHONE (Include Area Code) ( )

COMPLIANCE GUIDELINE

NUCC on IN5

NUCC recommends that the phone number not be reported.

Item Number 6: Patient's Relationship to Insured In IN 6, enter the patient's relationship to the insured who is listed in IN 4. Choosing *self* indicates that the insured is the patient. *Spouse* indicates that the patient is the husband or wife or qualified partner as defined by the insured's plan. *Child* means that the patient is the minor dependent as defined by the insured's plan. *Other* means that the patient is someone other than the insured, the spouse, or the child, which may include employee, ward, or dependent as defined by the insured's plan.

If the patient is a dependent but has a unique Member Identification Number that the payer requires on the claim, report *Self*, because the patient is reported as the insured.

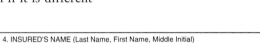

6. PATIENT RELATIONSHIP TO INSURED			
Self ☐	Spouse ☐	Child ☐	Other ☐

Item Number 7: Insured's Address The insured's address refers to the insured's permanent residence, which may be different from the patient's address (IN 5). Enter the address of

7. INSURED'S ADDRESS (No., Street)	
CITY	STATE
ZIP CODE	TELEPHONE (Include Area Code) ( )

the person who is listed in IN 4. For most payers, if the insured's address is the same as the patient's enter SAME. Do not report the insured's telephone number, per the NUCC.

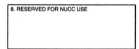

8. RESERVED FOR NUCC USE

Item Number 8: Reserved for NUCC Use This field is reserved for NUCC use. The previous use as "Patient Status" has been eliminated.

9. OTHER INSURED'S NAME (Last Name, First Name, Middle Initial)

Item Number 9: Other Insured's Name If Item Number 11d is marked yes, complete Item Numbers 9, 9a, and 9d; otherwise, leave blank. An entry in the other insured's name box indicates that there is a holder of another policy that may cover the patient. When additional group health coverage exists, enter the insured's name (the last name, first name, and middle initial of the enrollee in another health plan if it is different from that shown in IN 2).

Example

If a husband is covered by his employer's group policy and also by his wife's group health plan, enter the wife's name in IN 9. ◄

a. OTHER INSURED'S POLICY OR GROUP NUMBER

Item Number 9a: Other Insured's Policy or Group Number Enter the policy or group number of the other insurance plan. Do not use a hyphen or space as a separator with the policy or group number.

b. RESERVED FOR NUCC USE

Item Number 9b: Reserved for NUCC Use This field is reserved for NUCC use. The previous use for the date of birth and sex of the other insured indicated in IN 9 has been eliminated.

c. RESERVED FOR NUCC USE

Item Number 9c: Reserved for NUCC Use This field is reserved for NUCC use. The previous use for the name of the other insured's employer or school has been eliminated.

d. INSURANCE PLAN NAME OR PROGRAM NAME

Item Number 9d: Insurance Plan Name or Program Name Enter the other insured's insurance plan or program name. This box identifies the name of the plan or program of the other insured indicated in IN 9.

10. IS PATIENT'S CONDITION RELATED TO:

a. EMPLOYMENT? (Current or Previous)

☐ YES   ☐ NO

b. AUTO ACCIDENT?

PLACE (State)

☐ YES   ☐ NO

c. OTHER ACCIDENT?

☐ YES   ☐ NO

Item Numbers 10a–10c: Is Patient's Condition Related to: This information indicates whether the patient's illness or injury is related to employment, auto accident, or other accident. Choosing *employment* (current or previous) indicates that the condition is related to the patient's job or workplace. *Auto accident* means that the condition is the result of an automobile accident. *Other accident* means that the condition is the result of any other type of accident.

When appropriate, enter an X in the correct box to indicate whether one or more of the services described in IN 24 are for a condition or injury that occurred on the job or as a result of an automobile or other accident. The state postal code must be shown if YES is checked in IN 10b for Auto Accident. Any item checked YES indicates that there may be other applicable insurance coverage that would be primary, such as automobile liability insurance. Primary insurance information must then be shown in IN 11.

Item Number 10d: Claim Codes (Designated by NUCC) This IN identifies additional information about the patient's condition or the claim. When required by payers to include these codes, use the NUCC **condition codes** accessed on the NUCC website under Code Sets.

10d. CLAIM CODES (Designated by NUCC)

Item Number 11: Insured's Policy Group or FECA Number Enter the insured's policy or group number as it appears on the insured's health care identification card. If IN 4 is completed, this entry should also be completed.

11. INSURED'S POLICY GROUP OR FECA NUMBER

condition code Two-digit numeric or alphanumeric codes used to report a special condition or unique circumstance

The insured's policy group or FECA number is the alphanumeric identifier for the health, auto, or other insurance plan coverage. For workers' compensation claims, the workers' compensation carrier's alphanumeric identifier is used. The FECA (Federal Employees' Compensation Act) number is the nine-digit alphanumeric identifier assigned to a patient who is an employee of the federal government claiming work-related condition(s) under the Federal Employees Compensation Act.

Item Number 11a: Insured's Date of Birth/Sex The insured's date of birth and sex (gender) refer to the birth date and gender of the insured. Enter the insured's eight-digit birth date (MM/DD/CCYY) and sex.

a. INSURED'S DATE OF BIRTH	SEX
MM DD YY	M ☐ F ☐

Item Number 11b: Other Claim ID (Designated by NUCC) This IN is often used to report a claim number assigned by the payer. The NUCC designates applicable claim identifiers. The former use, the name of the insured's employer or the school attended by the insured, has been eliminated.

b. OTHER CLAIM ID (Designated by NUCC)

Item Number 11c: Insurance Plan Name or Program Name Enter the insurance plan or program name of the insured who is indicated in IN 1a. Note that some payers require an identification number of the primary insurer rather than the name in this field.

c. INSURANCE PLAN NAME OR PROGRAM NAME

Item Number 11d: Is There Another Health Benefit Plan? Select Yes if the patient is covered by additional insurance. If the answer is Yes, item numbers 9, 9a, and 9d must also be completed. If the patient does not have additional insurance, select No.

d. IS THERE ANOTHER HEALTH BENEFIT PLAN?
☐ YES ☐ NO *If yes*, complete items 9, 9a, and 9d.

Item Number 12: Patient's or Authorized Person's Signature Enter "Signature on File" or "SOF" if the patient/insured's signature is on file for the release of any medical or other informa-

READ BACK OF FORM BEFORE COMPLETING & SIGNING THIS FORM.
12. PATIENT'S OR AUTHORIZED PERSON'S SIGNATURE I authorize the release of any medical or other information necessary to process this claim. I also request payment of government benefits either to myself or to the party who accepts assignment below.

SIGNED _____ DATE _____

tion necessary to process the claim. Otherwise, this item number is for the legal signature. When legal signature is entered, also enter the date an authorization was signed in six-digit format (MM/DD/YY) or eight-digit format (MM/DD/CCYY). If there is no signature on file, leave blank or enter "No Signature on File."

COMPLIANCE GUIDELINE

Signatures on File

Before entering "Signature on File" or "SOF," make certain that, if a release is required, the release on file is current (signed within the last twelve months) and that it covers the release of information pertaining to all the services listed on the claim.

HEALTH INSURANCE CLAIM FORM

APPROVED BY NATIONAL UNIFORM CLAIM COMMITTEE (NUCC) 02/12

CARRIER →

| | | PICA | | | | | | | | | | PICA | | |

1. MEDICARE	MEDICAID	TRICARE	CHAMPVA	GROUP HEALTH PLAN	FECA BLK LUNG	OTHER	1a. INSURED'S I.D. NUMBER	(For Program in Item 1)
(Medicare#)	(Medicaid#)	(ID#/DoD#)	(Member ID#) [X]	(ID#)	(ID#)	(ID#)	GH331240789	

2. PATIENT'S NAME (Last Name, First Name, Middle Initial)	3. PATIENT'S BIRTH DATE MM DD YY	SEX M □ F □	4. INSURED'S NAME (Last Name, First Name, Middle Initial) CARUTHERS, ROBIN

5. PATIENT'S ADDRESS (No., Street)	6. PATIENT RELATIONSHIP TO INSURED Self [X] Spouse □ Child □ Other □	7. INSURED'S ADDRESS (No., Street) 167 CHEVY LANE

CITY	STATE	8. RESERVED FOR NUCC USE	CITY CLEVELAND	STATE OH

ZIP CODE	TELEPHONE (Include Area Code) ( )		ZIP CODE 44101	TELEPHONE (Include Area Code) ( )

9. OTHER INSURED'S NAME (Last Name, First Name, Middle Initial)	10. IS PATIENT'S CONDITION RELATED TO:	11. INSURED'S POLICY GROUP OR FECA NUMBER OH4071

a. OTHER INSURED'S POLICY OR GROUP NUMBER	a. EMPLOYMENT? (Current or Previous) □ YES [X] NO	a. INSURED'S DATE OF BIRTH MM DD YY 03 29 1985	SEX M □ F [X]

b. RESERVED FOR NUCC USE	b. AUTO ACCIDENT? □ YES [X] NO PLACE (State)	b. OTHER CLAIM ID (Designated by NUCC)

c. RESERVED FOR NUCC USE	c. OTHER ACCIDENT? □ YES [X] NO	c. INSURANCE PLAN NAME OR PROGRAM NAME ANTHEM BCBS PPO

d. INSURANCE PLAN NAME OR PROGRAM NAME	10d. CLAIM CODES (Designated by NUCC)	d. IS THERE ANOTHER HEALTH BENEFIT PLAN? □ YES [X] NO If yes, complete items 9, 9a, and 9d.

READ BACK OF FORM BEFORE COMPLETING & SIGNING THIS FORM.

12. PATIENT'S OR AUTHORIZED PERSON'S SIGNATURE I authorize the release of any medical or other information necessary to process this claim. I also request payment of government benefits either to myself or to the party who accepts assignment below.

SIGNED _SOF_   DATE _____

13. INSURED'S OR AUTHORIZED PERSON'S SIGNATURE I authorize payment of medical benefits to the undersigned physician or supplier for services described below.

SIGNED _SOF_

PATIENT AND INSURED INFORMATION →

FIGURE 7.2 Sample Completed CMS-1500, IN 1–13

---

13. INSURED'S OR AUTHORIZED PERSON'S SIGNATURE I authorize payment of medical benefits to the undersigned physician or supplier for services described below.

SIGNED _____

Item Number 13: Insured or Authorized Person's Signature This entry authorizes payment of medical benefits directly to the provider of the services listed on the claim. Enter "Signature on File," "SOF," or legal signature and the date signed, as appropriate. If there is no signature on the file, leave blank or enter "No Signature on File."

Physician or Supplier Information

The items in this part of the CMS-1500 claim form identify the health care provider, describe the services performed, and give the payer additional information to process the claim. Four types of providers may need to be reported: billing provider, pay-to provider, rendering provider, and referring provider.

The **billing provider** is a provider of health services, usually a physician practice. A **pay-to provider,** in contrast, is the person or organization that receives payment for the claim. The billing provider and the pay-to provider are very often the same. However, if a clearinghouse or billing service is authorized by the billing provider to transmit claims and process payments on their behalf, these service organizations are the pay-to providers. A **rendering provider** is a physician or other entity such as a lab that has provided the care. Again, it is possible that the rendering provider is the same as the billing provider. Finally, when another physician has sent the patient and needs to be identified as the *referring* provider (physician), the claim format allows for this data to be reported.

billing provider Person or organization sending a HIPAA claim.

pay-to provider Person or organization that will be paid for services on a HIPAA claim.

rendering provider Term used to identify an alternative physician or professional who provides the procedure on a claim.

COMPLIANCE GUIDELINE

Billing Provider Address

The billing provider's address must be a street address and may not be a PO Box or a lock box. Physicians who want payments sent to another address should use the pay-to address fields.

Item Number 14: Date of Current Illness, Injury, or Pregnancy (LMP) Enter the six-digit or eight-digit date for the first date of the present illness, injury, or pregnancy. For pregnancy, use the date of the last menstrual period (LMP) as the first date. This date refers to the first date of onset of illness, the actual date of injury, or the LMP for pregnancy.

14. DATE OF CURRENT ILLNESS, INJURY, or PREGNANCY (LMP)
MM   DD   YY   QUAL.

Item Number 15: Other Date Enter an "Other Date" related to the patient's condition or illness. The item number is asking whether the patient previously had a related condition. A previous pregnancy is not a similar illness. Leave blank if unknown.

15. OTHER DATE
QUAL.   MM   DD   YY

Item Number 16: Dates Patient Unable to Work in Current Occupation If the patient is employed and is unable to work in his or her current occupation, a six-digit or eight-digit date must be shown as the "from–to" dates that the patient is unable to work. "Dates patient unable to work in current occupation" refers to the time span the patient is or was unable to work. An entry in this field may indicate employment-related insurance coverage.

16. DATES PATIENT UNABLE TO WORK IN CURRENT OCCUPATION
MM   DD   YY   MM   DD   YY
FROM   TO

Item Number 17: Name of Referring Provider or Other Source Enter the name and credentials of the professional who referred, ordered, or supervised the service or supply on the claim.

17. NAME OF REFERRING PROVIDER OR OTHER SOURCE

Enter the applicable **qualifier,** which is a code indicating what the number stands for, to the left of the vertical dotted line. These can be listed: DN for referring provider, DK for ordering provider, or DQ for supervising provider.

qualifier Two-digit code for a type of provider identification number other than the NPI.

Item Number 17a and 17b (split field) The non-NPI ID number (for 17a) of the referring provider, ordering provider, or other source is the payer-assigned unique identifier of the physician or other health care provider. The non-NPI of the referring provider, ordering provider, or other source is put in IN 17a. The qualifier should also be reported above the dotted line on the left side of the box before the Other ID# is entered. The NUCC defines the qualifiers shown in Table 7.1. The NPI is entered in 17b.

17a.	
17b.	NPI

Item Number 18: Hospitalization Dates Related to Current Services The hospitalization dates related to current services refer to an inpatient stay and indicate the admission and discharge dates associated with the services on the claim.

18. HOSPITALIZATION DATES RELATED TO CURRENT SERVICES
MM   DD   YY   MM   DD   YY
FROM   TO

Table 7.1   Qualifiers for Non-NPI (Other ID) Numbers

Code	Definition
0B	State License Number
1G	Provider UPIN Number
G2	Provider Commercial Number
LU	Location Number (for supervising provider only)
N5	Provider Plan Network Identification Number
SY	Social Security Number (the SSN may not be used for Medicare)
X5	State Industrial Accident Provider Number
ZZ	Provider Taxonomy

If the services are needed because of a related hospitalization, enter the admission and discharge dates of that hospitalization in IN 18. For patients still hospitalized, the admission date is listed in the From box, and the To box is left blank.

19. ADDITIONAL CLAIM INFORMATION (Designated by NUCC)

Item Number 19: Additional Claim Information (Designated by NUCC) Refer to instructions from the payer regarding the use of this field. Some payers ask for certain identifiers in the field. If identifiers are reported in this field, the appropriate qualifiers describing the identifier should be used (see again Table 7.1).

claim attachment Documentation a provider sends a payer to support a claim.

This IN may be used to provide supplemental claim information, such as a **claim attachment** like a recovery plan, initial assessment, or immunization record.

20. OUTSIDE LAB?   **$ CHARGES**
☐ YES   ☐ NO

Item Number 20: Outside Lab? $ Charges "Outside lab? $ charges" indicates that services have been rendered by an independent provider as indicated in IN 32 and shows the related costs.

outside laboratory Purchased laboratory services.

Enter an X in No if no lab charges are reported. Complete this item when billing for laboratory services. Enter an X in Yes if the reported service was performed by an **outside laboratory.** If Yes is checked, enter the purchase price under "charges." A yes response indicates that the laboratory service was performed by an entity other than the entity billing for the service. When Yes is annotated, IN 32 must be completed. When billing for multiple purchased lab services, each service should be submitted on a separate claim.

21. DIAGNOSIS OR NATURE OF ILLNESS OR INJURY Relate A-L to service line below (24E)   ICD Ind.
A. _____   B. _____   C. _____   D. _____
E. _____   F. _____   G. _____   H. _____
I. _____   J. _____   K. _____   L. _____

Item Number 21: Diagnosis or Nature of Illness or Injury The *ICD Indicator* reports which version of ICD codes is being used, ICD-9-CM (code 9) or ICD-10-CM (code 0). Then the codes that describe the patient's condition are entered in priority order. The first code listed is the primary diagnosis. Additional codes for secondary diagnoses are used only when the diagnoses are directly related to the services being provided. Up to twelve codes can be entered. In 24E, relate lines A through L to the lines of service (see 24E below).

COMPLIANCE GUIDELINE

Diagnosis Code Required

A claim that does not report at least one diagnosis code will be denied.

22. RESUBMISSION CODE   **ORIGINAL REF. NO.**

Item Number 22: Resubmission and/or Original Reference Number Resubmission means the code and original reference number assigned by the destination payer or receiver to indicate a previously submitted claim or encounter. List the original reference number for resubmitted claims. Please refer to the most current instructions from the applicable public or private payer regarding the use of this field (e.g., code). When resubmitting a claim, enter the appropriate bill frequency code left justified in the left-hand side of the field.

BILLING TIP

Use the Period in Codes

Remember to enter the period when reporting diagnosis codes.

7- Replacement of prior claim

8- Void/cancel of prior claim

This Item Number is not intended for use for original claim submissions.

23. PRIOR AUTHORIZATION NUMBER

Item Number 23: Prior Authorization Number The prior authorization number refers to the payer-assigned number authorizing the service(s). Enter any of the following: prior authorization number or referral number, as assigned by the payer for the current service, or the Clinical Laboratory Improvement Amendments (CLIA) number or the mammography pre-certification number. Do not enter hyphens or spaces within the number.

Section 24 The term **service line information** describes section 24 of the claim, the part that reports the procedures—that is, the services—performed for the patient. Each item of service line information has a procedure code and a charge, with additional information as detailed below.

24. A. DATE(S) OF SERVICE From MM DD YY	To MM DD YY	B. PLACE OF SERVICE	C. EMG	D. PROCEDURES, SERVICES, OR SUPPLIES (Explain Unusual Circumstances) CPT/HCPCS	MODIFIER	E. DIAGNOSIS POINTER	F. $ CHARGES	G. DAYS OR UNITS	H. EPSDT Family Plan	I. ID. QUAL.	J. RENDERING PROVIDER ID. #
1										NPI	
2										NPI	
3										NPI	
4										NPI	
5										NPI	
6										NPI	

The six service lines in section 24, which contains INs 24A through 24J, are divided horizontally to fit both the NPI and a non-NPI identifier when required, as well as to permit the submission of supplemental information to support the billed service. For example, when billing HCPCS codes for the products such as drugs, the payer may require an indicator (N4) and the National Drug Code. The non-NPI identifier or supplemental information is to be placed in the upper shaded section of 24C through 24J.

Item Number 24A: Date(s) of Service Date(s) of service indicate the actual month, day, and year the service was provided. "Grouping services" refers to a charge for a series of identical services without listing each date of service.

Enter the from and to date(s) of service: If there is only one date of service, enter that date under From. Leave To blank or reenter the From date. If grouping services, the place of service, procedure code, charges, and individual provider for each line must be identical for that service line. Grouping is allowed only for services on consecutive days. The number of days must correspond to the number of units in IN 24G.

Item Number 24B: Place of Service In 24B, enter the appropriate two-digit code from the place of service code list for each item used or service performed. A **place of service (POS)** code describes the location where the service was provided. It is also called the facility type code. Table 7.2 shows typical codes for medical office claims.

Table 7.2 Selected Place of Service Codes

Code	Definition
11	Office
12	Home
22	Outpatient hospital
23	Emergency room—hospital
24	Ambulatory surgical center
31	Skilled nursing facility
81	Independent laboratory

BILLING TIP

Deleted TOS Codes

IN 24C previously was "Type of Service," which is no longer used. TOS codes have been eliminated from the CMS-1500 claim.

BILLING TIP

How Many Pointers?

According to the NUCC, up to four diagnosis pointers can be listed per service line.

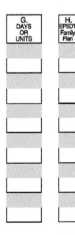

Item Number 24C: EMG   Item number 24C is EMG, for emergency indicator, as defined by federal or state regulations or programs, payer contracts, or HIPAA claim rules. Generally, an emergency situation is one in which the patient requires immediate medical intervention as a result of severe, life-threatening, or potentially disabling conditions. Check with the payer to determine whether the emergency indicator is necessary. If it is required, enter Y (yes) or N (no) in the unshaded bottom portion of the field.

Item Number 24D: Procedures, Services, or Supplies   Enter the CPT or HCPCS code(s) and modifier(s) (if applicable) from the appropriate code set in effect on the date of service. State-defined procedure and supply codes are needed for workers' compensation claims.

Item Number 24E: Diagnosis Pointer   The diagnosis pointer refers to the line letter from IN 21 that provides the link between diagnosis and treatment. In IN 24E, enter the diagnosis code reference letter A through L as shown in IN 21 to relate the date of service and the procedures performed to the primary diagnosis. When multiple diagnoses are related to one service, the reference letter for the primary diagnosis should be listed first; other applicable diagnosis reference letters should follow. Do not enter diagnosis codes in 24E.

Item Number 24F: $ Charges   Item number 24F lists the total billed charges for each service line in IN 24D. A charge for each service line must be reported. If the claim reports an encounter with no charge, such as a capitated visit, a value of zero (0) may be used.

The numbers should be entered without dollar signs and decimals. If the services are for multiple days or units, the number of days or units must be multiplied by the charge to determine the entry in IN 24F. This is done automatically when a PMP is used to create the claim.

Item Number 24G: Days or Units   The item *days or units* refers to the number of days corresponding to the dates entered in 24A or units as defined in CPT or HCPCS. Enter the number of days or units. This field is most commonly used for multiple visits, units of supplies, anesthesia units or minutes, or oxygen volume. If only one service is performed, the numeral 1 must be entered. Enter numbers left justified in the field. No leading zeros are required. If reporting a fraction of a unit, use the decimal point.

Item Number 24H: EPSDT Family Plan   The Medicaid EPSDT/family plan identifies certain services that may be covered under some state plans (see the Medicaid chapter).

Item Number 24I: ID Qualifier and 24J (Rendering Provider ID#) Item number 24I works together with IN 24J. These boxes are used to enter an ID number for the *rendering provider*—the individual who is providing the service. This identifier is required only if the rendering provider is not the billing provider shown in IN 33a and b.

If the number is an NPI, it goes in IN 24J in the nonshaded area next to the 24I NPI label. If the number is a non-NPI, the qualifier identifying the type of number goes in IN 24I next to the number in 24J. Refer back to Table 7.1 for the common qualifiers.

Item Number 25: Federal Tax ID Number Enter the billing provider's (IN 33) Employer Identification Number (EIN) or Social Security Number in IN 25. Mark the appropriate box (SSI or EIN). Do not use hyphens in numbers.

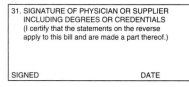

Item Number 26: Patient's Account No. Enter the patient account number used by the PMP to help identify the patient and post payments when working with RAs.

Item Number 27: Accept Assignment? Enter a capital X in the correct box. "Yes" means that the provider agrees to accept assignment, which is the mandated choice.

Item Number 28: Total Charge Item number 28 lists the total of all charges in item number 24F, lines 1 through 6. Do not use dollar signs or commas. If the claim is to be submitted on paper and there are more services to be billed, put *continued* here and put the total charge on the last claim form page.

Item Number 29: Amount Paid Enter the amount that the patient and/or other payers have paid toward this claim. Enter 00 in the cents area if the amount is a whole number.

Item Number 30: Reserved for NUCC Use This IN is reserved for NUCC use. The previous entry, "Balance Due," has been eliminated.

Item Number 31: Signature of Physician or Supplier Including Degrees or Credentials This feature no longer exists, leave IN 31 blank.

COMPLIANCE GUIDELINE

NUCC on IN 27

NUCC requires the YES answer for all payers.

Item Number 32, 32a, and 32b: Service Facility Location Information If the information in Item number 33 is different from Item number 32, enter the name, address, city, state, and nine-digit Zip code of the location where the services were rendered. In 32a, enter the NPI of the service facility location. In 32b, enter the two-digit qualifier for a non-NPI number. IN 32 allows for reporting another location for the service, such as a hospital.

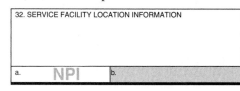

Physicians who are billing for purchased diagnostic tests or radiology services must identify the supplier's name, address, Zip code, and NPI in IN 32a.

Enter the payer-assigned identifying non-NPI number of the service facility in IN 32b with its qualifier (see Table 7.1).

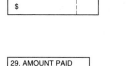

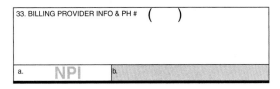

FIGURE 7.3 Sample Completed CMS-1500, INs 14–33

Item Number 33, 33a, and 33b: Billing Provider Information and Phone Number

IN 33 identifies the provider that is requesting to be paid for the services rendered and should always be completed.

Enter the provider's or supplier's billing name, address, ZIP code, phone number, NPI, and any non-NPI number with an appropriate qualifier. Note that no punctuation is used in the address, other than the hyphen for the nine-digit Zip code. Also, no space or hyphen is used as a separator within the phone number or between the qualifier and non-NPI identifier. The NPI should be placed in IN 33a. Enter the identifying non-NPI number of the billing provider in box 33b. The appropriate qualifier describing that the number is a non-NPI identifier is reported to the left of the non-NPI number in IN 33b. If the billing provider is a group, then the rendering provider NPI goes in IN24J. If the billing provider is a solo practitioner, then Item number 24J is left blank. The referring provider NPI goes in IN 17b.

taxonomy code Administrative code set used to report a physician's specialty.

A Note on Taxonomy Codes

Other ID number may be completed with a **taxonomy code** as well as a legacy number. (If two numbers are reported, they should be separated by three blank spaces.) A taxonomy code is a ten-digit number that stands for a physician's medical specialty. The type of specialty may affect the physician's pay, usually because of the payer's contract with the physician. For example, nuclear medicine is usually a higher-paid specialty than is internal medicine. An internist who is also certified in nuclear medicine would report the nuclear medicine taxonomy code when billing for that service and use the internal medicine taxonomy code when reporting internal medicine claims. Most PMPs store a taxonomy-code database.

All Administrative Code Sets for HIPAA Transactions

www.wpc-edi.com/codes/codes/Codes.asp

administrative code set
Required codes for various data elements.

Summary of Claim Information

Table 7.3 on the next two pages summarizes the information that is required for the correct completion of the CMS-1500 claim.

Exercise 7.1 Completing a CMS-1500 Form

Generate a claim for Ann Ingram's visit with Dr. Clarke.

Follow the steps at www.mhhe.com/newbycarr to complete the exercise at connect.mcgraw-hill.com on your own once you have watched the demo and tried the steps with prompts in practice mode. Use the information provided in the scenario to complete the exercise.

connect™ (plus+)

Exercise 7.2 Completing a CMS-1500 Form for a Dependent

Sarina Bell had a visit with Dr. Clarke. She is covered as a dependent under Herbert Bell's plan. Generate a claim for her visit.

Follow the steps at www.mhhe.com/newbycarr to complete the exercise at connect.mcgraw-hill.com on your own once you have watched the demo and tried the steps with prompts in practice mode. Use the information provided in the scenario to complete the exercise.

connect™ (plus+)

THINKING IT THROUGH 7.3

1. A patient who had a minor automobile accident was treated in the emergency room and released. What place of service code is reported?

2. If a physician practice uses a billing service to prepare and transmit its health care claims, which entity is the pay-to provider and which is the billing provider?

Table 7.3 Summary of CMS-1500 Claim Completion

Item Number	Content
1	**Medicare, Medicaid, TRICARE, CHAMPVA, Group Health Plan, FECA Black Lung, Other:** Enter the type of insurance.
1a	**Insured's ID Number:** The insurance identification number that appears on the insurance card of the policyholder.
2	**Patient's Name:** As it appears on the insurance card. Report only if different from the Insured.
3	**Patient's Birth Date/Sex:** Date of birth in eight-digit format; appropriate selection for male or female.
4	**Insured's Name:** The full name of the person who holds the insurance policy (the insured). If the patient is a dependent, the insured may be a spouse, parent, or other person.
5	**Patient's Address:** Address includes the number and street, city, state, and ZIP code. Report only if different from the Insured.
6	**Patient's Relationship to Insured:** Self, spouse, child, or other. *Self* means that the patient is the policyholder.
7	**Insured's Address:** Address of the person listed in IN 4.
8	**Reserved for NUCC Use:** Leave blank.
9	**Other Insured's Name:** If there is additional insurance coverage, the insured's name.
9a	**Other Insured's Policy or Group Number:** The policy or group number of the other insurance plan.
9b & c	**Reserved for NUCC Use:** Leave blank.
9d	**Insurance Plan Name or Program Name:** Other insured's insurance plan or program name.
10a–10c	**Is Patient Condition Related to:** To indicate whether the patient's condition is the result of a work injury, an automobile accident, or another type of accident.
10d	**Claim Codes (Designated by NUCC):** Report condition codes when applicable.
11	**Insured's Policy Group or FECA Number:** As it appears on the insurance identification card.
11a	**Insured's Date of Birth/Sex:** The insured's date of birth and sex.
11b	**Other Claim ID (Designated by NUCC):** Leave blank.
11c	**Insurance Plan Name or Program Name:** Of the insured.
11d	**Is There Another Health Benefit Plan?** Yes if the patient is covered by additional insurance. If yes, IN 9, 9a, and 9d must also be completed.
12	**Patient's or Authorized Person's Signature:** If the patient's or authorized person's signature is on file authorizing the release of information, enter "Signature on File," "SOF," or a legal signature. When legal signature, enter date signed in 6-digit format (MMDDYY) or 8-digit format (MMDDCCYY). Leave blank or enter "No Signature on File" if there is no signature on file.
13	**Insured or Authorized Person's Signature:** Enter "Signature on File," "SOF," or legal signature to indicate there is a signature on file authorizing payment of medical benefits. If there is no signature on file, leave blank or enter "No Signature on File."
14	**Date of Current Illness, Injury, or Pregnancy (LMP):** The date that symptoms first began for the current illness, injury, or pregnancy. For pregnancy, enter the date of the patient's last menstrual period (LMP).
15	**Other Date:** Enter an "Other Date" related to the patient's condition or treatment. Leave blank if unknown.

| Table 7.3 | *Continued* |

16	**Dates Patient Unable to Work in Current Occupation:** Dates the patient has been unable to work.
17	**Name of Referring Physician or Other Source:** Name and credentials of the physician or other source who referred the patient to the billing provider.
17a	**ID Number of Referring Physician:** Identifying number(s) for the referring physician.
18	**Hospitalization Dates Related to Current Services:** If the services provided are needed because of a related hospitalization, the admission and discharge dates are entered. For patients still hospitalized, the admission date is listed in the From box, and the To box is left blank.
19	**Additional Claim Information (Designated by NUCC):** Refer to instructions from the payer regarding this field.
20	**Outside Lab? $ Charges:** Completed if billing for outside lab services. Enter an X in No if no lab charges are reported on the claim.
21	**Diagnosis or Nature of Illness or Injury:** ICD-9-CM or ICD-10-CM indicator and up to twelve diagnosis codes in priority order.
22	**Resubmission and/or Original Reference Number:** List the original reference number for resubmitted claims.
23	**Prior Authorization Number:** If required by payer, report the assigned number.
24A	**Dates of Service:** Date(s) service was provided.
24B	**Place of Service:** A place of service (POS) code describes the location at which the service was provided.
24C	**EMG:** For emergency claims only.
24D	**Procedures, Services, or Supplies:** CPT or HCPCS codes and applicable modifiers for services provided.
24E	**Diagnosis Pointer:** Using the letters (A through L) listed to the left of the diagnosis codes in IN 21, enter the diagnoses for each service listed in IN 24D.
24F	**$ Charges:** For each service listed in IN 24D, enter charges without dollar signs and decimals.
24G	**Days or Units:** The number of days or units.
24H	**EPSDT Family Plan:** Medicaid-specific.
24I and 24J	**ID Qualifier and Rendering Provider ID Number:** Only report when different from IN 33A.
25	**Federal Tax ID Number:** Billing provider's (IN33) Employer Identification Number (EIN) or Social Security number.
26	**Patient's Account No.:** Patient account number used by the practice's accounting system.
27	**Accept Assignment?** Select Yes.
28	**Total Charge:** Total of all charges in IN 24F.
29	**Amount Paid:** Amount of the payments received for the services listed on this claim from patients and payers.
30	**Reserved for NUCC Use:** Leave blank.
31	**Signature of Physician or Supplier Including Degrees or Credentials:** Leave blank.
32	**Service Facility Location Information:** Complete if different from the billing provider information in IN 33.
33	**Billing Provider Information:** Billing office name, address, 9-digit Zip code, phone number, and ID numbers.

7.4 The HIPAA Claim

Most of the information reported on the CMS-1500 is also used to complete the HIPAA claim. PMPs are set up to automatically supply the various items of information for electronic claims. There are some different terms used in instructions for the HIPAA claim, though, and some additional data must be relayed to the payer. This section covers those terms and data items as it presents the basic organization of the HIPAA claim.

Claim Organization

data element Smallest unit of information in a HIPAA transaction.

The HIPAA claim contains many **data elements.** Examples of data elements are a patient's first name, middle name or initial, and last name. Although these data elements are essentially the same as those used to complete a CMS-1500, they are organized in a different way. This organization is efficient for electronic transmission, rather than for use on a paper form.

The elements are structured in the five major sections, or levels, of the claim:

1. Provider.
2. Subscriber (guarantor, insured, policyholder) and patient (the subscriber or another person).
3. Payer.
4. Claim details.
5. Services.

The levels are set up as a hierarchy, with the provider at the top, so that when the claim is sent electronically, the only data elements that have to be sent are those that do not repeat previous data. For example, when the provider is sending a batch of claims, provider data are sent once for all of them. If the subscriber and the patient are the same, then the patient data are not needed. But if the subscriber and the patient are different people, information about both is transmitted.

There are four types of data elements:

1. Required (R) data elements: For required data elements, the provider must supply the data element on every claim, and payers must accept the data element.
2. Required if applicable (RIA) data elements: These situational data elements are conditional on specific situations. For example, if the insured differs from the patient, the insured's name must be entered.
3. Not required unless specified under contract (NRUC): These elements are required only when they are part of a contract between a provider and a payer or when they are specified by state or federal legislation or regulations.
4. Not required (NR): These elements are not required for submission and/or receipt of a claim or encounter.

Table 7.4 shows all the data elements that can be reported. Review this table as you read the rest of this section.

Provider Information

COMPLIANCE GUIDELINE

Report Codes for Date of Service

The correct medical code sets are those valid at the time the health care is provided. The correct administrative code sets are those valid at the time the transaction—such as the claim—is started.

Like the CMS-1500, the HIPAA claim requires data on these types of providers, as applicable:

▶ Billing provider.
▶ Pay-to provider.
▶ Rendering provider.
▶ Referring provider.

For each provider, an NPI and possibly non-NPI numbers with the qualifiers as were shown in Table 7.1 are reported. The billing provider contact name and telephone number are required data elements.

Table 7.4 HIPAA Claim Data Elements

PROVIDER, SUBSCRIBER, PATIENT, PAYER

Billing Provider

Last or Organization Name
   First Name
   Middle Name
   Name Suffix
Primary Identifier: NPI
Address 1
Address 2
City Name
State/Province Code
Zip Code
Country Code
Secondary Identifiers, such as
   State License Number
Contact Name
Communication Numbers
   Telephone Number
   Fax
   E-mail
   Telephone Extension
Taxonomy Code
Currency Code

Pay-to Provider

Last or Organization Name
   First Name
   Middle Name
   Name Suffix
Primary Identifier: NPI
Address 1
Address 2

City Name
State/Province Code
Zip Code
Country Code
Secondary Identifiers, such as
   State License Number
Taxonomy Code

Subscriber

Insured Group or Policy Number
Group or Plan Name
Insurance Type Code
Claim Filing Indicator Code
Last Name
First Name
Middle Name
Name Suffix
Primary Identifier
   Member Identification Number
   National Individual Identifier
   IHS/CHS Tribe Residency Code
Secondary Identifiers
   IHS Health Record Number
   Insurance Policy Number
   SSN
Patient's Relationship to
   Subscriber
Other Subscriber Information
Birth Date
Gender Code
Address Line 1
Address Line 2

City Name
State/Province Code
Zip Code
Country Code

Patient

Last Name
First Name
Middle Name
Name Suffix
Primary Identifier
   Member ID Number
   National Individual Identifier
Address 1
Address 2
City Name
State/Province Code
Zip Code
Country Code
Birth Date
Gender Code
Secondary Identifiers
   IHS Health Record Number
   Insurance Policy Number
   SSN
Death Date
Weight
Pregnancy Indicator

Responsible Party

Last or Organization Name
First Name

Middle Name
Suffix Name
Address 1
Address 2
City Name
State/Province Code
Zip Code
Country Code

Payer

Payer Responsibility Sequence
   Number Code
Organization Name
Primary Identifier
   Payer ID
   National Plan ID
Address 1
Address 2
City Name
State/Province Code
Zip Code
Secondary Identifiers
   Claim Office Number
   NAIC Code
   TIN
Assignment of Benefits
Release of Information Code
Patient Signature Source Code
Referral Number
Prior Authorization Number

CLAIM

Claim Level

Claim Control Number (Patient
   Account Number)
Total Submitted Charges
Place of Service Code
Claim Frequency Code
Provider Signature on File
Medicare Assignment Code
Participation Agreement
Delay Reason Code
Onset of Current Symptoms or
   Illness Date
Similar Illness/Symptom Onset
   Date
Last Menstrual Period Date
Admission Date
Discharge Date

Patient Amount Paid
Claim Original Reference
   Number
Investigational Device Exemption
   Number
Medical Record Number
Note Reference Code
Claim Note
Diagnosis Code 1–12
Accident Claims
   Accident Cause
      Auto Accident
      Another Party Responsible
      Employment Related
      Other Accident
Auto Accident State/Province
   Code

Auto Accident Country Code
Accident Date
Accident Hour

Rendering Provider

Last or Organization Name
First Name
Middle Name
Name Suffix
Primary Identifier: NPI
Taxonomy Code
Secondary Identifiers

Referring/PCP Providers

Last or Organization Name
First Name
Middle Name

Name Suffix
Primary Identifier: NPI
Taxonomy Code
Secondary Identifiers
Proc

Service Facility Location

Type Code
Last or Organization Name
Primary Identifier: NPI
Address 1
Address 2
City Name
State/Province Code
Zip Code
Country Code
Secondary Identifiers

SERVICE LINE INFORMATION

Procedure Type Code
Procedure Code
Modifiers 1–4
Line Item Charge Amount
Units of Service/Anesthesia
   Minutes
Place of Service Code

Diagnosis Code Pointers 1–4
Emergency Indicator
Copay Status Code
Service Date Begun
Service Date End
Shipped Date
Onset Date

Similar Illness or Symptom Date
Referral/Prior Authorization
   Number
Line Item Control Number
Ambulatory Patient Group
Sales Tax Amount
Postage Claimed Amount

Line Note Text
Rendering/Referring/PCP
   Provider at the Service
   Line Level
Service Facility Location at the
   Service Line Level

Table 7.5 Claim Filing Indicator Codes

Table 7.5 Claim Filing Indicator Codes

Code	Definition
09	Self-pay
10	Central certification
11	Other nonfederal programs
12	Preferred provider organization (PPO)
13	Point of service (POS)
14	Exclusive provider organization (EPO)
15	Indemnity insurance
16	Health maintenance organization (HMO)
AM	Automobile medical
BL	Blue Cross and Blue Shield
CH	CHAMPUS (TRICARE)
CI	Commercial insurance company
DS	Disability
FI	Federal Employees Program
HM	Health maintenance organization
LM	Liability medical
MA	Medicare Part A
MB	Medicare Part B
MC	Medicaid
OF	Other federal program
TV	Title V
VA	Department of Veteran's Affairs plan
WC	Workers' compensation health claim
ZZ	Mutually Defined

Table 7.6 Relationship Codes

Code	Definition
01	Spouse
04	Grandfather or grandmother
05	Grandson or granddaughter
07	Nephew or niece
09	Adopted child
10	Foster child
15	Ward
17	Stepson or stepdaughter
19	Child
20	Employee
21	Unknown
22	Handicapped dependent
23	Sponsored dependent
24	Dependent of a minor dependent
29	Significant other
32	Mother
33	Father
34	Other adult
36	Emancipated minor
39	Organ donor
40	Cadaver donor
41	Injured plaintiff
43	Child where insured has no financial responsibility
53	Life partner
G8	Other relationship

Subscriber Information

subscriber The insured.

The HIPAA claim uses the term **subscriber** for the insurance policyholder or guarantor; this term is the same as insured on the CMS-1500 claim. The subscriber may be the patient or someone other than the patient. If the subscriber and patient are not the same person, data elements about the patient are also required. The name and address of any responsible party—an entity or person other than the subscriber or patient who has financial responsibility for the bill—are reported if applicable.

Claim Filing Indicator Code

claim filing indicator code
Administrative code that identifies the type of health plan.

A **claim filing indicator code** is an administrative code used to identify the type of health plan, such as a PPO. One of the claim filing indicator codes shown in Table 7.5 is reported. These codes are valid until a National Payer ID system becomes law.

Relationship of Patient to Subscriber

individual relationship code
Administrative code specifying the patient's relationship to the subscriber.

The HIPAA claim allows for a more detailed description of the relationship of the patient to the subscriber than does the CMS-1500. When the patient and the subscriber are not the same person, an **individual relationship code** is required to specify the patient's relationship to the subscriber. The current list of choices is shown in Table 7.6.

Other Data Elements

These situational data elements are required if another payer is known to potentially be involved in paying the claim:

► Other Subscriber Birth Date
► Other Subscriber Gender Code (F [female], M [male], or U [unknown])
► Other Subscriber Address

Payer Information

This section of the HIPAA claim contains information about the payer to whom the claim is going to be sent, called the **destination payer.** A payer responsibility sequence number code identifies whether the insurance carrier is the primary (P), secondary (S), or tertiary (T) payer. This code is used when more than one insurance plan is responsible for payment. The T code is used for the payer of last resort, such as Medicaid (see the chapter about Medicaid for an explanation of "payer of last resort").

destination payer Health plan receiving a HIPAA claim.

Claim Information

The claim information section of the HIPAA claim reports information related to just that particular claim. For example, an accident description is included if the patient's visit is the result of an accident. Data elements about the rendering provider—if not the same as the billing provider or the pay-to provider—are supplied. If another provider referred the patient for care, the claim reports data elements about the referring physician or primary care physician (PCP).

Claim Control Number

A **claim control number,** unique for each claim, is assigned by the medical office sending the claim. The maximum number of characters is twenty. The claim control number will appear on payments that come from payers, so it is very important for tracking purposes.

claim control number Unique number assigned to a claim by the sender.

Although sometimes called the patient account number, the claim control number should not be the same as the practice's account number for the patient. It may, however, incorporate the account number. For example, if the account number is A1234, a three-digit number might be added for each claim, beginning with A1234001.

Claim Frequency Code

The **claim frequency code**, also called the **claim submission reason code**, for physician practice claims indicates whether this claim is one of the following.

claim frequency code (claim submission reason code) Administrative code that identifies the claim as original, replacement, or void/cancel action.

Code	Definition
1	*Original Claim*—The initial claim sent for the patient, date of service, and procedure.
7	*Replacement of Prior Claim*—Used if an original claim is being replaced with a new claim.
8	*Void/Cancel of Prior Claim*—Used to completely eliminate a submitted claim.

The first claim is always a 1. Payers do not usually allow for corrections to be sent after a claim has been submitted; instead, an entire new claim is transmitted. However, some payers cannot process a claim with the frequency code 7 (replace a submitted claim). In this situation, submit a void/cancel of prior claim (frequency code 8) to cancel the original incorrect claim, and then submit a new, correct claim.

When a claim is replaced, the original claim number (Claim Original Reference Number) is reported.

Diagnosis Codes

The HIPAA claim permits up to twelve diagnosis codes to be reported. The order of entry is not regulated. Each diagnosis code must be directly related to the patient's treatment.

Up to four of these codes can be linked to each procedure code that is reported.

Claim Note

A claim note may be used when a statement needs to be included, such as to satisfy a state requirement or to provide details about a patient's medical treatment that are not reported elsewhere in the claim.

Service Line Information

The HIPAA claim has the same elements as the CMS-1500 at the service line level. Different information for a particular service line, such as a prior authorization number that applies only to that service, can be supplied at the service line level.

Diagnosis Code Pointers

A total of four diagnosis codes can be linked to each service line procedure. At least one diagnosis code must be linked to the procedure code. Codes two, three, and four may also be linked, in declining level of importance regarding the patient's treatment, to the service line.

Line Item Control Number

line item control number
Unique number assigned to each service line item reported.

A **line item control number** is a unique number assigned by the sender to each service line. Like the claim control number, it is used to track payments from the insurance carrier, but for a particular service rather than for the entire claim.

COMPLIANCE GUIDELINE

Attachments and PHI

A claim payer should receive only what is needed to process a claim. If an attachment has PHI related to another patient, those data must be marked over or deleted. Information about other dates of service or conditions not pertinent to the claim should also be crossed through or deleted.

Claim Attachments

A *claim attachment* is additional data in printed or electronic format sent to support a claim. Examples include lab results, specialty consultation notes, and discharge notes. A HIPAA transaction standard for electronic health care claim attachments is under development. When it is adopted, payers will be required to accept all attachments that are submitted by providers according to the standard. Until then, health plans can require providers to submit claim attachments in the format they specify.

THINKING IT THROUGH 7.4

1. A retiree is covered by his wife's insurance policy. His wife is still working and receives health benefits through her employer, which has a PPO plan.
   A. What code describes the spouse's relationship to the subscriber?
   B. What claim filing indicator code is reported?
   C. What claim filing indicator code is likely to be used if the insurance is TRICARE?
2. What type of code would show whether a claim is the original claim, a replacement, or being cancelled?
3. What is the purpose of a claim control number?
4. What is the purpose of a line item control number?

7.5 Health Care Claim Transmission

Claims are prepared for transmission after all required data elements have been posted to the PMP. The data elements that are transmitted are not seen physically, as they would be on a paper form. Instead, these elements are in a computer file.

Practices handle transmission of electronic claims—which may be called electronic media claims, or EMC—in a variety of ways. By far the most common method is to hire outside vendors—clearinghouses—to handle this task. The outside vendor is a business associate under HIPAA that must follow the practice's guidelines to ensure that patients' PHI remains secure and private.

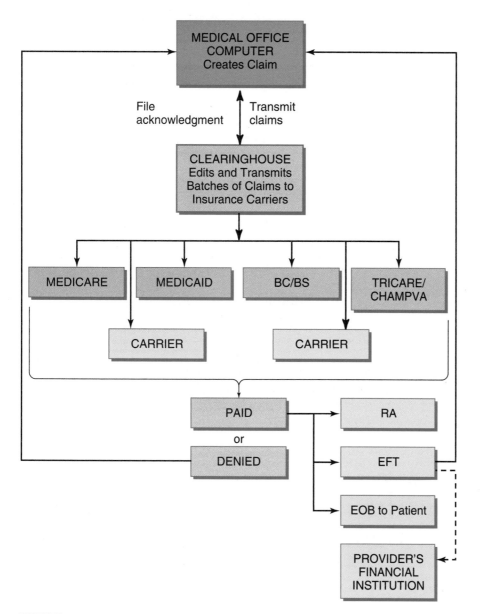

FIGURE 7.4 Claim Flow Using a Clearinghouse

There are three major methods of transmitting claims electronically: clearinghouse use, direct transmission, and direct data entry.

Use a Clearinghouse

The majority of providers use clearinghouses to send and receive data in correct EDI format. Under HIPAA, clearinghouses can accept nonstandard formats and translate them into the standard format. Clearinghouses must receive all required data elements from providers; they cannot create or modify data content. The typical flow of a claim ready for transmission is shown in Figure 7.4. Note that in some cases both the sender and the receiver have clearinghouses, so the provider's clearinghouse transmits to the payer's clearinghouse.

After a PMP-created file is sent, the clearinghouse correlates, or "maps," the content of each Item Number or data element to the HIPAA 837 transaction based on the payer's instructions. When the PMP has sent the claims, a report provides a summary of what was sent. Later, the receiver will send back an electronic response showing that the transmission was received.

Transmit Claims Directly

In the direct transmission approach, providers and payers exchange transactions directly without using a clearinghouse. To do this requires special technology. The provider must supply all the HIPAA data elements and follow specific EDI formatting rules.

Use Direct Data Entry (DDE)

Some payers offer online direct data entry (DDE) to providers. DDE involves using an Internet-based service into which employees key the standard data elements. Although the data elements must meet the HIPAA standards regarding content, they do not have to be formatted for standard EDI. Instead, they are loaded directly into the health plans' computers.

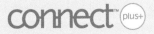

Exercise 7.3 Submitting Claims Electronically

Prepare a batch of electronic claims for transmission to a clearinghouse and review the Claim Edits Report.

Follow the steps at www.mhhe.com/newbycarr to complete the exercise at connect.mcgraw-hill.com on your own once you have watched the demo and tried the steps with prompts in practice mode. Use the information provided in the scenario to complete the exercise.

THINKING IT THROUGH 7.5

1. Based on Figure 7.4, what are the key functions of a clearinghouse?

7.6 Billing Secondary Payers

The practice has a schedule for transmitting claims, such as daily or every other day, which is followed. Claims are then received and processed by the *primary* payer—the plan that is the patient's primary insurance—which sends back an RA (*remittance advice*) detailing the reasons for the payment that is made. When a patient is covered by more than one health plan, the second and any other plans must be sent claims. These **secondary claims** (and, occasionally, **tertiary claims**) report what the primary payer paid on the claim. This fact is used by the secondary payer to calculate what, if anything, its payment obligations are.

secondary claim Claim sent to a secondary payer.

tertiary claim Claim sent to a tertiary payer.

Electronic Claims

The medical assistant transmits a claim to the secondary payer with the primary RA, sent either electronically or on paper, according to the payer's procedures. The secondary payer determines whether additional benefits are due under the policy's coordination of benefits (COB) provisions and sends payment with another RA to the billing provider. This flow is shown in Figure 7.5a.

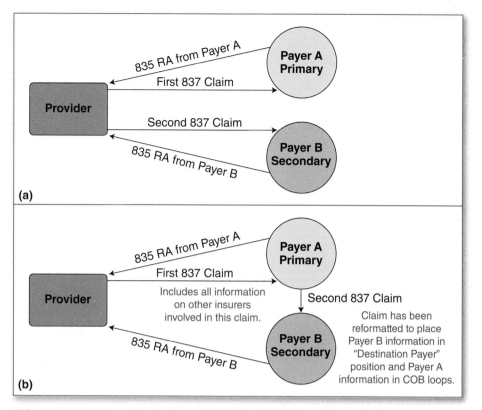

FIGURE 7.5 (a) Provider-to-Payer COB Model, (b) Provider-to-Payer-to-Payer COB Model

The practice does not send a claim to the secondary payer when the primary payer handles the coordination of benefits transaction. In this case, the primary payer electronically sends the COB transaction, which is the same HIPAA 837 that reports the primary claim, to the secondary payer. This flow is shown in Figure 7.5b.

When the primary payer forwards the COB transaction, a message appears on the primary payer's RA. For example, on a Medicare RA, COB is indicated by the phrase "CLAIM INFORMATION FORWARDED TO," followed by the name of the secondary payer, such as Anthem BCBS/CT State Retirement, Benefit Planners, and so forth. Medicare has a consolidated claims crossover process that is managed by a special coordination of benefits contractor (COBC). Plans that are supplemental to Medicare sign one national crossover agreement.

Paper Claims

If a paper RA is received, the procedure is to use the CMS-1500 to bill the secondary health plan that covers the beneficiary. The medical assistant completes the claim form and sends it with the primary RA attached.

THINKING IT THROUGH 7.6

1. In your opinion, is it more efficient to process secondary claims when paper claims are used or if electronic transactions are in place?

Chapter Summary

Learning Outcomes	Key Concepts/Examples
7.1 Outline the benefits of using practice management programs to prepare health care claims. Pages 146–148	Practice management programs (PMPs) increase efficiency by storing repeatedly used information in a database that can be accessed quickly. The major databases in PMPs are • Provider • Patient/Guarantor • Insurance Carriers • Diagnosis Codes • Procedure Codes • Transactions
7.2 Distinguish between the electronic and paper-based claim transactions. Pages 148–149	• The HIPAA mandated electronic transaction for claims is often called the "HIPAA claim" or the "837P claim" and is based on the CMS-1500, which is a paper claim form. • The information on the electronic transaction and paper form is the same, with a few exceptions.
7.3 Complete a CMS-1500 form. Pages 149–163	• The CMS claim form contains thirty-three item numbers, or information boxes. • Item numbers 1 through 13 refer to the patient and the patient's insurance coverage. • This information is found on the patient information form and the patient insurance card. • Item numbers 14 through 33 contain information about the provider, the patient's diagnosis, procedures performed, and the charge for services. • This information is often located on the patient's encounter form.
7.4 Discuss the data elements entered in the five sections of the HIPAA 837 claim transaction. Pages 164–168	The HIPAA claim contains data elements that are structured in the five major sections of the HIPAA 837 transaction. These five major sections include • Provider information • Subscriber information • Payer information • Claim information • Service line information
7.5 State the three major methods of electronic claim transmission. Pages 168–170	Practices handle the transmission of electronic claims with three major methods: • The majority of providers use clearinghouses to send and receive data in correct EDI format. • In the direct transmission approach, providers and payers exchange transactions directly without using a clearinghouse. • Some payers offer online direct data entry (DDE) to providers, which involves using an Internet-based service into which employees key the standard data elements.
7.6 Explain the process for billing secondary payers. Pages 170–171	• Secondary claims are submitted after the primary payer issues an RA (remittance advice) detailing how the claim was processed. • Secondary claims can be submitted electronically or on paper with the primary RA. • When the primary payer handles the coordination of benefits (COB) the practice does not submit a claim to the secondary payer.

Using Terminology

Match the key terms in the left column with the definitions in the right column.

_____ 1. [LO 7.3] Billing provider

_____ 2. [LO 7.4] Claim control number

_____ 3. [LO 7.4] Destination payer

_____ 4. [LO 7.4] Line item control number

_____ 5. [LO 7.3] Pay-to provider

_____ 6. [LO 7.3] POS code

_____ 7. [LO 7.6] Secondary claim

_____ 8. [LO 7.3] Rendering provider

_____ 9. [LO 7.4] Subscriber

_____ 10. [LO 7.3] Taxonomy code

A. Unique number assigned by the sender to a claim.

B. Unique number assigned by the sender to each service line on a claim.

C. Claim sent to a secondary carrier after the primary carrier has paid on a claim.

D. Stands for the type of provider specialty.

E. Entity providing patient care for this claim if other than the billing or pay-to provider.

F. Entity that is to receive payment for the claim.

G. Stands for the type of facility in which services reported on the claim were provided.

H. Insurance carrier that is to receive the claim.

I. Entity that is sending the claim to the payer.

J. The insurance policyholder or guarantor for the claim.

Checking Your Understanding

Write the letter of the choice that best completes the statement or answers the question.

1. **[LO 7.3]** If a physician uses a billing service to prepare and transmit its health care claims, which entity is the pay-to provider? _____
   A. Billing service
   B. Physician
   C. Referring provider
   D. Rendering provider

2. **[LO 7.1])** Medical PMPs store information such as patients' names in _____.
   A. Transactions
   B. Audit/edit reports
   C. Databases
   D. Taxonomy codes

3. **[LO 7.5]** What is the most common method used to submit health care claims? _____
   A. Using a clearinghouse
   B. Direct data entry
   C. Direct transmission
   D. Patient assistance

4. **[LO 7.2]** The name of the paper claim form is _____.
   A. HIPAA 837
   B. CMS-1492
   C. CMS-1500
   D. 837P

connect (plus+)

Enhance your learning at mcgrawhillconnect.com!
- Practice Exercises   • Worksheets
- Activities   • Integrated eBook

5. **[LO 7.2]** Which organization is in charge of the content of claims? _____
   A. CMS
   B. NUCC
   C. HIPAA
   D. PMP

6. **[LO 7.4]** On a HIPAA claim, the line item control number is in the _____.
   A. Claim information section
   B. Provider information section
   C. Services section
   D. Payer information section

7. **[LO 7.4]** If the subscriber and the patient are not the same person, what type of code describes this? _____
   A. Relationship code
   B. Place of service code
   C. National Payer ID
   D. Taxonomy code

8. **[LO 7.3]** Which type of code describes the medical specialty of a provider? _____
   A. Pay-to code
   B. Taxonomy code
   C. Relationship code
   D. POS code

9. **[LO 7.3]** What is the minimum number of diagnosis codes that must appear for each service line? _____
   A. Zero
   B. One
   C. Two
   D. Four

10. **[LO 7.3]** The correct medical code sets are those valid at the time the health care is provided. The correct _____ are those valid at the time the transaction—such as the claim—is started.
    A. Diagnosis code sets
    B. Administrative code sets
    C. Taxonomy code sets
    D. POS code sets

Applying Your Knowledge

[LO 7.4] Case 7.1

Joan McNavish, a sixty-one-year-old retiree, is covered by her husband's insurance policy. Her husband Ray is still working and receives health benefits through his employer, Rockford Valley Concrete, which has a PPO plan. In this case, who is the subscriber and who is the patient?

[LO 7.3, 7.4] Case 7.2

Sherry Denise Cleaver is a patient in the medical office where you work. This information appears on her patient information and encounter forms:

Name: Sherry Denise Cleaver

Established Patient

Birth Date: July 1, 2009

Marital Status: Single

Responsible Person: James T. Cleaver

Relationship to Patient: Father

Insured's Plan: BMA PPO

connect (plus+)

Enhance your learning at mcgrawhillconnect.com!
- Practice Exercises
- Worksheets
- Activities
- Integrated eBook

Diagnosis of otitis media, left ear, on May 13, 2016; the charge is $22 for a CPT 99211. The medical office collected a copayment of $10 and waits for payment directly from the insurance companies on assigned claims.

Supply the following data elements:

Subscriber:

Patient:

Relationship of Patient to Subscriber:

Claim Filing Indicator Code:

Total Charge:

Amount Collected:

Place of Service Code:

Diagnosis Code:

Date of Service:

Procedure Code/Charge:

[LO 7.3, 7.4] Case 7.3

The following information appears on a series of encounter forms for patient Daniel M. Williams. You are preparing a claim for the three encounters.

Patient: Daniel M. Williams (EP)

Insurance: Aetna POS

Insured: Marla Y. Jones (grandmother)

Date: 6-14-16

T-101 P-90 R-18 BP 132/76 WT 175

CC: Swollen neck glands, fever, headache, general malaise since this morning.

Dx: Epidemic parotitis.

Rx: Rest, fluids, Tylenol for headache prn. Return in 5 days for recheck.

Services and Charges: Office visit, problem-focused history and exam, straightforward decision making: $65.

Date: 6-19-16

T-101 P-88 R-18 BP 130/60

CC: Fever, pain, and swelling of right testicle.

Dx: Orchitis, complication of epidemic parotitis.

Rx: Ampicillin 500 mg. #16; IM Ampicillin 500 mg. Return 2 days for recheck.

Services and Charges: Office visit, problem-focused history and exam, straightforward decision making: $65.

Intramuscular (IM) administration of antibiotic (Ampicillin) 500 mg, $20.

Date: 6-21-16

T-98.8 P-80 R-16 BP 132/74

Rx: Recheck, improvement, continue meds, recheck in 2 weeks.

Dx: Orchitis.

Services and Charges: Office visit, problem-focused history and exam, straightforward decision making: $65.

Supply the following data elements:

Subscriber:

Patient:

Relationship:

connect™ plus+

Enhance your learning at mcgrawhillconnect.com!
• Practice Exercises   • Worksheets
• Activities   • Integrated eBook

Claim Filing Indicator Code:

Total Charge:

Place of Service Code:

Diagnosis Codes:

Service Line Information:

Date of Service:

Procedure Code/Charge:

Diagnosis:

Date of Service:

Procedure Codes/Charges:

Diagnosis:

Date of Service:

Procedure Code/Charge:

Diagnosis:

[LO 7.3, 7.4] Case 7.4

The following information is in the file of patient Martha M. Butler. You are preparing a claim for the encounters.

Name: Martha M. Butler (EP)

Insurance Medicare Part B

Date: 4-19-2016

T-98.8 P-68 R-15 BP 178/98 WT 155

CC: This a.m. while going to get mail pt. fell on sidewalk; a neighbor brought her in c/o pain and disability in left hip area, SOB, chest pain.

Exam: Pt. in distress, X-ray L hip two views—negative, ECG T-wave inversion.

Lab: Cardiac enzymes, electrolytes.

Dx: Sprained L hip, essential hypertension, R/O angina pectoris.

Rx: Injection 2.0 cc Norflex IM, moist heat, Norflex tablets #12, Inderal capsules 80 mg #30.

Return in 3 days for lab results and recheck.

Date: 4-22-2016

T-98.6 P-68 R-15 BP 150/88

Lab Results: Within normal limits.

Exam: Hip improving, ECG negative.

Dx: Essential hypertension, angina pectoris.

Rx: Continue prescribed meds. Nitrostat tablets, one tab dissolved under tongue at first sign of angina attack.

List of Fees for Service:

Date: 4-19-2016

Dx: Sprained L hip, essential hypertension.

Services and Charges:

Office visit, detailed history and detailed exam, decision making of moderate complexity: $80.

X-ray L hip, complete, two views, $90.

Therapeutic Intramuscular Injection 2.0 cc Norflex IM, $12.

ECG routine, 12 leads, interpretation and report, $55.

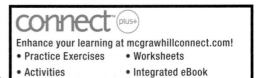

connect plus+

Enhance your learning at mcgrawhillconnect.com!
- Practice Exercises
- Worksheets
- Activities
- Integrated eBook

Date: 4-22-2016

Dx: Essential hypertension, angina pectoris.

Services and Charges: Office visit, problem-focused history and exam, straightforward decision making: $65.

Supply the following data elements:

Subscriber/Patient:

Claim Filing Indicator Code:

Total Charge:

Place of Service Code:

Diagnosis Codes:

Service Line Information:

Date of Service:

Procedure Code/Charge:

Diagnosis:

Date of Service:

Procedure Code/Charge:

Diagnosis:

Date of Service:

Procedure Code/Charge:

Diagnosis:

Date of Service:

Procedure Code/Charge:

Diagnosis:

Date of Service:

Procedure Code/Charge:

Diagnosis:

connect™ plus+

Enhance your learning at mcgrawhillconnect.com!
- Practice Exercises
- Worksheets
- Activities
- Integrated eBook

KEY TERMS

BlueCard
BlueCross BlueShield Association (BCBS)
carve out
Consolidated Omnibus Budget
    Reconciliation Act (COBRA)
credentialing
elective surgery
Employee Retirement Income Security
    Act of 1974 (ERISA)
family deductible
Federal Employees Health Benefits
    (FEHB) program
Flexible Blue
group health plan (GHP)
home plan
host plan
individual deductible
individual health plan (IHP)
late enrollee
maximum benefit limit
monthly enrollment list
open enrollment period
precertification
rider
self-insured health plan
stop-loss provision
utilization review
utilization review organization (URO)
waiting period

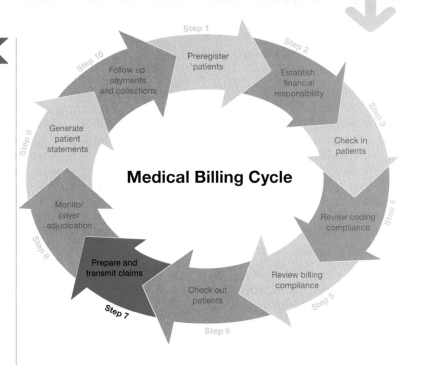

Medical Billing Cycle

Step 1 Preregister patients
Step 2 Establish financial responsibility
Step 3 Check in patients
Step 4 Review coding compliance
Step 5 Review billing compliance
Step 6 Check out patients
Step 7 Prepare and transmit claims
Step 8 Monitor payer adjudication
Step 9 Generate patient statements
Step 10 Follow up payments and collections

Learning Outcomes

After studying this chapter, you should be able to:

8.1 Compare group and individual health plans.

8.2 Differentiate among major private payers.

8.3 Support billing decisions using payment and billing guidelines.

8.4 Prepare accurate private payer claims.

8.5 Explain how to manage billing for capitated services.

Medical assistants must become knowledgeable about the billing rules of the private plans in which the practice participates. It is also important to know the features of the patients' private insurance plans and how they affect coverage of services and financial responsibility.

8.1 Private Insurance

People who are not covered by entitlement programs such as government-sponsored health insurance are often covered by private insurance. Many employers offer their employees the opportunity to become covered under an employee health care benefit plan. Sponsorship of medical insurance is an important benefit to employees that also gives employers federal income tax advantages.

Employer-Sponsored Medical Insurance

Many employees have medical insurance coverage under **group health plans (GHP)** that their employers sponsor. Human resources departments manage these health care benefits, negotiating with payers and then selecting a number of plans to offer employees. Both basic plans and riders that employees may buy and add to their policies are offered. **Riders,** also called options, are often offered for vision and dental services. Another popular rider is for complementary health care, covering treatments such as chiropractic/manual manipulation, acupuncture, massage therapy, dietetic counseling, and vitamin and minerals. Employers may also **carve out** certain benefits—that is, change a plan's standard coverage or providers—during negotiations to reduce the employer's price.

During specified periods (usually once a year) called **open enrollment periods,** employees choose the plan they prefer for the coming benefit period (see Figure 8.1). The employer provides tools (often Web-based) and information to help employees match their personal and family needs with the best-priced plan. Employees can customize their policies by choosing to accept various levels of premiums, deductibles, and other costs.

Federal Employees Health Benefits Program

The largest employer-sponsored health program in the United States is the **Federal Employees Health Benefits (FEHB) program,** which covers more than 8 million federal employees, retirees, and their families through over 250 health plans from a number of carriers. FEHB is administered by the federal government's Office of Personnel Management (OPM), which receives and deposits premiums and remits

group health plan (GHP) Plan of an employer or employee organization to provide health care to employees, former employees, or their families.

rider Document modifying an insurance contract.

carve out Part of a standard health plan changed under an employer-sponsored plan.

open enrollment period Time when a policyholder selects from offered benefits.

Link for All State Departments of Insurance

www.healthinsurance.com/
insurance_departments.html

Federal Employees Health Benefits (FEHB) Program Covers employees of the federal program.

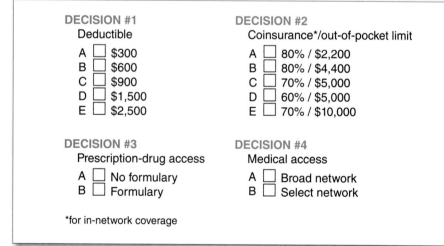

DECISION #1
Deductible

A ☐ $300
B ☐ $600
C ☐ $900
D ☐ $1,500
E ☐ $2,500

DECISION #2
Coinsurance*/out-of-pocket limit

A ☐ 80% / $2,200
B ☐ 80% / $4,400
C ☐ 70% / $5,000
D ☐ 60% / $5,000
E ☐ 70% / $10,000

DECISION #3
Prescription-drug access

A ☐ No formulary
B ☐ Formulary

DECISION #4
Medical access

A ☐ Broad network
B ☐ Select network

*for in-network coverage

FIGURE 8.1 Example of Selecting Benefits During Open Enrollment

payments to the carriers. Each carrier is responsible for furnishing identification cards and benefits brochures to enrollees, adjudicating claims, and maintaining records.

Self-Insured Health Plans

self-insured health plan
Organization that pays for health insurance directly and sets up a fund from which to pay.

To save money, some large employers cover the costs of employee medical benefits themselves, rather than buying insurance from carriers or managed care organizations. They create **self-insured health plans** that do not pay a premium to an insurance carrier or a managed care organization. Instead, self-insured health plans "insure themselves" and assume the risk of paying directly for medical services, setting aside funds with which they pay benefits. The employer establishes the benefit levels and the plan types offered to employees. Self-insured health plans may set up their own provider networks or, more often, lease the use of managed care organizations' networks. They may also buy other types of insurance—like a vision package—instead of insuring the benefit themselves. Self-insured health plans (in contrast to employer-sponsored "fully insured plans") are regulated by the federal **Employee Retirement Income Security Act of 1974 (ERISA)** instead of state laws. ERISA is run by the federal Department of Labor's Pension and Welfare Benefits Administration (EBSA).

Employee Retirement Income Security Act of 1974 (ERISA)
Law providing incentives and protection for companies with employee health and pension plans.

Benefit Eligibility under Group Health Plans

The group health plan specifies the rules for eligibility and the process of enrolling and disenrolling members. Rules cover employment status, such as full-time, part-time, disabled, and laid-off or terminated employees, as well as the conditions for enrolling dependents.

Waiting Period

waiting period Amount of time that must pass before an employee/dependent may enroll in a health plan.

Many plans have a **waiting period,** an amount of time that must pass before a newly hired employee or a dependent is eligible to enroll. The waiting period, which varies with the plan, is the time between the date of hire and the date the insurance becomes effective.

Late Enrollees

late enrollee Category of enrollment that may have different eligibility requirements.

The plan may impose different eligibility rules on a **late enrollee,** an individual who enrolls in a plan at a time other than the earliest possible enrollment date or a special enrollment date. For example, special enrollment may occur when a person becomes a new dependent through marriage.

Premiums and Deductibles

As explained in the first chapter, most plans require annual premiums. Although employers used to pay the total premiums as a benefit for employees, currently they pay an average of 80 percent of the cost.

individual deductible Fixed amount that must be met periodically by each individual of an insured/dependent group.

Many health plans also have a deductible that is due per time period. Noncovered services under the plan that the patient must pay out-of-pocket do not count toward satisfying a deductible. Some plans require an **individual deductible** that must be met for each person—whether the policyholder or a covered dependent—who has an encounter. Others have a **family deductible** that can be met by the combined payments of any covered members of the insured's family.

family deductible Fixed, periodic amount that must be met by the combined payments of an insured/dependent group before benefits begin.

Benefit Limits

maximum benefit limit
Amount an insurer agrees to pay for lifetime covered expenses.

Plans often have a **maximum benefit limit** (also called a lifetime limit), a monetary amount after which benefits end, and may also impose a condition-specific lifetime limit. For example, the plan may have a $500,000 lifetime limit on all benefits covered under the plan for any policyholder and a $2,000 limit on benefits provided for a specific health condition of an individual policy holder. Some plans may also have an annual benefit limit that restricts the amount payable in a given year.

COBRA

The **Consolidated Omnibus Budget Reconciliation Act (COBRA)** (1985; amended 1986) gives an employee who is leaving a job the right to continue health coverage under the employers' plan for a limited time at his or her own expense. COBRA participants usually pay more than do active employees, since the employer usually pays part of the premium for an active employee, while a COBRA participant generally pays the entire premium. However, COBRA is ordinarily less expensive than individual health coverage.

Individual Health Plans

Individual health plans (IHP) are also available for purchase; almost 10 percent of people with private health insurance have individual plans. People often elect to enroll in individual plans, although coverage is expensive, in order to continue their health insurance between jobs. Purchasers also include self-employed entrepreneurs, students, recent college graduates, and early retirees. Individual insurance plans have basic benefits without the riders or additional features associated with group health plans.

THINKING IT THROUGH 8.1

1. If a GHP has a ninety-day waiting period, on what day does health coverage become effective?

2. In terms of enrollment in a health plan, what is the status of an infant born to a subscriber in the plan?

3. A patient pays for a cosmetic procedure that is not medically necessary under the terms of the plan. Does this payment count toward the deductible?

4. Why is it important to verify a patient's eligibility for benefits? Can you think of events, like job-status change, that might affect coverage?

8.2 Major Private Payers and the Bluecross Blueshield Association

A small number of large insurance companies dominate the national market and offer employers all types of health plans, including self-funded plans. Local or regional payers are often affiliated with a national plan or with the BlueCross BlueShield Association.

Private payers supply complete insurance services, such as:

▶ Contracting with employers and with individuals to provide insurance benefits.
▶ Setting up physician, hospital, and pharmacy networks.
▶ Establishing fees.
▶ Processing claims.
▶ Managing the insurance risk.

Many large insurers own specialty companies that have insurance products in related areas. They may handle behavioral health, dental, vision, and life insurance. Many also work as federal government contractors for Medicare and Medicaid programs and handle prescription management divisions.

Major Payers and Accrediting Groups

The major national payers are listed below. Note that the BlueCross BlueShield Association (BCBS), which has both for-profit and nonprofit members, is not a payer;

Consolidated Omnibus Budget Reconciliation Act (COBRA) Law requiring employers with over twenty employees to allow terminated employees to pay for coverage for eighteen months.

individual health plan (IHP) Medical insurance plan purchased by an individual.

BILLING TIP

Timely Payments

Group health plans must follow states' Clean Claims Act and/or Prompt Payment Act and pay claims they accept for processing on a timely basis. ERISA (self-insured) plans are obligated to follow similar rules from the federal Dept. of Labor.

it is an association of more than forty payers. Its national scope, however, means that knowing about its programs is important for all medical assistants.

- *WellPoint, Inc.:* WellPoint is the nation's largest health insurer in terms of enrollment. It is also the largest owner of BlueCross and BlueShield plans (see the discussion of the BlueCross BlueShield Association below).
- *UnitedHealth Group:* UnitedHealth Group is another large health insurer that runs plans under its UnitedHealthcare subsidiary and also owns other major regional insurers.
- *Aetna:* With more than 44 million members, Aetna has a full range of products, including health care, dental, pharmacy, group life, behavioral health, disability and long-term care benefits.
- *CIGNA Health Care:* CIGNA is a large health insurer with strong enrollment in the Northeast and the West.
- *Kaiser Permanente:* The largest nonprofit HMO, Kaiser Permanente is a prepaid group practice that offers both health care services and insurance in one package. It runs physician groups, hospitals, and health plans in western, midwestern, and southeastern states plus Washington, D.C.
- *Health Net:* Health Net operates health plans in the West and has group, individual, Medicare, Medicaid, and TRICARE programs.
- *Humana Inc.:* Humana is particularly strong in the South and Southeast. It offers both traditional and consumer-driven products. Humana handles TRICARE operations in the Southeast.
- *Coventry:* Coventry Health Care is a national managed health care company based in Bethesda, Maryland, operating health plans, insurance companies, network rental/managed care services companies, and workers' compensation services companies. It provides a full range of risk and fee-based managed care products and services.

Outside agencies accredit and rate private payers. The major accrediting organizations are summarized in Table 8.1. Payers are also monitored by industry groups such as the National Association of Insurance Commissioners.

BlueCross BlueShield Association

BlueCross BlueShield Association (BCBS) Licensing agency of BCBS plans.

Founded in the 1930s to provide low-cost medical insurance, the **BlueCross BlueShield Association (BCBS)** is a national organization of independent companies and a Federal Employee Program that insures nearly 100 million people. All offer a full range of health plans, including consumer-driven health plans, to individuals, small and large employer groups, senior citizens, federal government employees, and others. In addition to major medical and hospital insurance, the "Blues" also have freestanding dental, vision, mental health, prescription, and hearing plans.

Subscriber Identification Card

Since BCBS offers local and national programs through many individual plans, BlueCross and BlueShield subscriber identification cards are used to determine the type of plan a person is covered by. Most BCBS cards list the following information:

Plan name.

Type of plan (a PPO in a suitcase is the logo for BCBS PPO members; the empty suitcase is the logo for Traditional, POS, or HMO members).

Subscriber name.

Subscriber identification number (the subscriber's Social Security number has been replaced with a unique ID) which can be a total of 17 characters, a three-position alphabetic prefix that identifies the plan and 14 alphanumeric characters.

Table 8.1 Plan Accrediting Organizations

- *National Committee for Quality Assurance (NCQA):* An independent nonprofit organization, NCQA is the leader in accrediting HMOs and PPOs. Working with the health care industry, NCQA developed a group of performance measures called HEDIS (Health Plan Employer Data and Information Set). HEDIS provides employers and consumers with information about each plan's effectiveness in preventing and treating disease, about policyholders' access to care, about documentation, and about members' satisfaction with care. NCQA's guidelines on the process by which plans select physicians and hospitals to join their networks, called **credentialing,** include performance measures. NCQA requires plans to review the credentials of all providers in their plans every two years to ensure that the providers continue to meet appropriate standards of professional competence.

- *Utilization Review Accreditation Commission (URAC):* URAC, also known as the American Accreditation Healthcare Commission, is another leading accrediting group. Like NCQA, it is a nonprofit organization that establishes standards for managed health care plans. URAC has accreditation programs addressing both the security and privacy of health information as required by HIPAA.

- *The Joint Commission (formerly the Joint Commission on Accreditation of Healthcare Organizations or JCAHO):* TJC sets and monitors standards for many types of patient care. TJC is made up of members from the American College of Surgeons, the American College of Physicians, the American Medical Association, the American Hospital Association, and the American Dental Association. TJC verifies compliance with accreditation standards for hospitals, long-term care facilities, psychiatric facilities, home health agencies, ambulatory care facilities, and pathology and clinical laboratory services. TJC works with NCQA and the American Medical Accreditation Program to coordinate the measurement of the quality of health care across the entire health care system.

- *American Medical Accreditation Program (AMAP):* AMAP helps alleviate the pressures facing physicians, health plans, and hospitals by reducing cost and administrative effort while simultaneously documenting quality. As a comprehensive program, AMAP measures and evaluates individual physicians against national standards, criteria, and peer performance in five areas: credentials, personal qualifications, environment of care, clinical performance, and patient care.

- *Accreditation Association for Ambulatory Health Care, Inc. (AAAHC):* AAAHC has accredited managed care organizations for more than twenty years. Its program emphasizes an assessment of clinical records, enrollee and provider satisfaction, provider qualifications, utilization of resources, and quality of care.

credentialing Periodic verification that a provider or facility meets professional standards.

Effective date of coverage.

BCBS plan codes and coverage codes.

Participation in reciprocity plan with other BCBS plans.

Copayments, coinsurance, and deductible amounts.

Information about additional coverage, such as prescription medication and mental health care.

Information about preauthorization requirements.

Claim submission address.

Contact phone numbers.

Types of Plans

An indemnity BCBS plan has an individual and family deductible and a coinsurance payment. Individual annual deductibles may range from as little as $100 to as much as $2,500 or more. The family deductible is usually twice the amount of the individual deductible. Once the deductible has been met, the plan pays a percentage of the charges, usually 70, 80, or 90 percent, until an annual maximum out-of-pocket amount has been reached. After that, the plan pays 100 percent of approved charges until the end of the benefit year. At the beginning of the new benefit year, the out-of-pocket amount resets, and 100 percent reimbursement does not occur until the out-of-pocket maximum for the new year has been met. Once the cap has been met, charges by nonparticipating providers are paid at 100 percent of the allowed amount. If the charges exceed the allowed amount, the patient must pay the balance to the provider, even though the annual cap has been met.

BCBS plans also offer many types of managed care programs, including the following:

- ▶ **HMO:** A patient must choose a primary care physician who is in the BCBS network. HMO has an Away From Home Care Program that provides emergency room coverage if the subscriber needs care when traveling. Many BlueCross and BlueShield plans also have a Guest Membership through the Away From Home Care Program. A Guest Membership is a courtesy enrollment for members who are temporarily residing outside of their home HMO service area for at least ninety days.
- ▶ **POS:** Members of a POS plan may receive treatment from a provider in the network, or they may choose to see a provider outside the network and pay a higher fee. Depending on the particular plan, a patient may or may not have a primary care provider.
- ▶ **PPO:** Physicians and other health care providers sign participation contracts with BCBS agreeing to accept reduced fees in exchange for membership in the network. As network members, providers are listed in a provider directory and receive referrals from other network members. PPO subscribers have an icon with the letters PPO inside of a suitcase on their Blue ID cards. A patient may choose to see a network provider or, for higher fees, a nonnetwork provider.

BlueCard Program

BlueCard Program that provides benefits for subscribers who are away from their local areas.

The **BlueCard** program is a nationwide program that makes it easy for patients to receive treatment when outside their local service area and also makes it easy for a provider to receive payment when treating patients enrolled in plans outside the provider's service area. The program links participating providers and independent BCBS plans throughout the nation with a single electronic claim processing and reimbursement system. It works as follows:

1. A subscriber who requires medical care while traveling outside the service area presents the subscriber ID card to a BCBS participating provider.
2. The provider verifies the subscriber's membership and benefit coverage by accessing the payer's website or by calling the BlueCard eligibility number. Only the required copayment can be collected; the provider cannot ask the patient to pay any other fees.
3. After providing treatment, the provider submits the claim to the local BCBS plan in his or her service area, which is referred to as the **host plan.**
4. The host plan sends the claim via modem to the patient's **home plan** (the plan in effect when the patient is at home), which processes the claim and sends it back to the host plan.
5. The host plan pays the provider according to local payment methods, and the home plan sends the remittance advice. For example, if a subscriber from New Jersey requires treatment while traveling in Delaware, the provider in Delaware can treat the patient, file the claim, and collect payment from the Delaware plan.

host plan Participating provider's local BCBS plan.

home plan BCBS plan in the subscriber's community.

Flexible Blue Plan

Flexible Blue BCBS consumer-driven health plan.

BlueCross and BlueShield companies also offer a consumer-driven health plan called **Flexible Blue.** This plan combines a comprehensive PPO plan with either an HSA, an HRA, or a FSA. Also part of the CDHP are online decision-support resources.

1. Jan Wommelsdorf, of Fargo, North Dakota, was on vacation in Portland, Oregon, when she became ill. She has BCBS BlueCard insurance, so she telephoned the BlueCard toll-free number to find a provider near her in Portland. She was examined by Dr. Vijay Sundaram and provided with a special diet to follow until she returns home and visits her regular physician.

   A. Who submits the claim, Jan Wommelsdorf or Dr. Sundaram?

   B. Is the claim submitted to Jan's local BCBS plan in North Dakota or to Dr. Sundaram's local plan in Oregon?

8.3 Billing Guidelines under Participation Contracts

Providers, like employers and employees, must evaluate health plans. They judge which plans to participate in based primarily on the financial arrangements that are offered. Because managed care organizations are the predominant health care delivery systems, most medical practices have a number of contracts with plans in their area.

Contract Provisions

When a participation contract is being considered by a practice's contract evaluation team, an experienced medical administrative assistant may be asked to assist. The team is usually led by a practice manager or by a committee of physicians; an outside attorney typically reviews the contract as well. The managed care organization's business history, accreditation standing, and licensure status are reviewed.

The major question to be answered is whether participation in the plan is a good financial opportunity. All plans pay less than the physicians' fees schedules, so there is less revenue for each procedure. Some plans pay fees that are very low, and even gaining many more patients who have this plan may not make it profitable. The evaluation team checks the fees the plan pays for the CPT codes that the practice's providers most often bill. If the plan reduces payment for these services too much, the evaluation team may decide not to join, even though participation would bring more patients.

Other aspects of the plan, such as its medical necessity guidelines, are also considered. Some physicians do not accept certain plans because, in their view, complying with the plans' health care protocols will limit their professional medical judgment in treating patients.

The main parts of participation contracts are the following:

▶ Introductory section (often called "recitals" and "definitions")
▶ Contract purpose and covered medical services
▶ Physicians' responsibilities
▶ Managed care plan obligations
▶ Compensation and billing guidelines

Physicians' Responsibilities

When the practice decides to participate, it must follow the rules of the contract, including these points:

▶ *Covered services:* The types of services that the provider must offer to plan members.
▶ *Acceptance of plan members:* Whether providers must see all plan members who wish to use their services or some percentage or specific number of members.

► *Referrals:* Whether providers must refer patients to other participating providers only. It also covers the conditions under which the referral rules do not apply, such as in an emergency.

► *Preauthorization:* If the provider is responsible for securing preauthorization for the patient, as is the case in most HMOs, this is stated.

► *Quality assurance/utilization review:* Providers typically must agree to allow access to certain records for the payer's quality assurance and utilization review (QA/UR) activities. **Utilization review** refers to the payer's process for determining medical necessity—whether the review is conducted before or after the services are provided.

► *Other provisions:* Providers' credentials, health plan protocols, HIPAA privacy policies, record retention, and other guidelines from the payer's medical review program are covered.

utilization review   Payer's process for determining medical necessity.

Plan Obligations

Similarly, the participation contract stipulates some responsibilities of the plan toward the provider, including:

► Identification of enrolled patients: The plan's method of identifying enrolled patients should be specified. Usually, this is with an identification card like the one shown in Figure 8.2. In this example, the provider network, the schedule of

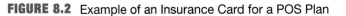

PHYSICIANS
HEALTH SERVICE

NETWORK:	003	SCHEDULE: C77	OFC: $15
SUBSCRIBER:	GEORGE HERKER		
GROUP:	POS		
CONTRACT:	CHARTER POS		
RIDERS:	P, CM, C2, PS		

IDENTIFICATION

100329712   For Pharmacy Questions 877-747-9378

BILLING CODE	NAME
01	GEORGE A.
02	MARY B.
03	ANDREW E.
04	PETER E.

AdvanceRx

Front

Physicians Health Services

PLEASE BE SURE TO CARRY THIS CARD AND PRESENT IT AT THE TIME OF SERVICE
If you have questions, call PHS Customer Relations at (800) 555-1000
E-mail Address: member@phs.com   Internet Address: http://www.phs.com

MEMBERS: Medical Services provided by a non-PHS physician will be subject to deductibles and coinsurance. Please refer to your plan documents to determine what services are covered and/or may require prior authorization.
EMERGENCIES: You are covered for emergencies worldwide. If the situation is life-threatening, go to the nearest hospital or call 911. If not life-threatening, but urgent, attempt to contact your PHS physician first. If you are away from home and are admitted to an out-of-area hospital, call PHS as soon as possible at (800) 555-1000.

Mail Claims To: PHS Claims Dept., P.O. Box 981, Randall CT 06691-0981
For electronic claims submission information call the Claims EDI Dept at (800) 555-1001
This Card Does Not Guarantee Coverage

Back

FIGURE 8.2 Example of an Insurance Card for a POS Plan

benefits, the office visit copayment, the name of the policyholder, the group, the type of contract, the patient's identification number, and the patient's dependents are listed.

▶ Payments: A claim turnaround time is specified in the contract. This tells how long it will take for a physician to be paid for services.

▶ Protection against loss: If the provider is assuming financial risk for the cost of care, as happens under capitation, the contract should have a **stop-loss provision.** This clause limits the provider's costs if there is an unexpectedly high use of services. Stop-loss provisions state a dollar amount over which the provider will be repaid.

stop-loss provision Protection against large losses or severely adverse claims experience.

Billing Guidelines

Participation contracts other than for capitated plans often state the basis for the payer's allowed amounts. A payer may base allowed amounts on a percentage of the Medicare Physician Fee Schedule (MPFS) or a discounted fee-for-service arrangement.

Compiling Billing Data

Practices generally bill out from their normal fee schedules, rather than billing the contracted fees, even if they are known. Writing off the differences between normal fees and payments under the participation contract is done when the RA is processed. Billing this way permits the practice to track how much revenue is lost by participating in a particular contract, which is valuable information for future contract negotiations.

Physician's Fee Schedule for CPT 99211 $25

Contract Fee for PAR Providers for CPT 99211 $18

Loss of Revenue per Visit for CPT 99211 $7

Service Performed 3,500 Visits Annually

Annual Lost Revenue for This CPT Code $3,500

A record can be kept of lost revenue per each commonly billed CPT code. To negotiate higher fees, a practice may compare the difference in payer accounts over a year for its commonly billed procedures and use this comparison when negotiating contract renewal and reviewing fees.

Billing for No-Shows

The contract determines whether a participating provider can charge a patient for a product used to set up a procedure when the patient cancels. Often, a physician may bill only for a rendered service, not for a service that is not delivered, including cancellations and no-shows. In nonparticipating situations, have patients agree in writing to pay before scheduling procedures. Follow the practice's financial policy for billing for no-shows or cancellations.

Collecting Copayments

Payers vary as to the copayment(s) required. Some plans require a copayment only when an E/M service is provided, and others require it when the patient visits an office for any procedure or service. Copayment amounts may also vary according to the service performed. Some plans have different copayment amounts for office visits, emergency room visits, ambulance services, and preventive services. When two services, such as an E/M service and a billable procedure, are performed on the same date of service, either one or two copayments may be required, again depending on the payer.

Another variable in collecting copayments involves primary and secondary plans. Medical assistants should verify whether a copayment is to be collected under the

COMPLIANCE GUIDELINE

Collect Copays

The practice is obligated to follow payer copayment guidelines. Routinely waiving copays and deductibles may be fraudulent under participation contracts. This should be stated in the financial policy that patients are given.

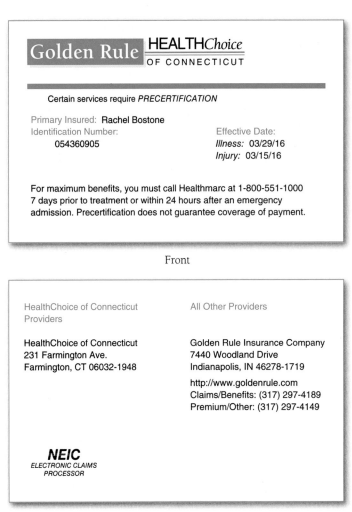

Front

Back

FIGURE 8.3 Example of an Insurance Card Showing Precertification Requirement

secondary plan. Usually it is not, unless the primary plan does not cover the service or if the member is satisfying a deductible for the primary plan.

Billing Surgical Procedures

Most managed care plans have rules for authorizing emergency surgical procedures and elective surgery. Emergency surgery usually must be approved within a specified period, such as forty-eight hours, after admission was required. **Elective surgery** is a procedure that can be scheduled ahead of time, but which may or may not be medically necessary. It usually requires preauthorization during a specified period before the service is performed. The preauthorization requirement is usually shown on the patient's insurance card. Many plans require preauthorization for out-of-network services even though they are covered under the plan. The practice must send a completed preauthorization form or online application for review in advance of the admission.

Some elective surgical procedures are done on an inpatient basis, so the patient is admitted to the hospital; others are done on an outpatient basis. The following are common outpatient surgeries:

▶ Abdominal hernia
▶ Bunionectomy

elective surgery Nonemergency surgical procedure.

- ▶ Carpal tunnel
- ▶ Destruction of cutaneous vascular proliferative lesions
- ▶ Knee arthroscopy
- ▶ Otoplasty
- ▶ Sclerotherapy

For a major course of treatment, such as surgery, chemotherapy, and radiation for a patient with cancer, many private payers use the services of a **utilization review organization (URO).** The URO is hired by the payer to evaluate the medical necessity of planned procedures. When a provider (or a patient) requests preauthorization for a treatment plan, the URO issues a report of its findings. The patient and provider are both notified of the results. If the planned services are not covered, the patient should agree to pay for them before the treatment begins.

utilization review organization (URO) Organization hired by a payer to evaluate medical necessity.

BILLING TIP

The Term *Precertification*

Precertification ("precert") is another term for preauthorization. It is usually applied to hospital admissions and outpatient surgery. Both terms have the same meaning.

precertification Preauthorization for hospital admission or outpatient procedures.

THINKING IT THROUGH 8.3

1. Read the following preauthorization policy from a typical PPO plan and answer the questions that follow:

> *Preauthorization is the process of collecting information prior to inpatient admissions and selected ambulatory procedures and services. The process permits advance eligibility verification, determination of coverage, and communication with the physician and/or member. It also allows the PPO to coordinate the member's transition from the inpatient setting to the next level of care (discharge planning), or to register members for specialized programs like disease management, case management, or maternity management programs. In some instances, preauthorization is used to inform physicians, members, and other health care providers about cost effective programs and alternative therapies and treatments.*
>
> *Certain health care services require preauthorization under this plan. When a service requires preauthorization, the provider is responsible to preauthorize those services prior to treatment. However, if the patient's plan covers self-referred services to network providers or self-referrals to out-of-network providers, and the patient is able to self-refer for covered benefits, it is the member's responsibility to contact the plan to preauthorize those services.*

A. What does the plan state are the purposes of preauthorization?

B. In your own words, define *self-refer.*

C. Under what circumstances is it the patient's responsibility to get preauthorization approval?

8.4 Private Payer Claims

General claim completion guidelines for CMS-1500 forms follow the NUCC guidelines. Note that "group" is checked for group health plans and "other" for individual plans. Figure 8.4 shows a completed claim for a patient with an employer-sponsored group health plan from a BlueCross BlueShield member plan.

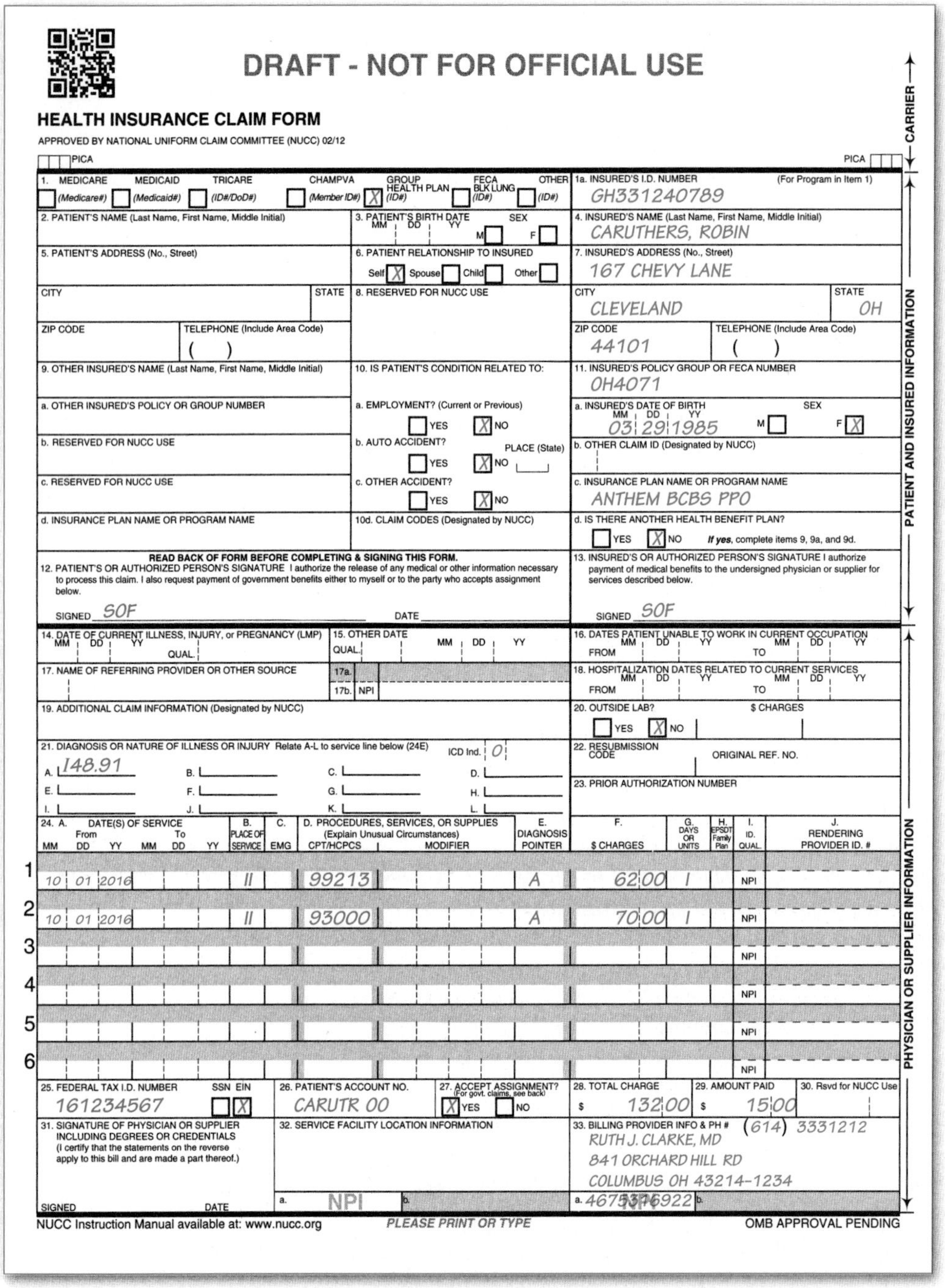

FIGURE 8.4 CMS-1500 (02/12) Completion for Private Payers

Exercise 8.1 — Completing a Primary Private Payer Claim

Patient Alan J. Harcar has insurance coverage under a CIGNA plan. Create a claim for his recent visit with Dr. Clarke.

Follow the steps at www.mhhe.com/newbycarr to complete the exercise at connect.mcgraw-hill.com on your own once you have watched the demo and tried the steps with prompts in practice mode. Use the information provided in the scenario to complete the exercise.

Exercise 8.2 Creating a BCBS Claim

Patient Diana E. O'Keefe has insurance coverage under a BCBS plan. Create a claim for her recent visit with Dr. Clarke.

Follow the steps at www.mhhe.com/newbycarr to complete the exercise at connect.mcgraw-hill.com on your own once you have watched the demo and tried the steps with prompts in practice mode. Use the information provided in the scenario to complete the exercise.

connect plus+

THINKING IT THROUGH 8.4

1. On Figure 8.4, why do INs 2 and 5 contain no data?

8.5 Capitation Management

When the practice has a capitated contract, careful attention must be paid to patient eligibility, referral requirements, encounter reports, claim write-offs, and billing procedures.

Patient Eligibility

Under most capitated agreements with primary care physicians, providers receive monthly payments that cover the patients who chose them as their PCPs for that month. The **monthly enrollment list** that the plan sends with the payment should list the current members. This list, also called a "provider patient listing" or "roster," contains patients' names, identification numbers, dates of birth, type of plan or program, and effective date of registration to the PCP. At times, however, the list is not up-to-date. To be sure that the patient is eligible for services, the insurance coverage is always verified.

The plan's contract with the provider lists the services and procedures that are covered by the cap rate. For example, a typical contract with a primary care provider might include the following services:

▶ Preventive care: well-child care, adult physical exams, gynecological exams, eye exams, and hearing exams.
▶ Counseling and telephone calls.
▶ Office visits.
▶ Medical care: medical care services such as therapeutic injections and immunizations, allergy immunotherapy, electrocardiograms, and pulmonary function tests.
▶ Local treatment of first-degree burns, application of dressings, suture removal, excision of small skin lesions, removal of foreign bodies or cerumen from external ear.

monthly enrollment list
Document of eligible members of a capitated plan for a monthly period.

Referral Requirements

An HMO may require a PCP to refer a patient to an in-network provider or to get authorization from the plan to refer a patient to an out-of-network provider. Patients who self-refer to nonparticipating providers may be balance-billed for those services. Both PCPs and specialists may be required to keep logs of referral activities.

Encounter Reports and Claim Write-offs

Most HMOs require capitated providers to submit encounter reports for patient encounters. Some do not require regular procedural coding and charges on the reports; the payer's form may just list "office visit" to be checked off. However, some plans do require the use of a regular claim with CPT codes. The practice management program is set up so that charges for service under capitated plans are written off as an adjustment to the patient's account. The billing staff knows not to expect additional payment based on a claim for a capitated-plan patient. If the service charges were not written off, the PMP would double-count the revenue for these patient encounters—once at the beginning of the month when the capitated payment was entered for a patient, and then again when a claim was created for a patient who has had an encounter during the month. Thus, the regular charges for the services that are included in the cap rate are written off by the biller. Only the monthly capitated payment remains on the patient's account—unless the patient has incurred charges beyond those items.

Billing for Excluded Services

Under a capitated contract, providers bill patients for services not covered by the cap rate. Medical insurance specialists need to organize this information for billing. For example, a special encounter form for the capitated plan might list the CPTs covered under the cap rate and then list the CPTs that can be billed. The plan's summary grid should indicate the plan's payment method for the additional services to be balance-billed, such as discounted fee-for-service.

THINKING IT THROUGH 8.5

1. Refer to the description of services covered under a PCP's cap rate above. Under this agreement, would the provider be permitted to bill the patient for a flu shot? A Pap test? A PSA test?

Chapter Summary

Learning Outcomes	Key Concepts/Examples
8.1 Compare group and individual health plans. Pages 179–181	• Group health plans are established and regulated by the employer. • Employers decide on basic plan coverage and optional riders, eligibility requirements, and premiums and deductibles. • Individual health plans provide coverage to those not covered under a group health plan. • Individual insurance plans have basic benefits.
8.2 Differentiate among major private payers. Pages 181–185	• A small number of large insurance companies dominate the national market. • WellPoint Inc. • United Health Group. • Aetna. • CIGNA Health Care. • Kaiser Permanente. • Health Net. • Humana Inc. • Coventry. • BlueCross BlueShield Association is a national organization of independent companies and a Federal Employee Program that insure nearly 100 million people.
8.3 Support billing decisions using payment and billing guidelines. Pages 185–189	• Insurance contracts are evaluated to determine if participation will be financially beneficial to the physician's practice. • Contract rules that must be followed specify the physician's responsibility as a participating provider and the plan's responsibilities toward the participating provider. • Managed care contracts outline compensation and billing guidelines that include the fees that can be charged by the provider, billing rules, and the patient's financial responsibilities.

Learning Outcomes	Key Concepts/Examples
8.4 Prepare accurate private payer claims. Pages 189–191	• Claims are prepared in accordance with the payer's billing and claims guidelines. • Indicate GROUP if the patient is covered by an employer sponsored plan. • Indicate OTHER if the patient is covered by an individual health plan.
8.5 Explain how to manage billing for capitated services. Pages 191–192	• Insurance coverage must be verified before services are provided to patients enrolled in capitated plans. • Regular services provided under the plan are written off. • Services not covered by the capitation rate can be billed.

Using Terminology

Match the key terms in the left column with the definitions in the right column.

_____ 1. **[LO 8.2]** Host plan

_____ 2. **[LO 8.2]** Credentialing

_____ 3. **[LO 8.3]** Stop-loss provision

_____ 4. **[LO 8.1]** Rider

_____ 5. **[LO 8.1]** Carve out

_____ 6. **[LO 8.1]** Consolidated Omnibus Budget Reconciliation Act (COBRA)

_____ 7. **[LO 8.5]** Monthly enrollment list

_____ 8. **[LO 8.3]** Utilization review organization

_____ 9. **[LO 8.3]** Precertification

_____ 10. **[LO 8.2]** Home plan

A. Review performed to ensure that a provider has met the appropriate standards of professional competence.

B. Document of eligible members of a capitated plan for a monthly period.

C. Authorization of hospital admission or outpatient surgery.

D. Options, such as dental or vision services, that are added to a health plan.

E. Hired by the payer to evaluate the medical necessity of planned procedures.

F. BlueCross and BlueShield plan that the patient has contracted with for coverage.

G. Changes made to a plan's standard coverage.

H. Often found in a capitated managed care contract, this clause protects the provider if there is an unexpected high use of services.

I. Allows for continuation of coverage under an employer's health plan.

J. The local BlueCross and BlueShield plan in the provider's service area.

Checking Your Understanding

Write the letter of the choice that best completes the statement or answers the question.

1. **[LO 8.1]** The largest employer sponsored health program in the United States is _____.
   A. Medicare
   B. Medicaid
   C. Federal Employees Health Benefits program
   D. Workers' compensation

2. **[LO 8.1]** In employer-sponsored health plans, employees may choose their plan during the _____.
   A. Carve out   C. Contract period
   B. Open enrollment period   D. Utilization review

connect™ (plus+)

Enhance your learning at mcgrawhillconnect.com!
• Practice Exercises   • Worksheets
• Activities   • Integrated eBook

3. **[LO 8.2]** BlueCross BlueShield Association member plans offer _____.
    A. All major types of health plans
    B. Only consumer-driven health plans
    C. Only HMO plans
    D. Only Indemnity plans

4. **[LO 8.5]** Under a capitated HMO plan, the physician practice receives _____.
    A. An encounter report
    B. Precertification for services
    C. A monthly enrollment list
    D. A secondary insurance identification number

5. **[LO 8.3]** Elective surgery is a procedure that _____.
    A. Is done to improve a patient's appearance
    B. Is always covered under a health plan
    C. Usually requires preauthorization
    D. Is only performed in an emergency

6. **[LO 8.2]** Which organization was founded to provide low cost medical insurance? _____
    A. The Joint Commission
    B. BlueCross BlueShield Association
    C. Centers for Medicare and Medicaid services
    D. American Medical Association

7. **[LO 8.3]** What document is researched to determine private payers' compensation and billing guidelines? _____
    A. ERISA   C. HIPAA guidelines
    B. Participation contract   D. CMS-1500

8. **[LO 8.4]** According to NUCC guidelines, what is checked on the CMS-1500 for individual health plans? _____
    A. Group   C. Private
    B. Individual   D. Other

9. **[LO 8.3]** Emergency surgery usually requires _____.
    A. A deductible paid to the hospital or clinic
    B. Precertification (preauthorization) within a specified time after the procedure
    C. A referral before the procedure
    D. Credentialing for the procedure

10. **[LO 8.2]** Which credentialing agency is made up of members from the American Medical Association and the American Hospital Association? _____
    A. NCQA   C. TJC
    B. AAAHC   D. AMAP

Applying Your Knowledge

[LO 8.4] Case 8.1

Audit the private-payer primary claim below. What problems do you find in the preparation of the claim? List the item numbers and the problems or questions you would raise.

1. _____

2. _____

3. _____

4. _____

5. _____

6. _____

7. _____

8. _____

9. _____

DRAFT - NOT FOR OFFICIAL USE

HEALTH INSURANCE CLAIM FORM

APPROVED BY NATIONAL UNIFORM CLAIM COMMITTEE (NUCC) 02/12

□□□ PICA

CARRIER

| 1. MEDICARE (Medicare#) | MEDICAID (Medicaid#) | TRICARE (ID#/DoD#) | CHAMPVA (Member ID#) | GROUP HEALTH PLAN (ID#) [X] | FECA BLK LUNG (ID#) | OTHER (ID#) | 1a. INSURED'S I.D. NUMBER (For Program in Item 1) |

2. PATIENT'S NAME (Last Name, First Name, Middle Initial)
BELLINI, JIMMY

3. PATIENT'S BIRTH DATE MM 03 DD 04 YY 2007 SEX M [X] F □

4. INSURED'S NAME (Last Name, First Name, Middle Initial)
BELLINI, GEORGE, I

5. PATIENT'S ADDRESS (No., Street)
4144 BARKER AVE

6. PATIENT RELATIONSHIP TO INSURED
Self □ Spouse □ Child □ Other □

7. INSURED'S ADDRESS (No., Street)
SAME

CITY **JACKSONVILLE** STATE **FL**

8. RESERVED FOR NUCC USE

CITY STATE

ZIP CODE **35000** TELEPHONE (Include Area Code) ( )

ZIP CODE TELEPHONE (Include Area Code) ( )

9. OTHER INSURED'S NAME (Last Name, First Name, Middle Initial)

10. IS PATIENT'S CONDITION RELATED TO:

11. INSURED'S POLICY GROUP OR FECA NUMBER
21B

a. OTHER INSURED'S POLICY OR GROUP NUMBER

a. EMPLOYMENT? (Current or Previous) □ YES [X] NO

a. INSURED'S DATE OF BIRTH MM DD YY SEX M [X] F □

b. RESERVED FOR NUCC USE

b. AUTO ACCIDENT? □ YES [X] NO PLACE (State)

b. OTHER CLAIM ID (Designated by NUCC)

c. RESERVED FOR NUCC USE

c. OTHER ACCIDENT? □ YES [X] NO

c. INSURANCE PLAN NAME OR PROGRAM NAME
AETNA WORLD PLAN

d. INSURANCE PLAN NAME OR PROGRAM NAME

10d. CLAIM CODES (Designated by NUCC)

d. IS THERE ANOTHER HEALTH BENEFIT PLAN? □ YES [X] NO *If yes*, complete items 9, 9a, and 9d.

READ BACK OF FORM BEFORE COMPLETING & SIGNING THIS FORM.
12. PATIENT'S OR AUTHORIZED PERSON'S SIGNATURE I authorize the release of any medical or other information necessary to process this claim. I also request payment of government benefits either to myself or to the party who accepts assignment below.

SIGNED *George Bellini* DATE **3/15/2016**

13. INSURED'S OR AUTHORIZED PERSON'S SIGNATURE I authorize payment of medical benefits to the undersigned physician or supplier for services described below.

SIGNED _____

14. DATE OF CURRENT ILLNESS, INJURY, or PREGNANCY (LMP) MM DD YY QUAL.

15. OTHER DATE QUAL. MM DD YY

16. DATES PATIENT UNABLE TO WORK IN CURRENT OCCUPATION FROM MM DD YY TO MM DD YY

17. NAME OF REFERRING PROVIDER OR OTHER SOURCE 17a. 17b. NPI

18. HOSPITALIZATION DATES RELATED TO CURRENT SERVICES FROM MM DD YY TO MM DD YY

19. ADDITIONAL CLAIM INFORMATION (Designated by NUCC)

20. OUTSIDE LAB? □ YES [X] NO $ CHARGES

21. DIAGNOSIS OR NATURE OF ILLNESS OR INJURY Relate A-L to service line below (24E) ICD Ind. **O**

A. **Z00.129** B. **Z23** C. D.
E. F. G. H.
I. J. K. L.

22. RESUBMISSION CODE ORIGINAL REF. NO.

23. PRIOR AUTHORIZATION NUMBER

PATIENT AND INSURED INFORMATION

24. A. DATE(S) OF SERVICE From MM DD YY	To MM DD YY	B. PLACE OF SERVICE	C. EMG	D. PROCEDURES, SERVICES, OR SUPPLIES (Explain Unusual Circumstances) CPT/HCPCS / MODIFIER	E. DIAGNOSIS POINTER	F. $ CHARGES	G. DAYS OR UNITS	H. EPSDT Family Plan	I. ID. QUAL.	J. RENDERING PROVIDER ID. #
1	03 15 2016				99382	A	132 00	I		NPI	1212343456
2	03 15 2016				90707	B	82 00	I		NPI	1212343456
3	03 15 2016				90701	B	70 00	I		NPI	1212343456
4	03 15 2016				90471	B	20 00	I		NPI	1212343456
5	03 15 2016				90472	B	20 00	I		NPI	1212343456
6										NPI	

25. FEDERAL TAX I.D. NUMBER **214809186** SSN □ EIN [X]

26. PATIENT'S ACCOUNT NO. **BEI20**

27. ACCEPT ASSIGNMENT? (For govt. claims, see back) □ YES □ NO

28. TOTAL CHARGE $ **314 00**

29. AMOUNT PAID $ **15 00**

30. Rsvd for NUCC Use

31. SIGNATURE OF PHYSICIAN OR SUPPLIER INCLUDING DEGREES OR CREDENTIALS (I certify that the statements on the reverse apply to this bill and are made a part thereof.)

SIGNED _____ DATE _____

32. SERVICE FACILITY LOCATION INFORMATION

a. NPI b.

33. BILLING PROVIDER INFO & PH # ( )
841 ORCHARD HILL RD
COLUMBUS OH 43214-1234

a. **4675316922** b.

PHYSICIAN OR SUPPLIER INFORMATION

NUCC Instruction Manual available at: www.nucc.org *PLEASE PRINT OR TYPE* OMB APPROVAL PENDING

---

connect™ plus+

Enhance your learning at mcgrawhillconnect.com!
- Practice Exercises   • Worksheets
- Activities   • Integrated eBook

9

MEDICARE

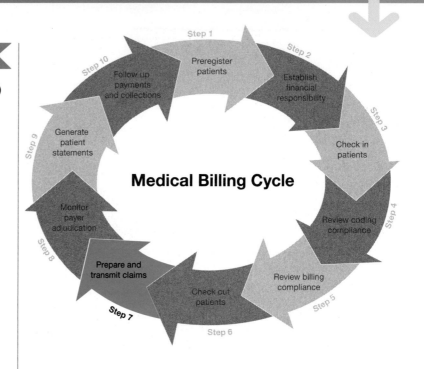

Medical Billing Cycle

Learning Outcomes

After studying this chapter, you should be able to:

9.1 Differentiate among Medicare Parts A, B, C, and D.

9.2 Compare the Original Medicare Plan and Medicare Advantage Plans.

9.3 Calculate fees for participating physicians and for nonparticipating physicians when they do and do not accept assignment.

9.4 Complete an advance beneficiary notice of noncoverage (ABN).

9.5 Determine whether Medicare is the primary or secondary payer in a given situation.

9.6 Prepare accurate Medicare claims.

Medicare is a federal medical insurance program established in 1965 under Title XVIII of the Social Security Act. The Medicare program is managed by the Centers for Medicare and Medicaid Services (CMS) under the Department of Health and Human Services (HHS). Although it has just four parts, it is arguably the most complex program that medical practices deal with, involving numerous rules and regulations that must be followed for claims to be paid. To complicate matters, these rules change frequently, and keeping up with the changes is a challenge for providers and medical assistants alike.

9.1 Medicare Overview

The federal health insurance program for people who are sixty-five or older is known as **Medicare.** Medicare also provides benefits to people with some disabilities and end-stage renal disease (ESRD), which is permanent kidney failure. A person covered by Medicare is called a **Medicare beneficiary.** Some beneficiaries qualify through the Social Security Administration. Others are eligible through the Railroad Retirement System.

The federal government does not pay Medicare claims directly. Instead, it contracts with insurance organizations to process claims on its behalf. Insurance companies that process claims are known as **Medicare administrative contractors (MACs).** Providers are assigned to a MAC based on the state in which they are physically located. DME MACs handle claims for durable medical equipment, supplies, and drugs billed by physicians (see the procedural coding chapter).

Medicare Federal health insurance program for people who are sixty-five or older.

Medicare beneficiary Person covered by Medicare.

Medicare administrative contractor (MAC) Contractor who handles claims and related functions.

Medicare Part A

Medicare Part A helps pay for inpatient hospital services, care in a skilled nursing facility, home health care, and hospice care. Fees paid by Medicare Part A for inpatient hospital services are based on groupings of diagnoses. Hospital cases across the country have been analyzed to arrive at the fixed fees Medicare pays for hospital services. The payment is based on the principal diagnosis. These topics are covered in more depth later in this text.

People who are eligible for Social Security benefits are automatically enrolled in Medicare Part A. They do not have to pay insurance premiums. Although people age sixty-five or older who do not qualify for Social Security benefits have the option of enrolling in Part A, technically they must pay premiums to get benefits. Most people, in fact, do not pay a premium for Part A because they or their spouse has 40 or more quarters of Medicare-covered employment.

Medicare Part A Program that pays for hospitalization, care in a skilled nursing facility, home health care, and hospice care.

Medicare Part B

Medicare Part B helps pay for physician services, outpatient hospital services, durable medical equipment, medical services, clinical laboratory services, home health care, and blood supply. Many preventive services are also covered. Every year, more preventive services are included, as the provisions of the Affordable Care Act are implemented gradually.

All Medicare providers must file claims on behalf of patients at no cost to the patients. Medical assistants file claims under Part B for physician services, even if the services are performed in hospital settings. They do not usually file claims for Part A benefits.

Part B coverage is optional. Everyone who is eligible for Part A may choose to enroll in Part B by paying monthly premiums (usually deducted automatically from Social Security retirement benefit payments). They are also subject to an annual deductible and coinsurance, which are established by federal law. The two basic

Medicare Part B Program that pays for physician services, outpatient hospital services, durable medical equipment, and other services and supplies.

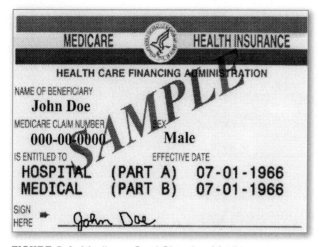

FIGURE 9.1 Medicare Card Showing Medicare Eligibility and Medicare Health Insurance Claim Number

types of plans available under Medicare Part B—the Original Medicare Plan and Medicare Advantage plans—are discussed below.

Medicare Part C

Medicare Part C (originally called Medicare + Choice) is available to individuals who are eligible for Part A and enrolled in Part B. Under Part C, private health insurance companies can contract with CMS to offer Medicare benefits through their own policies. In 2003, under the Medicare Prescription Drug, Improvement, and Modernization Act (commonly called the *Medicare Modernization Act, or MMA*), **Medicare Advantage** became the new name for Medicare + Choice plans, and certain rules were changed to give Part C enrollees better benefits and lower costs.

Medicare Part D

Medicare Part D, authorized under the MMA, provides voluntary Medicare prescription drug plans that are open to people who are eligible for Medicare. All Medicare prescription drug plans are private insurance plans, and most participants pay monthly premiums to access discounted prices. A prescription drug plan has a list of drugs it covers, called a **formulary,** often structured in payment tiers.

Medicare Insurance Card

Each Medicare enrollee receives a health insurance card (see Figure 9.1). This card lists the beneficiary's name, sex, and Medicare number and the effective dates for Part A and Part B coverage. The Medicare number, called the Medicare **health insurance claim number (HICN),** is assigned by CMS and usually consists of the Social Security number followed by a numeric or alphanumeric ending. The letter at the end provides additional information about the patient. For example, *A* stands for wage earner, *B* for spouse's number, and *D* for widow or widower.

When the beneficiary's card shows a prefix (such as A, MA, WA, or WD) instead of a suffix, the patient is eligible for railroad retirement benefits, and claims must be submitted to the Railroad Medicare Part B claim office:

Palmetto GBA (Government Benefits Administrator)

Railroad Retirees Benefits Medicare Claim Office

PO Box 10066

Augusta, GA 30999-0001

1-800-833-4455

www.palmettoGBA.com

Medicare Part C Managed care health plans under the Medicare Advantage program.

Medicare Advantage Medicare plans other than the Original Medicare Plan.

Medicare Part D Medicare prescription drug reimbursement plans.

formulary List of a plan's selected drugs and their proper dosages.

health insurance claim number (HICN) Medicare beneficiary's identification number.

BILLING TIP

Use Exact Name and HICN

Be sure to use the patient's name and HICN exactly as they appear on the Medicare card. This information must match Medicare's Common Working File (CWF), the Medicare claim processing system.

Wrong Information on Card

Advise patients who insist that their cards are not correct to contact the local Social Security field office or to use online access to get a correct card.

THINKING IT THROUGH 9.1

1. Research the current year's Medicare Part B premium and deductible. Are higher-income beneficiaries subject to a surcharge?

9.2 Part B Plans and Medigap Plans

Medicare Part B beneficiaries can choose from among a number of insurance plans and "gap" plans.

Original Medicare Plan

Medicare beneficiaries who enroll in the Medicare fee-for-service plan (referred to by Medicare as the **Original Medicare Plan**) can choose any licensed physician certified by Medicare. They must pay the premium, the coinsurance (which is 20 percent), and the annual deductible specified each year by the Medicare law, which is voted on by Congress. What amount of a patient's medical bills has been applied to the annual deductible is shown on the **Medicare Remittance Notice (MRN),** which is the RA that the office receives, and also on the **Medicare Summary Notice (MSN)** that the patient receives. Each time a beneficiary receives services, a fee is billable. Because of Medicare rules, most offices bill the patient for any balance due after the MRN is received, rather than at the time of the appointment.

BILLING TIP

Collecting the Medicare Deductible

Each calendar year, beginning January 1 and ending December 31, Medicare enrollees must satisfy a deductible for covered services under Medicare Part B. Can this be collected before the claim is filed with Medicare?

The date of service generally determines when expenses are incurred, but expenses are allocated to the deductible in the order in which Medicare receives and processes the claims. If the enrollee's deductible has previously been collected by another office, this could cause the enrollee an unnecessary hardship in raising this excess amount. Medicare advises providers to file their claim first and wait for the remittance advice before collecting any deductible.

Medicare Advantage Plans

Medicare also offers Medicare Advantage plans, as explained earlier. Beneficiaries can choose to enroll in one of the following types of plans instead of in the Original Medicare Plan:

1. Medicare coordinated care plans (CCPs)
2. Medicare private fee-for-service plans
3. Medical Savings Accounts (MSAs)

Medicare Coordinated Care Plans

Many Medicare beneficiaries are enrolled in Medicare Advantage coordinated care plans. A coordinated care plan includes providers who are under contract to deliver the benefit package approved by CMS. Many CCPs are run by the same major payers that offer private (commercial) coverage. CCPs may use features to control utilization, such as requiring referrals from primary care providers (PCP), and may use methods of paying providers to encourage high-quality and cost-effective care. A plan may require the patient to receive treatment within the plan's network. If a patient goes out of the network for services, the plan will not pay; the patient must pay the entire bill at the time of service. This restriction does not apply to emergency treatment (which may be provided anywhere in the United States) and **urgently needed care** (care provided while temporarily outside the plan's network area). CCP plans include HMOs, generally capitated, with or without

Original Medicare Plan Medicare fee-for-service plan.

Medicare Remittance Notice (MRN) RA the office receives from Medicare.

Medicare Summary Notice (MSN) Remittance advice from Medicare to beneficiaries.

urgently needed care Beneficiary's unexpected illness or injury requiring immediate treatment.

a point-of-service option, POSs, which are the Medicare version of independent practice associations (IPAs), PPOs, special needs plans (SNPs), and religious fraternal benefits plans (RFBs).

To maintain uniform coverage within a geographic area, CMS requires managed care plans to provide all of the Medicare benefits available in the service area. Beyond that restriction, plans are free to offer coverage for additional services not covered under fee-for-service plans, such as prescription drugs, preventive care (including physical examinations and inoculations), eyeglasses and hearing aids, dental care, and care for treatment received while traveling overseas.

Medicare Private Fee-for-Service (PFFS)

Under a Medicare private fee-for-service plan, patients receive services from Medicare-approved providers or facilities of their choosing. The plan is operated by a private insurance company that contracts with Medicare but pays on a fee-for-service basis.

Medical Savings Accounts

Medical Savings Account (MSA) Medicare health savings account program.

The **Medical Savings Account (MSA)** is similar to a private medical savings account. It combines a high-deductible fee-for-service plan with a tax-exempt trust to pay for qualified medical expenses. The maximum annual MSA plan deductible is set by law. CMS pays premiums for the insurance policies and makes a contribution to the MSA; the beneficiary puts in the rest of the fund. Beneficiaries use the money in their MSAs to pay for their health care before the high deductible is reached. At that point, the Medicare Advantage plan offering the MSA pays for all expenses for covered services.

Medigap Plans for Original Medicare Plan Beneficiaries

Individuals enrolled in the Original Medicare Plan often have additional insurance, either Medigap insurance they purchase or insurance provided by a former employer. These plans frequently pay the patient's Part B deductible and additional procedures that Medicare does not cover. If Medicare does not pay a claim because of lack of medical necessity, Medigap and supplemental carriers are not required to pay the claim either.

Medigap Plan offered by a private insurance carrier to supplement coverage.

Medigap is private insurance that beneficiaries may purchase to fill in some of the gaps—unpaid amounts—in Medicare coverage. These gaps include the annual deductible, any coinsurance, and payment for some noncovered services. Even though private insurance carriers offer Medigap plans, coverage and standards are regulated by federal and state law.

Medigap policyholders pay monthly premiums. There are a number of standard plans with varying coverage; however, they must all cover certain basic benefits. Generally, subscribers in gap plans that are "retired"— that is, closed to new beneficiaries—can keep their plans, which then do not accept new members. Monthly premiums vary widely across the different plan levels, as well as within a single plan level, depending on the insurance company selected.

COMPLIANCE GUIDELINE

The Medicare Advantage program is administered by the Center for Beneficiary Choices, a department of CMS.

THINKING IT THROUGH 9.2

1. In exchange for their increased coverage, what types of restrictions do Medicare Advantage CCP plans place on their beneficiaries?

9.3 Medicare Charges

The *Medicare Physician Fee Schedule (MPFS)* is the basis for payments for all Original Medicare Plan services. This national system is based on the Resource-Based Relative Value Scale (RBRVS) system using cost factors that represent the physician's time and how much it costs to run a practice (see the chapter about payment methods and checkout procedures).

Medicare Learning Network
www.cms.gov/MLNGenInfo

CMS Online Manual System
www.cms.gov/manuals

Participation

Annually, physicians choose whether they want to participate in the Medicare program. Participating physicians agree to accept assignment for all Medicare claims and to accept Medicare's allowed charge according to the Medicare Physician Fee Schedule as payment in full for services. A PAR physician may bill the patient for coinsurance and deductibles but may not collect amounts higher than the Medicare amount allowed by the fee schedule. Medicare is responsible for paying 80 percent of this allowed charge (after patients have met their annual deductibles). Patients are responsible for the other 20 percent. The physician may bill the patient for services not covered by Medicare.

An important online resource is the **Medicare Learning Network (MLN)** site. The MLN is a collection of articles that explain all Medicare topics. It is searchable by topic or by year. Another key resource is the Medicare **Internet-Only Manuals,** a collection of manuals that have day-to-day operating instructions, policies, and procedures based on statutes and regulations.

Medicare Learning Network (MLN) Online collection of articles explaining all Medicare topics.

Internet-Only Manuals (IOM) Medicare's collection of manuals.

Example

A Medicare PAR provider has a usual charge of $200 for a diagnostic flexible sigmoidoscopy (CPT 45330), and the Medicare-allowed charge is $84. The provider must write off the difference between the two charges. The patient is responsible for 20 percent of the allowed charge, not of the provider's usual charge:

Provider's usual fee:	$200.00
Medicare allowed charge:	$ 84.00
Medicare pays 80 percent:	$ 67.20
Patient pays 20 percent:	$ 16.80

The total the provider can collect is $84. The provider must write off the $116 difference between the usual fee and the allowed charge. ◄

Nonparticipation

Nonparticipating physicians decide whether to accept assignment on a claim-by-claim basis. Providers who elect not to participate in the Medicare program but who accept assignment on a claim are paid 5 percent less for their services than PAR providers. For example, if the Medicare-allowed amount for a service is $100, the PAR provider receives $80 (80 percent of $100), and the nonPAR provider receives $76 ($80 minus 5 percent). NonPAR providers who do not accept assignment are subject to Medicare's charge limits. They may not charge a Medicare patient more than 115 percent of the amount listed in the Medicare nonparticipating fee schedule. This amount—115 percent of the fee listed in the nonPAR MFS—is called the **limiting charge.**

For a claim that is not assigned, the provider can collect the full payment of the limiting charge from the patient at the time of the visit. The claim is then submitted to Medicare. If approved, Medicare will pay 80 percent of the allowed amount on the nonPAR fee schedule—not the limiting amount. Medicare sends this payment directly to the patient, since the physician has already been paid.

limiting charge Highest fee nonparticipating physicians may charge for a particular service.

Example

This example illustrates the different fee structures for PARs, nonPARs who accept assignment, and nonPARs who do not accept assignment.

Participating Provider

Physician's standard fee	$120.00
Medicare fee	$ 60.00
Medicare pays 80% ($60.00 × 80%)	$ 48.00
Patient or supplemental plan pays 20% ($60.00 × 20%)	$ 12.00
Provider adjustment (write-off) ($120.00 − $60.00)	$ 60.00

Nonparticipating Provider (Accepts Assignment)

Physician's standard fee	$120.00
Medicare nonPAR fee ($60.00 − 5%)	$ 57.00
Medicare pays 80% ($57.00 × 80%)	$ 45.60
Patient or supplemental plan pays 20% ($57.00 × 20%)	$ 11.40
Provider adjustment (write-off) ($120.00 − $57.00)	$ 63.00

Nonparticipating Provider (Does Not Accept Assignment)

Physician's standard fee	$120.00
Medicare nonPAR fee ($60.00 − 5%)	$ 57.00
Limiting charge (115% × $57.00)	$ 65.55
Patient billed	$ 65.55
Medicare pays patient (80% × $57.00)	$ 45.60
Total provider can collect	$ 65.55
Patient out-of-pocket expense ($65.55 − $45.60)	$ 19.95 ◄

COMPLIANCE GUIDELINE

Diagnostic Lab Billing

Physicians must accept assignment for clinical diagnostic laboratory services (generally, procedures with CPT codes in the 80000s). A physician may not bill Medicare patients for these services. If the physician does not accept Medicare assignment for them, the right to bill the patient is forfeited. The physician may accept assignment for laboratory services only and refuse to accept assignment for other services. In this case, two separate claims may be filed. One claim accepts assignment for laboratory services, and the other refuses assignment for other services.

Medicare's Correct Coding Initiative and Medically Unlikely Edits

Medicare's National Correct Coding Council develops correct coding guidelines in order to control improper procedural coding in Part B claims. This council issues policies, called the **Correct Coding Initiative (CCI),** to correct two types of errors: (1) unintentional coding errors resulting from a misunderstanding of coding, and (2) intentional incorrect coding done to increase payments. CCI guidelines are part of the automatic edits for electronic claims.

CCI, updated every quarter, has many thousands of CPT code combinations called **CCI edits** that are used by computers in the Medicare system to check claims. The CCI edits are available on a CMS website. CCI edits apply to claims that bill for more than one procedure performed on the same patient (Medicare beneficiary), on the same date of service, by the same performing provider. Claims are denied when codes reported together do not "pass" an edit.

Correct Coding Initiative (CCI) Computerized Medicare system that prevents overpayment.

CCI edits CPT code combinations used to check Medicare claims.

CCI prevents billing two procedures that, according to Medicare, could not possibly have been performed together. Here are examples:

▶ Reporting the removal of an organ both through an open incision and with laparoscopy.
▶ Reporting female- and male-specific codes for the same patient.

CCI edits also test for unbundling. A claim should report a bundled procedure code instead of multiple codes that describe parts of the complete procedure. For example, since a single code is available to describe removal of the uterus, ovaries, and fallopian tubes, physicians should not use separate codes to report the removal of the uterus, ovaries, and fallopian tubes individually.

CCI requires physicians to report only the more extensive version of the procedure performed and disallows reporting of both extensive and limited procedures. For example, only a deep biopsy should be reported if both a deep biopsy and a superficial biopsy are performed at the same location. Since CCI has been in place, Medicare claim rejections have multiplied. Selecting the correct codes to be reported on claims saves the medical office time and money in resubmitting rejected claims.

CMS has also established units of service edits, referred to as **medically unlikely edits (MUEs),** in order to lower the Medicare fee-for-service paid claims error rate. MUEs are intended to reduce the number of health care claims that are sent back simply because of clerical or practice management program errors.

MUEs are edits that test a claim for the same beneficiary, CPT code, date of service, and billing provider against Medicare's rule. The initial set of MUEs is based on anatomical considerations. An example is an edit that rejects a claim for a hysterectomy on a male patient. MUEs also automatically reject claim items containing units of service billed in excess of Medicare allowances.

Correct Coding Initiative Updates
www.cms.gov/
NationalCorrectCodInitEd/
Medically Unlikely Edits
www.cms.gov/
NationalCorrectCodInitEd/08_
MUE.asp

medically unlikely edits (MUEs) Units of service edits used in order to lower the Medicare fee-for-service paid claims error rate.

Incentives and Fraud Initiatives

Physician Quality Reporting System (PQRS)

The **Physician Quality Reporting System (PQRS)** is a voluntary quality reporting program established by CMS in which physicians or other eligible professionals collect and report their practice data in relation to a set of patient-care performance measures that are established annually. The program's goal is to determine best practices, define measures, support improvement, and improve systems. Physicians who successfully report are eligible for an additional 1.5 percent payment from CMS. The PQRS incentive is an all-or-nothing lump-sum payment. The provider must meet the basic requirement of reporting at least 80 percent of the time on up to three measures applicable to the professionals' practice. If more than three quality measures are applicable, the professional need only report on three.

Physician Quality Reporting System (PQRS) Voluntary reporting program in which physicians or other professionals collect and report their practice data.

Medicare Integrity Program

The Medicare program makes about $500 billion in payments per year and has a significant amount of improper payments. The Centers for Medicare and Medicaid Services' (CMS) **Medicare Integrity Program (MIP)** is designed to identify and address fraud, waste, and abuse, which are all causes of improper payments. The MIP has a number of initiatives related to review of documentation and billing.

Medicare Integrity Program (MIP) Designed to identify and address fraud, waste, and abuse.

THINKING IT THROUGH 9.3

1. Medicare Part B covers a screening Pap smear for women for the early detection of cervical cancer but will not pay for an E/M service for the same patient on the same day. Would this payment rule be part of MUEs or CCI edits?

9.4 Using the ABN

Medicare does not provide coverage for certain services and procedures. Claims will be denied for services that are not considered reasonable and necessary for the patient and for services that are excluded by Medicare.

BILLING TIP

ABNs

- Via the ABN, beneficiaries may choose to receive an item/service and pay for it out of pocket, rather than have a Medicare claim submitted.
- The ABN must be specific to the service and date, signed and dated by the patient, and filed.
- Use the GY modifier to speed Medicare denials so the amount due can be collected from the patient (or a secondary payer).

Participating physicians agree to not bill patients for services that Medicare declares as being not reasonable and necessary unless the patients were informed ahead of time in writing and agreed to pay for the services. **Local coverage determinations (LCDs)** and **national coverage determinations (NCDs)** issued by Medicare help sort out medical necessity issues. LCDs (formerly called Local Medicare Review Policies, or LMRPs) and NCDs contain detailed and updated information about the coding and medical necessity of specific services, including:

local coverage determination (LCD) Notices sent to physicians with information about the coding and medical necessity of a service.

- ▶ A description of the service.
- ▶ A list of indications (instances in which the service is deemed medically necessary).
- ▶ The appropriate CPT/HCPCS code.
- ▶ The appropriate ICD-10-CM code.
- ▶ A bibliography containing recent clinical articles to support the Medicare policy.

national coverage determination (NCD) Policy stating whether and under what circumstances a service is covered.

Mandatory ABNs

If a provider thinks that a procedure will not be covered by Medicare because it is not reasonable and necessary, the patient is notified of this before the treatment by means of a standard **advance beneficiary notice of noncoverage (ABN)** from CMS (see Figure 9.2). A filled-in form is given to the patient to review and sign. The ABN form is designed to:

advance beneficiary notice of noncoverage (ABN) Form used to inform patients that a service is not likely to be reimbursed.

- ▶ Identify the service or item that Medicare is unlikely to pay for.
- ▶ State the reason Medicare is unlikely to pay.
- ▶ Show the patient an estimate of how much the service or item will cost the beneficiary if Medicare does not pay.

The purpose of the ABN is to help the beneficiary make an informed decision about services that might have to be paid out-of-pocket. A provider who could have been expected (by Medicare) to know that a service would not be covered and who performed the service without informing the patient could be liable for the charges.

When provided, the ABN must be verbally reviewed with the beneficiary or his/her representative and questions posed during that discussion must be answered before the form is signed. The form must be provided in advance to allow the beneficiary or representative time to consider options and make an informed choice. The ABN may be delivered by employees or subcontractors of the provider, and is not required in an emergency situation. After the form has been completely filled in and signed, a copy is given to the beneficiary or his or her representative. In all cases, the provider must retain the original notice on file.

COMPLIANCE GUIDELINE

The ABN must be provided in advance of the service to allow the beneficiaries or their representatives time to consider options and make an informed choice.

A. Notifier:_____

B. Patient Name:_____   **C. Identification Number:**_____

Advance Beneficiary Notice of Noncoverage (ABN)

NOTE: If Medicare doesn't pay for **D.**_____ below, you may have to pay.
Medicare does not pay for everything, even some care that you or your health care provider have good reason to think you need. We expect Medicare may not pay for the **D.**_____ below.

D.	E. Reason Medicare May Not Pay:	F. Estimated Cost

WHAT YOU NEED TO DO NOW:
- Read this notice, so you can make an informed decision about your care.
- Ask us any questions that you may have after you finish reading.
- Choose an option below about whether to receive the **D.**_____ listed above.
   Note: If you choose Option 1 or 2, we may help you to use any other insurance that you might have, but Medicare cannot require us to do this.

G. Options: Check only one box. We cannot choose a box for you.
☐ **OPTION 1.** I want the **D.**_____ listed above. You may ask to be paid now, but I also want Medicare billed for an official decision on payment, which is sent to me on a Medicare Summary Notice (MSN). I understand that if Medicare doesn't pay, I am responsible for payment, but **I can appeal to Medicare** by following the directions on the MSN. If Medicare does pay, you will refund any payments I made to you, less co-pays or deductibles.
☐ **OPTION 2.** I want the **D.**_____ listed above, but do not bill Medicare. You may ask to be paid now as I am responsible for payment. **I cannot appeal if Medicare is not billed**.
☐ **OPTION 3.** I don't want the **D.**_____ listed above. I understand with this choice I am **not** responsible for payment, and **I cannot appeal to see if Medicare would pay.**

H. Additional Information:

This notice gives our opinion, not an official Medicare decision. **If you have other questions on this notice or Medicare billing, call** 1-800-MEDICARE **(1-800-633-4227/**TTY: **1-877-486-2048).**
Signing below means that you have received and understand this notice. You also receive a copy.

I. Signature:	J. Date:

Form CMS-R-131 (03/11)   Form Approved OMB No. 0938-0566

FIGURE 9.2 Advance Beneficiary Notice of Noncoverage (ABN)

Voluntary ABNs

Participating providers may bill patients for services that are not covered by the Medicare program, such as routine physicals and many screening tests. Giving a patient written notification that Medicare will not pay for a service before providing it is a good policy, although it is not required. When patients are notified ahead of time, they understand their financial responsibility to pay for the service. The ABN form may be used for this type of voluntary notification. In this case, the purpose of the ABN is to advise beneficiaries, before they receive services that are not Medicare benefits, that Medicare will not pay for them and to provide beneficiaries with an estimate of how much they may have to pay.

How to Complete the ABN

The ABN has five sections and ten blanks:

▶ Header (Blanks A–C)
▶ Body (Blanks D–F)
▶ Options Box (Blank G)
▶ Additional Information (Blank H)
▶ Signature Box (Blanks I–J)

Section 1: Header

Blanks (A–C) Header. This section must be completed by the notifier (the provider) before the form is given to the patient.

Blank (A) Notifier. Enter the provider's name, address, and telephone number. If the billing and notifying entities are not the same, the name of more than one entity may be given in the notifier area as long as the Additional Information (H) section below on the form states who should be contacted for questions.

Blank (B) Patient Name. Enter the beneficiary's name as it appears on the beneficiary's Medicare (HICN) card. The ABN will not be invalidated by a misspelling or missing initial, as long as the beneficiary or representative recognizes the name listed on the notice as that of the beneficiary.

Blank (C) Identification Number. Use of this field is optional. A practice may choose to enter an identification number for the beneficiary, such as medical record number, that helps link the notice with a related claim. Medicare numbers (HICNs) or Social Security numbers must not appear on the notice.

Section 2: Body

Blank (D) the Descriptors. The following types of descriptors may be used in the header of Blank (D):

▶ Item
▶ Service
▶ Laboratory test
▶ Test
▶ Procedure
▶ Care
▶ Equipment

The notifier must list the specific items or services believed to be noncovered under the header of Blank (D). General descriptions of specifically grouped supplies are permitted. For example, "wound care supplies" would be a sufficient description of a group of items used to provide this care. An itemized list of each supply is generally not required.

When a reduction in service occurs, this needs to be made clear to the beneficiary. For example, entering "wound care supplies decreased from weekly to monthly" would be appropriate to describe a decrease in frequency for this category of supplies; just writing "wound care supplies decreased" is insufficient.

Blank (E) Reason Medicare May Not Pay. In this blank, notifiers must explain, in beneficiary-friendly language, why they believe the items or services described in Blank (D) may not be covered by Medicare. Three commonly used reasons for noncoverage are:

▶ "Medicare does not pay for this test for your condition."
▶ "Medicare does not pay for this test as often as this (denied as too frequent)."
▶ "Medicare does not pay for experimental or research use tests."

To be a valid ABN, there must be at least one reason applicable to each item or service listed in Blank (D); it can be the same reason for all items.

Blank (F) Estimated Cost. Notifiers must complete Blank (F) to ensure the beneficiary has all available information to make an informed decision about whether or not to obtain potentially noncovered services. Notifiers must make a good-faith effort to insert a reasonable estimate for all of the items or services listed in Blank (D).

Section 3: Options Box

Blank (G) Options. This section, to be filled in by the patient, has three choices:

▶ OPTION 1 allows the beneficiary to receive the items and/or services at issue and requires the notifier to submit a claim to Medicare. This will result in a payment decision that can be appealed. Note: Beneficiaries who need to obtain an official Medicare decision in order to file a claim with a secondary insurance should choose Option 1.

▶ OPTION 2 allows the beneficiary to receive the noncovered items and/or services and pay for them out of pocket. No claim will be filed and Medicare will not be billed. Thus, there are no appeal rights associated with this option.

▶ OPTION 3 means the beneficiary does not want the care in question. By checking this box, the beneficiary understands that no additional care will be provided, and thus there are no appeal rights associated with this option.

The beneficiary must choose only one of the three options listed in Blank (G). If there are multiple items or services listed in Blank (D) and the beneficiary wants to receive some, but not all, of the items or services, the notifier can accommodate this request by using more than one ABN. The notifier can furnish an additional ABN listing the items/services the beneficiary wishes to receive with the corresponding option. If the beneficiary cannot or will not make a choice, the notice should be annotated, for example: "beneficiary refused to choose an option."

Section 4: Additional Information

Blank (H) Additional Information. This information may be used by the provider to provide additional clarification that the provider believes will be of use to beneficiaries, such as a statement advising the beneficiary to notify the provider about certain tests that were ordered, but not received, and information on other insurance coverage for beneficiaries, such as a Medigap policy.

Section 5: Signature Box

Once the beneficiary reviews and understands the information contained in the ABN, the Signature Box can be completed by the beneficiary (or representative). This box cannot be completed in advance of the rest of the notice. The beneficiary (or representative) must sign and date the notice to indicate that he or she has received the notice and understands its contents. If a representative signs on behalf of a beneficiary, he or she should write out "representative" in parentheses after his or her signature. The representative's name should be clearly legible or noted in print. The disclosure statement in the footer of the notice is required to be included on the document.

Modifiers for ABNs

A selection of modifiers may be appended to CPT/HCPCS codes on Medicare claims when an ABN has been signed. These modifiers indicate whether an ABN is on file or was considered needed.

▶ Modifier GZ means that the provider believes a service will be denied as not medically necessary but does not have an ABN due to circumstances. It may also mean that the physician did not determine that Medicare will not pay until the service is rendered, so it is too late to get the patient to sign an ABN. This modifier cannot be reported along with GX.

▶ Modifier GA means "waiver of liability statement issued as required by payer policy." This modifier is used only when a mandatory ABN was issued for a service. Medicare's claim processing system automatically denies claim lines with GA and assigns beneficiary liability for the charge.

▶ Modifier GY means that the provider considers the service excluded and did not complete an ABN, as none was required.

▶ Modifier GX means "notice of liability issued, voluntary under payer policy." This is the modifier for voluntary ABNs. Medicare's claim processing system automatically denies lines submitted with GX appended to noncovered charges, and assigns beneficiary liability for the charge.

THINKING IT THROUGH 9.4

1. A physician provides routine foot care and, wanting to be sure the patient understands that this is not a covered Medicare benefit, has the patient sign a filled-in ABN. What modifier is used with the procedure code for the foot care?

9.5 Medicare Secondary Payer

In general, if a patient has additional insurance coverage, after the primary payer's RA has been posted, the next step is billing the second payer. The primary claim, of course, gave that payer information about the patient's secondary insurance policy. The secondary payer now needs to know what the primary payer paid on the claim in order to coordinate benefits.

Benefits for a patient who has both Medicare and other coverage are coordinated under the rules of the **Medicare Secondary Payer (MSP)** program. The Medicare coordination of benefits contractor receives inquiries regarding Medicare as second payer and has information on a beneficiary's eligibility for benefits and the availability of other health insurance that is primary to Medicare.

The medical assistant is responsible for identifying the situations where Medicare is the secondary payer and for preparing appropriate primary and secondary claims. A form for this purpose is used to gather and validate information about Medicare patients' primary plans during the patient check-in process.

If a beneficiary has Medigap insurance, Medicare is the *primary payer*. That means that Medicare pays first, and then the Medigap carrier determines its obligations. File the claim with Medicare first. After a MAC processes a claim for a patient with Medigap coverage, the MAC automatically forwards the claim to the Medigap payer, indicating the amount Medicare approved and paid for the procedures. Once the Medigap carrier adjudicates the claim, the provider is paid directly, eliminating the need for the practice to file a separate Medigap claim. The beneficiary receives copies of the Medicare Summary Notices that explain the charges paid and due.

Some individuals are eligible for both Medicaid and Medicare (**Medi-Medi beneficiary**). Claims for these patients are first submitted to Medicare. Then they are sent to Medicaid along with the Medicare Remittance Notice. Most Medicare carriers transmit these **crossover claims** to the state Medicaid payer automatically.

In some situations, Medicare is the *secondary payer*. Generally, these situations are related to accidents or job-related illnesses or injuries. Medicare is a secondary payer when:

▶ The patient is covered through an employer's group health plan or the spouse's employer's group health plan.

Medicare Secondary Payer (MSP) Federal law requiring private payers to be the primary payers for Medicare beneficiaries' claims.

Medi-Medi beneficiary Person eligible for both Medicare and Medicaid.

crossover claims Claims for a Medicare or Medicaid beneficiary.

► The services are for treatment of a work-related illness or injury covered by workers' compensation or federal black lung benefits.

► No-fault insurance or liability insurance covers the services, such as those for illness or injury resulting from an automobile accident.

► A patient with end-stage renal disease is covered by an employer's group health plan. In this case, Medicare is the secondary payer for the first eighteen months.

THINKING IT THROUGH 9.5

1. Ron Polonsky is a seventy-one-year-old retired distribution manager. He and his wife Sandra live in Lincoln, Nebraska. Sandra is fifty-seven and is employed as a high-school science teacher. She has family coverage through a group health insurance plan offered by the state of Nebraska. Ron is covered as a dependent on her plan. The Medicare Part B carrier for Nebraska is the regional MAC. Which carrier is Ron's primary insurance carrier? Why?

9.6 Claim Completion

Physicians who treat Medicare beneficiaries must file claims for their patients even if they do not participate and do not accept assignment on the claims. CMS mandates electronic transmission of Medicare claims using the HIPAA 837 format, except by very small practices.

Timely Filing

Medicare law sets specific guidelines for **timely filing** of claims for benefits. The health reform law (Patient Protection and Affordable Care Act, or PPACA) required a change in Medicare timely filing of claims for Part B providers. Previously, Medicare law required the claim to be filed no later than the end of the calendar year following the year in which the service was furnished. The new law requires claims to be filed within one calendar year after the date of service. When filing a late claim, be sure to include an explanation of the reason for the late filing and have evidence to support it. Late claims may be paid if the lateness is due to a good cause, such as a Medicare administrative error, unavoidable delay, or accidental record damage.

timely filing Medicare law requiring claims to be filed within one calendar year.

Paper Claim Instructions

In the rare case when a CMS-1500 claim is required, follow the instructions shown in Table 7.3 (pages 162–163). Figure 9.3 shows a completed Medicare claim.

Exercise 9.1 Completing a Medicare Claim

Patient George O. Ahmadian has insurance coverage under an Original Medicare plan. Create a claim for his recent visit with Dr. Clarke.

Follow the steps at www.mhhe.com/newbycarr to complete the exercise at connect.mcgraw-hill.com on your own once you have watched the demo and tried the steps with prompts in practice mode. Use the information provided in the scenario to complete the exercise.

connect™ (plus+)

DRAFT - NOT FOR OFFICIAL USE

HEALTH INSURANCE CLAIM FORM

APPROVED BY NATIONAL UNIFORM CLAIM COMMITTEE (NUCC) 02/12

☐☐ PICA   PICA ☐☐

1. MEDICARE	MEDICAID	TRICARE	CHAMPVA	GROUP HEALTH PLAN	FECA BLK LUNG	OTHER	1a. INSURED'S I.D. NUMBER (For Program in Item 1)
☒ (Medicare#)	☐ (Medicaid#)	☐ (ID#/DoD#)	☐ (Member ID#)	☐ (ID#)	☐ (ID#)	☐ (ID#)	456221234A

2. PATIENT'S NAME (Last Name, First Name, Middle Initial)

3. PATIENT'S BIRTH DATE MM | DD | YY   SEX M ☐ F ☐

4. INSURED'S NAME (Last Name, First Name, Middle Initial)
NAPJER, JOHN, D

5. PATIENT'S ADDRESS (No., Street)

6. PATIENT RELATIONSHIP TO INSURED
Self ☒ Spouse ☐ Child ☐ Other ☐

7. INSURED'S ADDRESS (No., Street)
47 CARRIAGE DR

CITY   STATE

8. RESERVED FOR NUCC USE

CITY CHESHIRE   STATE CO

ZIP CODE   TELEPHONE (Include Area Code) ( )

ZIP CODE 80034   TELEPHONE (Include Area Code) ( )

9. OTHER INSURED'S NAME (Last Name, First Name, Middle Initial)

10. IS PATIENT'S CONDITION RELATED TO:

11. INSURED'S POLICY GROUP OR FECA NUMBER

a. OTHER INSURED'S POLICY OR GROUP NUMBER

a. EMPLOYMENT? (Current or Previous) ☐ YES ☒ NO

a. INSURED'S DATE OF BIRTH MM | DD | YY 05 | 05 | 1944   SEX M ☒ F ☐

b. RESERVED FOR NUCC USE

b. AUTO ACCIDENT? ☐ YES ☒ NO   PLACE (State)

b. OTHER CLAIM ID (Designated by NUCC)

c. RESERVED FOR NUCC USE

c. OTHER ACCIDENT? ☐ YES ☒ NO

c. INSURANCE PLAN NAME OR PROGRAM NAME

d. INSURANCE PLAN NAME OR PROGRAM NAME

10d. CLAIM CODES (Designated by NUCC)

d. IS THERE ANOTHER HEALTH BENEFIT PLAN?
☐ YES ☐ NO If yes, complete items 9, 9a, and 9d.

READ BACK OF FORM BEFORE COMPLETING & SIGNING THIS FORM.
12. PATIENT'S OR AUTHORIZED PERSON'S SIGNATURE I authorize the release of any medical or other information necessary to process this claim. I also request payment of government benefits either to myself or to the party who accepts assignment below.

SIGNED SOF   DATE

13. INSURED'S OR AUTHORIZED PERSON'S SIGNATURE I authorize payment of medical benefits to the undersigned physician or supplier for services described below.

SIGNED

14. DATE OF CURRENT ILLNESS, INJURY, or PREGNANCY (LMP) MM | DD | YY 10 | 01 | 2016 QUAL.

15. OTHER DATE QUAL. MM | DD | YY

16. DATES PATIENT UNABLE TO WORK IN CURRENT OCCUPATION FROM MM | DD | YY TO MM | DD | YY

17. NAME OF REFERRING PROVIDER OR OTHER SOURCE

17a.
17b. NPI

18. HOSPITALIZATION DATES RELATED TO CURRENT SERVICES FROM MM | DD | YY TO MM | DD | YY

19. ADDITIONAL CLAIM INFORMATION (Designated by NUCC)

20. OUTSIDE LAB? ☐ YES ☒ NO $ CHARGES

21. DIAGNOSIS OR NATURE OF ILLNESS OR INJURY Relate A-L to service line below (24E)   ICD Ind. 0
A. 50.9   B. 59.9   C.   D.
E.   F.   G.   H.
I.   J.   K.   L.

22. RESUBMISSION CODE   ORIGINAL REF. NO.

23. PRIOR AUTHORIZATION NUMBER

24. A. DATE(S) OF SERVICE					B. PLACE OF SERVICE	C. EMG	D. PROCEDURES, SERVICES, OR SUPPLIES (Explain Unusual Circumstances) CPT/HCPCS	MODIFIER	E. DIAGNOSIS POINTER	F. $ CHARGES	G. DAYS OR UNITS	H. EPSDT Family Plan	I. ID. QUAL.	J. RENDERING PROVIDER ID. #
From MM	DD	YY	To MM	DD	YY										
1	10	03	2016				11		99203		A, B	95 00	1		NPI
2															NPI
3															NPI
4															NPI
5															NPI
6															NPI

25. FEDERAL TAX I.D. NUMBER 123459666   SSN ☐ EIN ☒

26. PATIENT'S ACCOUNT NO. NAP0123

27. ACCEPT ASSIGNMENT? (For govt. claims, see back) ☒ YES ☐ NO

28. TOTAL CHARGE $ 95 00

29. AMOUNT PAID $ 0 00

30. Rsvd for NUCC Use

31. SIGNATURE OF PHYSICIAN OR SUPPLIER INCLUDING DEGREES OR CREDENTIALS (I certify that the statements on the reverse apply to this bill and are made a part thereof.)

SIGNED   DATE

32. SERVICE FACILITY LOCATION INFORMATION

a. NPI   b.

33. BILLING PROVIDER INFO & PH # (614) 3331212
RUTH J. CLARKE, MD
841 ORCHARD HILL RD
COLUMBUS OH 43214-1234

a. 4675316922   b.

NUCC Instruction Manual available at: www.nucc.org   PLEASE PRINT OR TYPE   OMB APPROVAL PENDING

FIGURE 9.3 CMS-1500 (02/12) Completion for Medicare Primary Claims

Chapter Summary

Learning Outcomes	Key Concepts/Examples
9.1 Differentiate among Medicare Parts A, B, C, and D. Pages 197–198	• Medicare Part A provides coverage for care in hospitals, skilled nursing facilities, home health, and hospice care. • Part B provides outpatient medical coverage. • Part C offers plans provided by private health insurance companies called Medicare Advantage, as an option to coverage under the Original Medicare Plan. • Part D is a prescription drug plan.
9.2 Compare the Original Medicare Plan and Medicare Advantage Plans. Pages 199–200	• The Original Medicare Plan is a fee for service plan that allows beneficiaries the freedom to choose from any licensed provider or specialist certified by Medicare. • Patients are responsible for an annual deductible and a coinsurance. • Patients receive a Medicare Summary Notice (MSN) detailing their services and charges. • Under Medicare Advantage beneficiaries can enroll in a coordinated care plan (CCPs), private fee for service plan, or a medical savings account (MSA). • Individuals enrolled in the Original Medicare Plan often have Medigap insurance to pay for annual deductibles and coinsurance.
9.3 Calculate fees for participating physicians and for nonparticipating physicians when they do and do not accept assignment. Pages 201–203	• Participating providers agree to accept assignment for all Medicare claims and to accept Medicare's allowed charge according to the Medicare Physician Fee Schedule as payment in full for services. • Nonparticipating providers decide whether to accept assignment on a claim by claim basis. • Providers who elect not to participate in the Medicare program are paid 5 percent less than participating providers. • Nonparticipating providers who do not accept assignment are subject to Medicare's limiting charges.
9.4 Complete an advance beneficiary notice of noncoverage (ABN). Pages 204–208	The ABN has five sections and ten blanks. • Section 1 is the Header (Blanks A–C). • Section 2 is the Body (Blanks D–F). • Section 3 is the Options Box (Blank G). • Section 4 is for Additional Information (Blank H). • Section 5 is the Signature Box (Blanks I–J).
9.5 Determine whether Medicare is the primary or secondary payer in a given situation. Pages 208–209	Medicare is a secondary payer when • The patient is covered through an employer or a spouse's group health plan. • The services are for treatment covered by workers' compensation or federal black lung benefits. • No-fault insurance or liability insurance covers the services. • A patient with end stage renal disease is covered by an employer's group health plan.
9.6 Prepare accurate Medicare claims. Pages 209–210	• CMS mandates electronic transmission of Medicare claims. • Medicare law requires claims to be filed within one calendar year after the date of service.

Using Terminology

Match the key terms in the left column with the definitions in the right column.

_____ 1. **[LO 9.3]** Physician Quality Reporting System (PQRS)

_____ 2. **[LO 9.4]** Advance beneficiary notice of noncoverage (ABN)

_____ 3. **[LO 9.1]** Medicare administrative contractor (MAC)

_____ 4. **[LO 9.6]** Timely filing

_____ 5. **[LO 9.4]** Local coverage determination (LCD)

_____ 6. **[LO 9.1]** Medicare Advantage

_____ 7. **[LO 9.5]** Medicare Secondary Payer (MSP)

_____ 8. **[LO 9.2]** Medigap

_____ 9. **[LO 9.2]** Medicare Remittance Notice (MRN)

_____ 10. **[LO 9.2]** Medicare Summary Notice (MSN)

A. Medicare form used to notify a patient that an item or service may not be covered.

B. Federal law requiring private payers to be the primary payers for Medicare beneficiaries' claims.

C. Contains detailed and updated information about coding and medical necessity of services.

D. Insurance companies that process Medicare claims.

E. Sent to the patient to explain how benefits were applied.

F. Private insurance purchased as a supplement to the original Medicare Plan.

G. CMS program that provides incentives based on performance measurements.

H. Sent to the provider to explain how a claim was processed.

I. Medicare law requiring claims to be filed within one calendar year.

J. Medicare plans provided through private insurance companies.

Checking Your Understanding

Write the letter of the choice that best completes the statement or answers the question.

1. **[LO 9.1]** Medicare Part A covers _____.
   A. Physician services
   B. Prescription drugs
   C. Inpatient hospital services
   D. Durable medical equipment

2. **[LO 9.2]** The Original Medicare Plan requires a premium, deductible, and _____.
   A. Medigap
   B. Coinsurance
   C. Supplemental insurance
   D. A formulary

3. **[LO 9.4]** Which ABN modifier indicates that a service that was done is not covered when no ABN was signed? _____
   A. —AB
   B. —GA
   C. —GY
   D. —GZ

4. **[LO 9.4]** Which ABN modifier indicates that a signed ABN is on file? _____
   A. —GY
   B. —GA
   C. —GZ
   D. —AB

5. **[LO 9.3]** What percentage of the allowed amount does Medicare pay participating providers? _____
   A. 75%
   B. 80%
   C. 90%
   D. 100%

connect™ (plus+)

Enhance your learning at mcgrawhillconnect.com!
- Practice Exercises
- Worksheets
- Activities
- Integrated eBook

6. **[LO 9.1]** Medicare beneficiaries with a health insurance claim number that starts with a prefix are covered under _____.
   A. Medicare Advantage
   B. Medicare Part D
   C. Medicare Part C
   D. Railroad Medicare

7. **[LO 9.6]** Medicare claims must be submitted _____.
   A. Within 6 months of the date of service.
   B. By the end of the calendar year following the service.
   C. Within one calendar year of the service.
   D. Within 90 days of the service.

8. **[LO 9.5]** An individual eligible for both Medicaid and Medicare is known as a _____.
   A. Medicare administrative contractor (MAC)
   B. Medicare beneficiary
   C. Medigap beneficiary
   D. Medi-Medi beneficiary

9. **[LO 9.1]** Outpatient hospital services are billed to _____.
   A. Medicare Part A
   B. Medicare Part B
   C. Medicare Part C
   D. Medicare Part D

10. **[LO 9.3]** Nonparticipating providers who do not accept assignment are subject to a limiting charge of _____.
    A. 5%   C. 115%
    B. 20%   D. 80%

Applying Your Knowledge

[LO 9.3]   Case 9.1

The following information is presented on a patient's Medicare MSN. What does the patient owe?

BILL SUBMITTED BY: Dr. Anthony B. Starpish
29 Washington Square North
New York, NY 10011

Date	Services and Service Code	Medicare Charges	Approved
2-10-2016	1 Destruction of hemorrhoids (46934-78)	$325.00	$194.78*

(Note: *The approved amount is based on the fee schedule.)

Explanation:

Of the total charges, Medicare approved	$194.78	(The provider agreed to accept this amount.)
Your 20 percent	−$38.96	
The 80 percent Medicare pays	$155.82	

You have already met the deductible for 2016.

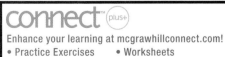

Enhance your learning at mcgrawhillconnect.com!
• Practice Exercises   • Worksheets
• Activities   • Integrated eBook

[LO 9.3] Case 9.2

Fill in the blanks in the following payment situations:

Participating Provider

Physician's standard fee	$210.00
Medicare fee	$115.00
Medicare pays 80%	$ _____
Patient or supplemental plan pays 20%	$ _____
Provider adjustment (write-off)	$ _____

Nonparticipating Provider (Accepts Assignment)

Physician's standard fee	$210.00
Medicare nonPAR fee	$109.25
Medicare pays 80%	$ _____
Patient/supplemental plan pays 20%	$ _____
Provider adjustment (write-off)	$ _____

Nonparticipating Provider (Does Not Accept Assignment)

Physician's standard fee	$210.00
Medicare nonPAR fee	$109.25
Limiting charge	$ _____
Patient billed	$ _____
Medicare pays patient	$ _____
Total provider can collect	$ _____
Patient out-of-pocket expense	$ _____

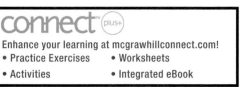

Enhance your learning at mcgrawhillconnect.com!
- Practice Exercises
- Worksheets
- Activities
- Integrated eBook

10

MEDICAID

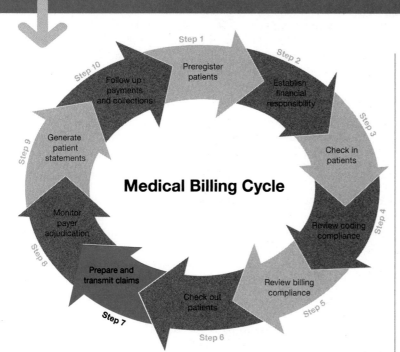

Medical Billing Cycle

- Step 1 Preregister patients
- Step 2 Establish financial responsibility
- Step 3 Check in patients
- Step 4 Review coding compliance
- Step 5 Review billing compliance
- Step 6 Check out patients
- Step 7 Prepare and transmit claims
- Step 8 Monitor payer adjudication
- Step 9 Generate patient statements
- Step 10 Follow up payments and collections

KEY TERMS

categorically needy
Children's Health Insurance Program (CHIP)
Early and Periodic Screening, Diagnosis, and Treatment (EPSDT)
Federal Medicaid Assistance Percentage (FMAP)
fiscal agent
Medicaid
MediCal
medically indigent
medically needy
payer of last resort
Temporary Assistance for Needy Families (TANF)
third-party liability
Welfare Reform Act

Learning Outcomes

After studying this chapter, you should be able to:

10.1 Identify two ways Medicaid programs vary from state to state.

10.2 Compare the Medicaid benefits that are determined by federal and by state laws.

10.3 Explain two broad classifications of people who are eligible for Medicaid assistance.

10.4 Explain factors that require special attention when filing Medicaid claims.

Medicaid is the nation's largest non-employer-sponsored health insurance program. Because Medicaid is run by states, rather than by the federal government, medical assistants refer to the laws and regulations of their state Medicaid programs to correctly process claims for these patients.

10.1 Introduction to Medicaid

Most of the claims that medical assistants file are for benefits due under health insurance plans. However, one government program that pays for health care services is actually an assistance program, not an insurance program.

Medicaid pays for health care services for people with incomes below the national poverty level. Both federal and state governments pay for the program, and in some areas local taxes support it as well. The federal government makes payments to states under the **Federal Medicaid Assistance Percentage (FMAP).** The amount of the payment is based on the state's average per capita income in relation to the national income average. States with high per capita incomes receive less federal funding than do states with low per capita incomes. In each state, Medicaid is administered by a **fiscal agent,** an organization that processes claims for a government program. The Center for Medicaid and State Operations, a department of the Centers for Medicare and Medicaid Services (CMS), oversees the programs that are administered by the states.

The first Medicaid programs were required by federal law as part of the Social Security Act of 1965. Under the legislation, the federal government determines which kinds of medical services are covered and paid for by the federal portion of the program. States participate in their Medicaid programs in two ways: (1) they may authorize additional kinds of services or make additional groups eligible, and (2) they determine eligibility within federal guidelines. Because of this participation by state governments, Medicaid programs change often and vary widely from state to state. Thus, this chapter gives only general information about Medicaid.

However, this variation is expected to be reduced as the Affordable Care Act (ACA) rules are implemented beginning in 2014. The ACA requires that people who are (1) not elderly and (2) have incomes below 133 percent of the poverty level will be eligible for Medicaid in 2014. The ACA ruling is expected to add 16 million people to Medicaid enrollment.

A physician may choose to participate in the Medicaid program or not to accept Medicaid patients. Participating in the Medicaid program means agreeing to accept Medicaid reimbursement for covered services as payment in full. The physician must write off the difference, if any, between fees charged for services and the amount reimbursed. The physician may not bill the patient for the difference. However, the physician may bill the patient for services not covered by Medicaid.

THINKING IT THROUGH 10.1

1. Research the Medicaid eligibility requirements, benefits, and limitations in your state.

10.2 Medicaid Coverage

According to federal guidelines, Medicaid pays for the following types of health care:

► Physician services.
► Laboratory and X-ray services.
► Inpatient hospital services.
► Outpatient hospital services.

Medicaid Pays for health care services for people with incomes below the national poverty level.

Federal Medicaid Assistance Percentage (FMAP) Basis for federal government Medicaid allocations to states.

fiscal agent Organization that processes claims for a government program.

COMPLIANCE GUIDELINE

HIPAA Rules Apply

The HIPAA Privacy Rule, Electronic Health Care Transaction and Code Sets standards, and Security Rule apply to physicians who are treating Medicaid patients.

Federal Medicaid Information
www.cms.gov/
MedicaidGenInfo/

- Rural health clinic services.
- Home health care.
- Family planning services.
- Federally qualified health-center (FQHC) services.
- Skilled care at a public nursing facility.
- Nurse-midwife services.
- Early and Periodic Screening, Diagnosis, and Treatment (EPSDT) services.
- Transportation to medical care.

Family planning services include counseling, diagnosis, treatment, drugs, and supplies related to planning the number and spacing of children. **Early and Periodic Screening, Diagnosis, and Treatment (EPSDT)** is a prevention, early-detection, and treatment program for children under the age of twenty-one who are enrolled in Medicaid. Covered services include medical history; physical exam; assessment of development and immunization status; and screening for anemia, lead absorption, tuberculosis, sickle cell trait and disease, and dental, hearing, and vision problems. States must pay for all services identified in an EPSDT exam, even if they do not pay for the services for other eligible individuals.

The **Children's Health Insurance Program (CHIP),** part of the Balanced Budget Act of 1997, requires states to develop and implement plans for health insurance coverage for uninsured children. The more than 5 million children served by CHIP come from low-income families whose incomes are not low enough to qualify for Medicaid. The program is funded jointly by the federal government and the states. It provides coverage for many preventive services and covers children up to age nineteen.

The Ticket to Work and Work Incentives Improvement Act of 1999 (TWWIIA) expands the availability of health care services for workers with disabilities. Previously, persons with disabilities often had to choose between health care and work. TWWIIA gives states the option of allowing individuals with disabilities to purchase Medicaid coverage that is necessary to enable them to maintain employment.

The state portion of a Medicaid program often includes a number of additional services under its federally funded Medicaid program. Some examples of extra assistance enacted by individual states include:

- Clinic services.
- Emergency room care.
- Ambulance services.
- Chiropractic services.
- Mental-health services.
- Certain cosmetic procedures.
- Allergy services.
- Dermatology services.
- Dental care.
- Home and community-based care to certain persons with chronic impairments.
- Podiatry services.
- Eyeglasses and eye refraction.
- Prescription drugs.
- Prosthetic devices.
- Private-duty nursing.
- Other diagnostic, screening, preventive, and rehabilitative services.

In recent years, however, because of large state budget deficits, state laws have cut back on some of these benefits—for example, prescription drug benefits and hearing, vision, and dental benefits for adults. Many states have also had to restrict eligibility for Medicaid and to reduce Medicaid payments to doctors, hospitals, nursing homes, and other providers.

Early and Periodic Screening, Diagnosis, and Treatment (EPSDT) Medicaid's prevention, early detection, and treatment program for eligible children under twenty-one.

Children's Health Insurance Program (CHIP) Offers health insurance coverage for uninsured children.

In each state, the Medicaid and/or social services agency can provide a list of services and any limits or preauthorization requirements for those services. Any additional services, such as those just listed, are paid entirely from state funds.

THINKING IT THROUGH 10.2

1. Explain the difference between the EPSDT program and the CHIP program.

10.3 Medicaid Eligibility and Plans

Generally, Medicaid recipients are people with low incomes who have children, or are over the age of sixty-five, are blind, or have permanent disabilities. Within federal guidelines, states determine income levels and other qualifications for eligibility.

Categorically Needy versus Medically Needy

categorically needy Person who receives assistance from government programs.

Welfare Reform Act Law that established TANF and tightened Medicaid eligibility requirements.

Temporary Assistance for Needy Families (TANF) Program that provides cash assistance for low-income families.

medically needy Classification for people with high medical expenses and low financial resources.

medically indigent Classification for people with high medical expenses and low financial resources.

MediCal California's Medicaid program.

One group of Medicaid recipients is known as **categorically needy.** Their needs are addressed under the Personal Responsibility and Work Opportunity Reconciliation Act of 1996 (P.L. 104–193), commonly known as the **Welfare Reform Act,** which created **Temporary Assistance for Needy Families (TANF).** Eligibility for TANF is determined at the county level. This program helps with living, as opposed to medical, expenses.

Some states extend Medicaid eligibility to include another group of people classified as **medically needy** or **medically indigent.** These individuals earn enough money to pay for basic living expenses, but they cannot afford high medical bills. In some cases, Medicaid recipients in the medically needy classification must pay deductibles before they receive benefits. Some Medicaid recipients in this category must pay coinsurance for medical services. States choose their own names for the programs. For example, California calls its program **MediCal.**

Once Medicaid eligibility is determined, the recipient gets an identification card or coupon explaining effective dates and additional information such as a coinsurance requirement, if any. Different states authorize coverage for different lengths of time. Some states issue cards twice a month, some once a month, and others every two months or every six months. Most states, however, are moving to electronic verification of eligibility under the Electronic Medicaid Eligibility Verification System (EMEVS). Eligibility should be checked each time a patient makes an appointment and before the patient sees the physician. Many states provide both online and telephone verification systems.

Medicaid Plans

In most states, Medicaid offers both fee-for-service and managed care plans.

Fee-for-Service

Medicaid clients enrolled in a fee-for-service plan may be treated by the provider of their choice, as long as that provider accepts Medicaid. The provider submits the claim to Medicaid and is paid directly by Medicaid.

Managed Care

Many states have shifted the Medicaid population from fee-for-service programs to managed care plans. Nationally, about half of Medicaid recipients are in managed care plans. Client enrollment in a managed care plan is either mandatory or voluntary, depending on state regulations. Medicaid managed care plans restrict patients to a network of physicians, hospitals, and clinics. Individuals enrolled in managed care plans must obtain all services and referrals through their primary care provider (PCP). The PCP is responsible for coordinating and monitoring the patient's care. If the patient needs to see a specialist, the PCP must provide a referral; otherwise, the managed care plan will not pay for the service.

Managed care plans offer Medicaid recipients several advantages. Some Medicaid patients experience difficulty finding a physician who will treat them, in part due to the lower fee structure. Under a managed care plan, individuals choose a primary care physician who provides treatment and manages their medical care. The patient also has access to specialists should the need arise. In addition, managed care programs offer greater access to preventive care such as immunizations and health screenings.

Fraud and Abuse in Medicaid

The Medicaid Alliance for Program Safeguards is committed to fighting fraud and abuse, which divert dollars that should be spent to safeguard the health and welfare of Medicaid clients. Although states are primarily responsible for policing fraud in the Medicaid program, CMS provides technical assistance, guidance, and oversight in these efforts. Fraud schemes often cross state lines, and CMS strives to improve information sharing among the Medicaid programs and other stakeholders.

Medicaid fraud can take many forms. Here are some of the more common schemes:

▶ Billing for "phantom patients" who did not really receive services.
▶ Billing for medical services or goods that were not provided.
▶ Billing for old items as if they were new.
▶ Billing for more hours than there are in a day.
▶ Billing for tests that the patient did not need.
▶ Paying kickbacks in exchange for referrals for medical services or goods.
▶ Charging Medicaid for personal expenses not related to caring for a Medicaid client.
▶ Overcharging for health care services or goods that were provided.
▶ Concealing ownership in a related company.
▶ Using false credentials.
▶ Double-billing for health care services or goods that were provided.

THINKING IT THROUGH 10.3

1. Distinguish between individuals who are categorically needy and those who are medically needy under Medicaid definitions.

10.4 Filing Medicaid Claims

Medicaid claims are filed in the patient's home state. Because Medicaid is covered by HIPAA, Medicaid claims are usually submitted using the HIPAA 837 claim (see the chapter covering health care claim preparation and transmission). In some situations, however, a paper claim using the CMS-1500 format may be used, or a state-specific form may be requested. If the CMS-1500 is required, follow the guidelines in

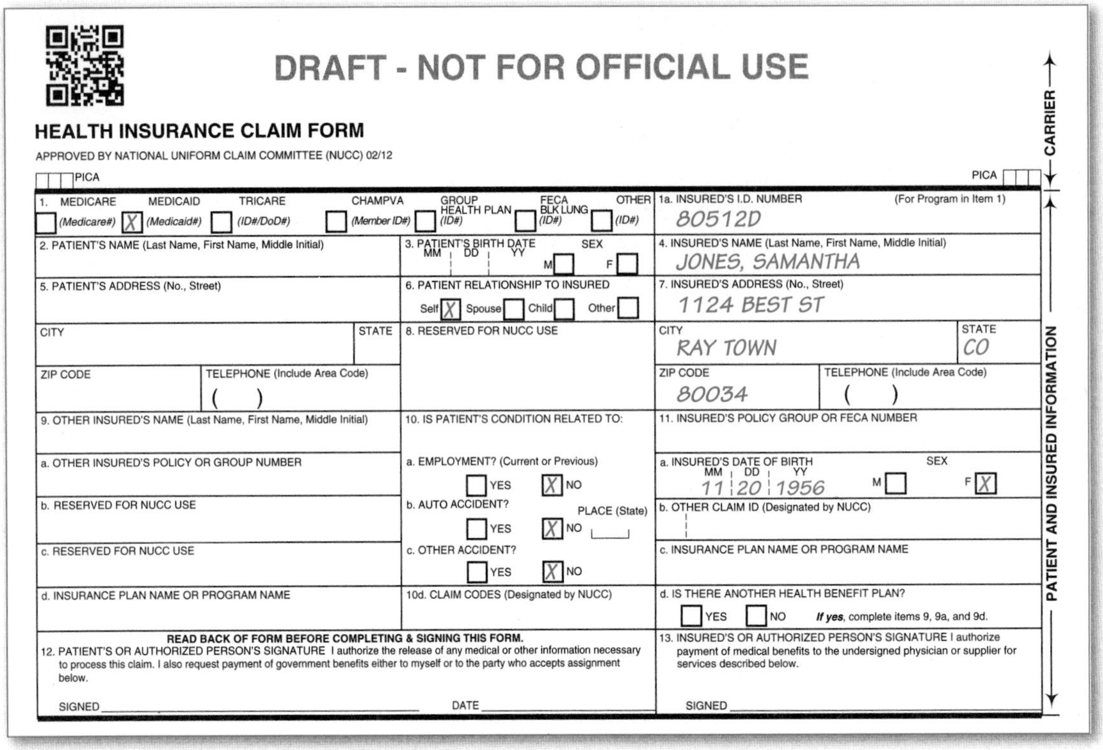

DRAFT - NOT FOR OFFICIAL USE

HEALTH INSURANCE CLAIM FORM

APPROVED BY NATIONAL UNIFORM CLAIM COMMITTEE (NUCC) 02/12

PICA | PICA

CARRIER

1. MEDICARE (Medicare#) | MEDICAID (Medicaid#) [X] | TRICARE (ID#/DoD#) | CHAMPVA (Member ID#) | GROUP HEALTH PLAN (ID#) | FECA BLK LUNG (ID#) | OTHER (ID#)

1a. INSURED'S I.D. NUMBER (For Program in Item 1): 80512D

2. PATIENT'S NAME (Last Name, First Name, Middle Initial)

3. PATIENT'S BIRTH DATE MM DD YY | SEX M F

4. INSURED'S NAME (Last Name, First Name, Middle Initial): JONES, SAMANTHA

5. PATIENT'S ADDRESS (No., Street)

6. PATIENT RELATIONSHIP TO INSURED: Self [X] Spouse Child Other

7. INSURED'S ADDRESS (No., Street): 1124 BEST ST

CITY | STATE

8. RESERVED FOR NUCC USE

CITY: RAY TOWN | STATE: CO

ZIP CODE | TELEPHONE (Include Area Code) ( )

ZIP CODE: 80034 | TELEPHONE (Include Area Code) ( )

9. OTHER INSURED'S NAME (Last Name, First Name, Middle Initial)

10. IS PATIENT'S CONDITION RELATED TO:

11. INSURED'S POLICY GROUP OR FECA NUMBER

a. OTHER INSURED'S POLICY OR GROUP NUMBER

a. EMPLOYMENT? (Current or Previous) YES NO [X]

a. INSURED'S DATE OF BIRTH MM DD YY: 11 20 1956 | SEX M F [X]

b. RESERVED FOR NUCC USE

b. AUTO ACCIDENT? YES NO [X] PLACE (State)

b. OTHER CLAIM ID (Designated by NUCC)

c. RESERVED FOR NUCC USE

c. OTHER ACCIDENT? YES NO [X]

c. INSURANCE PLAN NAME OR PROGRAM NAME

d. INSURANCE PLAN NAME OR PROGRAM NAME

10d. CLAIM CODES (Designated by NUCC)

d. IS THERE ANOTHER HEALTH BENEFIT PLAN? YES NO *If yes*, complete items 9, 9a, and 9d.

READ BACK OF FORM BEFORE COMPLETING & SIGNING THIS FORM.

12. PATIENT'S OR AUTHORIZED PERSON'S SIGNATURE I authorize the release of any medical or other information necessary to process this claim. I also request payment of government benefits either to myself or to the party who accepts assignment below.

SIGNED ______ DATE ______

13. INSURED'S OR AUTHORIZED PERSON'S SIGNATURE I authorize payment of medical benefits to the undersigned physician or supplier for services described below.

SIGNED ______

PATIENT AND INSURED INFORMATION

FIGURE 10.1 CMS-1500 (02/12) Claim Completion for Medicaid

Table 7.3 (on pages 162–163) and complete the form as shown in Figure 10.1. In each state, the fiscal agent provides the rules for submitting claims. The website for each state is shown in Table 10.1.

Medicaid managed care claims are filed differently than other Medicaid claims. Claims are sent to the managed care organization instead of to the state Medicaid department. Participating providers agree to the guidelines of the managed care organization, provided that they are in compliance with federal requirements.

BILLING TIP

Medicaid Claims

Since the patient is a Medicaid beneficiary, signatures in IN 12 and 13 are not required.

Claim Data

A number of special data elements may be required for completion of HIPAA-compliant Medicaid claims. The requirements are controlled by state guidelines. The following elements are reported:

- Whether family planning services were involved in the visit.
- Whether the services are the result of a screening referral (EPSDT).
- Whether the services involved a special program such as a special federal funding program.
- A Service Authorization Exception Code when a provider must receive authorization for specific services that could not be obtained because of such reasons as the need for emergency care.
- The physician's Medicaid number as a secondary identifier.

Out-of-State Filing

Sometimes a physician in one state treats a patient who lives in another state, either because the patient is traveling or because the patient lives near a state boundary and has easier access to physicians in the neighboring state. Since Medicaid is administered on a state-by-state basis, the Medicaid claim must be filed in the patient's home state. Nevertheless, most Medicaid programs have state-to-state agreements to cover each other's Medicaid patients. The fiscal agent in the patient's home state may be contacted to get forms and claim processing information.

Table 10.1 Medicaid Websites by State

State	Abbr.	Website
ALABAMA	AL	www.medicaid.state.al.us/
ALASKA	AK	www.hss.state.ak.us/dhcs/Medicaid/
ARIZONA	AZ	www.ahcccs.state.az.us/site/
ARKANSAS	AR	www.medicaid.state.ar.us/
CALIFORNIA	CA	www.dhs.ca.gov/mcs/
COLORADO	CO	www.chcpf.state.co.us/default.asp
CONNECTICUT	CT	www.ct.gov/dss/
DELAWARE	DE	www.dhss.delaware.gov/
DISTRICT OF COLUMBIA	DC	doh.dc.gov/doh/site/default.asp
FLORIDA	FL	www.fdhc.state.fl.us/Medicaid/
GEORGIA	GA	dch.georgia.gov
HAWAII	HI	med-quest.us/
IDAHO	ID	www.healthandwelfare.idaho.gov/
ILLINOIS	IL	www.hfs.illinois.gov/medical/
INDIANA	IN	www.state.in.us/
IOWA	IA	www.dhs.state.ia.us/
KANSAS	KS	da.state.ks.us/hpf/
KENTUCKY	KY	chfs.ky.gov
LOUISIANA	LA	www.dhh.state.la.us/
MAINE	ME	www.maine.gov/
MARYLAND	MD	www.dhmh.state.md.us/
MASSACHUSETTS	MA	www.mass.gov/
MICHIGAN	MI	www.Michigan.gov/mdch
MINNESOTA	MN	www.dhs.state.mn.us/
MISSISSIPPI	MS	www.medicaid.state.ms.us/
MISSOURI	MO	www.dss.mo.gov/
MONTANA	MT	www.dphhs.mt.gov
NEBRASKA	NE	hhs.state.ne.us/
NEVADA	NV	dhcfp.state.nv.us/
NEW HAMPSHIRE	NH	www.dhhs.state.nh.us/
NEW JERSEY	NJ	www.state.nj.us/
NEW MEXICO	NM	www.state.nm.us/
NEW YORK	NY	www.health.state.ny.us/
NORTH CAROLINA	NC	www.dhhs.state.nc.us/
NORTH DAKOTA	ND	www.nd.gov/humanservices/
OHIO	OH	jfs.ohio.gov/ohp/
OKLAHOMA	OK	www.ohca.state.ok.us/
OREGON	OR	www.oregon.gov/DHS/
PENNSYLVANIA	PA	www.dpw.state.pa.us/
RHODE ISLAND	RI	www.dhs.state.ri.us/
SOUTH CAROLINA	SC	www.dhhs.state.sc.us/
SOUTH DAKOTA	SD	www.state.sd.us/
TENNESSEE	TN	www.state.tn.us/tenncare/
TEXAS	TX	www.hhsc.state.tx.us/Medicaid/
UTAH	UT	health.utah.gov/medicaid/
VERMONT	VT	www.ovha.state.vt.us/medicaid.cfm
VIRGINIA	VA	www.dmas.virginia.gov/
WASHINGTON	WA	fortress.wa.gov/dshs/maa/
WEST VIRGINIA	WV	www.wvdhhr.org/bms/
WISCONSIN	WI	www.dhfs.state.wi.us/medicaid/
WYOMING	WY	wyequalitycare.acs-inc.com/

Claim Factors

When filing Medicaid claims for any state, the medical assistant should pay special attention to:

▶ *Eligibility*—Medicaid eligibility varies from month to month if the recipient's income fluctuates. Comply with the state's requirements for verifying eligibility. Check the patient's Medicaid identification card or coupon, and photocopy the front and back on each visit. Date the photocopy. Some states require this photocopy to be attached to the submitted claim form. An example of a Medicaid card is shown in Figure 10.2.

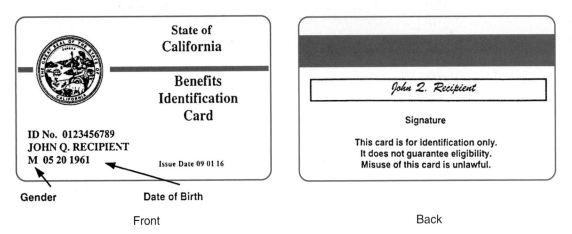

Gender	**Date of Birth**
Front	Back

FIGURE 10.2 Example of a Medicaid Identification Card

▶ *Preauthorization*—Most states require preauthorization for specified services. Check with the state's fiscal agent to find out how to get preauthorization by telephone and whether a written confirmation form must also be filed. If the state requires preauthorization, charges for services that did not get prior approval will not be paid. In emergencies, such as emergency room situations, authorization may be obtained after the treatment.

▶ *Filing Deadline*—The time line for filing a Medicaid claim ranges from two months to one year from the date of service. Find out the state's requirements, and file claims promptly.

▶ *Third-Party Liability*—**Third-party liability** is the obligation of a government program or insurance plan to pay all or part of a patient's medical costs. Before filing a claim with Medicaid, it is important to determine whether the patient has other insurance coverage.

Payer of Last Resort

If a patient who is eligible for Medicaid has additional health care coverage through an insurance plan or another government program such as Medicare, the patient's Medicaid eligibility does not relieve the other program or plan of its responsibility. In fact, the other program or insurance carrier is the primary carrier in these cases. Medicaid is the secondary carrier. File the claim first with the primary carrier, and file for Medicaid benefits last. Because of this sequence, Medicaid is referred to as the **payer of last resort.**

Dual-Eligibles

If a patient is covered by both Medicare and Medicaid (a Medi-Medi beneficiary or "dual-eligible"), Medicare is primary. The claim that is sent to Medicare is automatically crossed over to Medicaid for secondary payment.

Exercise 10.1 Completing a Medicaid Claim

Patient Isabella Neufield has coverage under Medicaid. Create a claim for her recent visit with Dr. Clarke.

Follow the steps at www.mhhe.com/newbycarr to complete the exercise at connect.mcgraw-hill.com on your own once you have watched the demo and tried the steps with prompts in practice mode. Use the information provided in the scenario to complete the exercise.

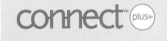

THINKING IT THROUGH 10.4

1. Why is it important to determine whether or not a patient has alternative insurance coverage before filing a claim with Medicaid?

Chapter Summary

Learning Outcomes	Key Concepts/Examples
10.1 Identify two ways Medicaid programs vary from state to state. Page 216	• States authorize additional services or groups eligible for coverage under their Medicaid program. • States determine eligibility within federal guidelines.
10.2 Compare the Medicaid benefits that are determined by federal and by state laws. Pages 216–218	• Early and Periodic Screening, Diagnosis, and Treatment (EPSDT) is a prevention, early detection, and treatment program for children under age twenty-one enrolled in Medicaid. • The Children's Health Insurance Program (CHIP) is a state program to provide health insurance coverage to uninsured children. • The Ticket to Work and Work Incentives Improvement Act of 1999 gives states the option to allow persons with disabilities to purchase Medicaid coverage and maintain employment.
10.3 Explain two broad classifications of people who are eligible for Medicaid assistance. Pages 218–219	• Medicaid recipients classified as categorically needy are eligible for Temporary Assistance for Needy Families. • Individuals with high medical expenses and limited financial resources are classified as medically needy or medically indigent.
10.4 Explain factors that require special attention when filing Medicaid claims. Pages 219–223	• Patients' eligibility and Medicaid identification cards need to be verified. • Preauthorization must be obtained for specified services. • Claims are subject to timely filing limits. • Third-party liability must be determined.

Using Terminology

Match the key terms in the left column with the definitions in the right column.

_____ 1. [LO 10.3] Medically indigent

_____ 2. [LO 10.2] Children's Health Insurance Program (CHIP)

_____ 3. [LO 10.3] Welfare Reform Act

_____ 4. [LO 10.2] Early and Periodic Screening, Diagnosis, and Treatment (EPSDT)

A. Program that offers uninsured children health insurance.

B. Program that provides financial assistance to low income families.

C. Private insurance plan or government program obligated to pay for a patient's medical costs.

D. An organization that processes claims for a government program.

E. Law that created Temporary Assistance for Needy Families (TANF).

F. Federal and state assistance program for health care services.

connect plus+

Enhance your learning at mcgrawhillconnect.com!
- Practice Exercises
- Worksheets
- Activities
- Integrated eBook

_____ **5.** **[LO 10.4]** Third-party liability

_____ **6.** **[LO 10.3]** Categorically needy

_____ **7.** **[LO 10.3]** Temporary Assistance for Needy Families (TANF)

_____ **8.** **[LO 10.3]** MediCal

_____ **9.** **[LO 10.1]** Fiscal agent

_____ **10.** **[LO 10.1]** Medicaid

G. California's Medicaid program.

H. Prevention, early detection, and treatment program for children under twenty-one.

I. Persons who are eligible for programs such as Temporary Assistance for Needy Families (TANF).

J. Individuals who qualify for Medicaid because of high medical bills and limited financial resources.

Checking Your Understanding

Write the letter of the choice that best completes the statement or answers the question.

1. **[LO 10.3]** Medicaid identification cards must be checked for eligibility _____.
   A. Once a year
   B. Every six months
   C. Only when there is a change in the patient's address
   D. Every time the patient receives services

2. **[LO 10.1]** Under the Federal Medicaid Assistance Program, the federal government makes payment directly to _____.
   A. States
   B. Individuals eligible to receive TANF
   C. Individuals who are blind or disabled
   D. Individuals who are categorically needy

3. **[LO 10.3]** Eligibility for TANF is determined _____.
   A. At the federal level
   B. At the state level
   C. At the county level
   D. At the national level

4. **[LO 10.3]** Applicants who qualify for Medicaid because they have high medical bills and limited income are classified as _____.
   A. Categorically needy
   B. Financially needy
   C. Medically needy
   D. Economically needy

5. **[LO 10.3]** More Medicaid recipients are being enrolled in _____.
   A. Supplemental plans
   B. Plans with a coinsurance
   C. Preventive care plans
   D. Managed care plans

6. **[LO 10.2]** The Ticket to Work and Work Incentives Improvement Act _____.
   A. Allows persons with disabilities to purchase Medicaid coverage
   B. Pays incentives to working Medicaid recipients
   C. Provides health insurance coverage to children
   D. Provides health insurance coverage to all working adults

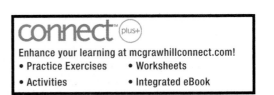

connect™ plus+

Enhance your learning at mcgrawhillconnect.com!
- Practice Exercises
- Activities
- Worksheets
- Integrated eBook

7. **[LO 10.3]** The Medicaid Alliance for Program Safeguards _____.
   A. Specifies civil and criminal penalties for fraudulent activities
   B. Audits state Medicaid payers on a regular basis
   C. Is a CMS program that came about as a result of the Welfare Reform Act
   D. Oversees states' fraud and abuse efforts

8. **[LO 10.4]** Claims for patients enrolled in a Medicaid managed care plan should be submitted to _____.
   A. The state Medicaid department
   B. Centers for Medicaid and Medicare services
   C. The managed care organization
   D. The department of social services

9. **[LO 10.4]** When treating a patient that has an out-of-state Medicaid plan claims are submitted to _____.
   A. The local Medicaid
   B. The patient's state Medicaid
   C. The department of social services in the patient's home state
   D. Centers for Medicaid and Medicare services

10. **[LO 10.4]** When a Medicaid patient has other coverage Medicaid _____.
    A. Pays Primary
    B. Is canceled
    C. Pays 80 percent of the allowed amount
    D. Is the payer of last resort

Applying Your Knowledge

Note: Refer to Chapter 7 to research place of service and claim filing indicator codes.

[LO 10.4] Case 10.1

Physician Information:
Name: Selena R. Rodez, MD
NPI: 8901234567
Medicaid PIN: HC29004

Patient Information Form:
Name: Grace B. Chin (New Patient)
Age: 47
Sex: Female
Birth Date: November 7, 1963
Social Security Number: 056-99-0034
Medicaid Eligibility: June 1-30, 2010 (*Note*: Copayment of $10 per office visit required.)
Medicaid Number: 056990034
Insurance Carrier: None

Patient's Encounter Form:
Date: 6-20-2016
T-98 BP 135/80
CC: Patient has a cut in the left eye, cause unknown. No visual problems. Reports some pain.
Dx: Ocular laceration without prolapse or loss of intraocular tissue, left eye.
Rx: Ophthalmic solution, 2 drops to left eye × 10 days.

connect plus+

Enhance your learning at mcgrawhillconnect.com!
• Practice Exercises   • Worksheets
• Activities   • Integrated eBook

List of Fees for Service:

Charges: Office visit, Level I, $35

Copayment collected

Supply the following data elements:

Billing Provider _____

Billing Provider's Primary Identifier _____

Billing Provider's Secondary Identifier _____

Subscriber/Patient _____

Subscriber's Primary Identifier _____

Claim Filing Indicator Code _____

Place of Service Code _____

Diagnosis Codes _____

Total Charge _____

Amount Collected _____

Service Line Information

Date of Service _____

Procedure Code/Charge _____

Diagnosis _____

[LO 10.4]   Case 10.2

Physician Information:

Name: Gloria A. Poyner, MD

NPI: 9012345678

Medicaid PIN: DC55289

Patient Information Form:

Name: George Eustis Kador (New Patient)

Sex: Male

Birth Date: November 27, 1948

Social Security Number: 033-45-7034

Medicaid Eligibility: July 1-31, 2016 (*Note*: Copayment of $7.50 per office visit required.)

Medicaid Number: 046971134

Insurance Carrier: None

Patient's Encounter Form:

Date: 7-7-2016

T-98 BP 135/80

CC: Patient presents with complaint of recent onset of palpitations. Reviewed social and medical history and records. Performed detailed system review and prescribed a twenty-four-hour electrocardiographic monitoring (a continuous original ECG waveform), supplying the monitor with hookup and recording; scanning analysis with report; reviewed and interpreted the analysis and report.

Dx: Palpitations

Date: 7-8-2016

Follow-up Office Visit: Diagnosed ectopic auricular beats. Discussed therapy with patient in this follow-up visit.

Dx: Atrial premature depolarization

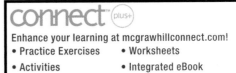

connect plus+

Enhance your learning at mcgrawhillconnect.com!
- Practice Exercises
- Worksheets
- Activities
- Integrated eBook

List of Fees for Services

7-7-2016

Services and Charges: Office visit, comprehensive history, comprehensive examination, moderately complex medical decision making, $65

ECG monitoring for twenty-four hours—recording, analysis/report, physician analysis and interpretation, $125

Copayment collected

7-8-2016

Services and Charges: Office visit, expanded history and examination, fifteen minutes with patient, $45

Copayment collected

Supply the following data elements:

Billing Provider _____

Billing Provider's Primary Identifier _____

Billing Provider's Secondary Identifier _____

Subscriber/Patient _____

Subscriber's Primary Identifier _____

Claim Filing Indicator Code _____

Place of Service Code _____

Diagnosis Codes _____

Total Charge _____

Amount Collected _____

Service Line Information

Date of Service _____

Procedure Code/Charge _____

Diagnosis _____

Date of Service _____

Procedure Code/Charge _____

Diagnosis _____

Date of Service _____

Procedure Code/Charge _____

Diagnosis _____

connect plus+

Enhance your learning at mcgrawhillconnect.com!
- Practice Exercises   • Worksheets
- Activities   • Integrated eBook

11

TRICARE AND CHAMPVA

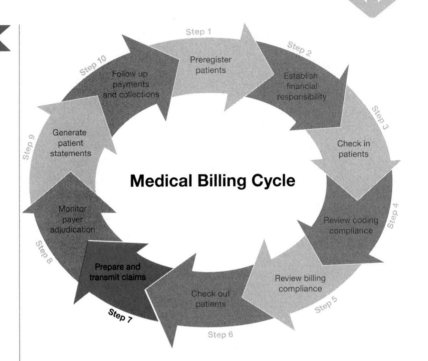

Learning Outcomes

After studying this chapter, you should be able to:

11.1 Discuss the eligibility requirements for TRICARE.

11.2 Compare TRICARE participating and nonparticipating providers.

11.3 Differentiate among the various TRICARE plans.

11.4 Explain the TRICARE for Life program.

11.5 Discuss the eligibility requirements for CHAMPVA.

11.6 Prepare accurate TRICARE and CHAMPVA claims.

The government's medical insurance programs for active-duty members, their families, and disabled veterans are served by participating providers in many parts of the country. Medical assistants become familiar with the benefits, coverage, and billing rules for these programs in order to correctly verify eligibility, collect payments, and prepare claims.

11.1 The TRICARE Program

TRICARE is the Department of Defense's health insurance plan for military personnel and their families. TRICARE, which includes managed care options, replaced the program known as the **Civilian Health and Medical Program of the Uniformed Services (CHAMPUS).** TRICARE is a regionally managed health care program that brings the resources of military hospitals together with a network of civilian facilities and providers to offer increased access to health care services. All military treatment facilities, including hospitals and clinics, are part of the TRICARE system. TRICARE also contracts with civilian facilities and physicians to provide more extensive services to beneficiaries.

Members of the following uniformed services and their families are eligible for TRICARE: the Army, Navy, Air Force, Marine Corps, Coast Guard, Public Health Service (PHS), and National Oceanic and Atmospheric Administration (NOAA). Reserve and National Guard personnel become eligible when on active duty for more than thirty consecutive days or when they retire from reserve status at age sixty. The uniformed services member is referred to as a **sponsor,** since the member's status makes other family members eligible for TRICARE coverage.

When a TRICARE patient arrives for treatment, the medical information specialist photocopies both sides of the individual's military ID card and checks the expiration date to confirm that coverage is still valid (see Figure 11.1). Decisions about eligibility are not made by TRICARE; the various branches of military service make them. Information about patient eligibility is stored in the **Defense Enrollment Eligibility Reporting System (DEERS).** Sponsors may contact DEERS to verify eligibility; providers may not contact DEERS directly because the information is protected by the Privacy Act.

TRICARE Government health program serving dependents of active-duty service members, military retirees and their families, some former spouses, and survivors of deceased military members.

Civilian Health and Medical Program of the Uniformed Services (CHAMPUS) Now the TRICARE program.

sponsor Uniformed service member in a family qualified for TRICARE or CHAMPVA.

Defense Enrollment Eligibility Reporting System (DEERS) Worldwide database of TRICARE and CHAMPVA beneficiaries.

THINKING IT THROUGH 11.1

1. TRICARE and CHAMPVA are government medical insurance plans primarily for families of members of the U.S. uniformed services. Special regulations apply to situations in which beneficiaries seek medical services outside of military treatment facilities. What are the best ways to find out about the rules and regulations pertaining to these patients?

BILLING TIP

Sponsor Information

Enter the sponsor's branch of service, status, and grade in the practice management program (PMP) when creating TRICARE patient cases.

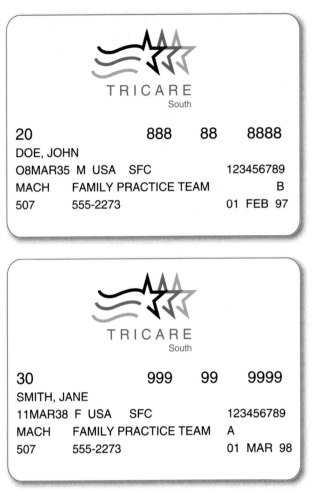

FIGURE 11.1 Sample Military (TRICARE) Identification Cards

11.2 Provider Participation and Nonparticipation

TRICARE pays only for services rendered by authorized providers. Authorized providers are certified by TRICARE regional contractors to have met specific educational, licensing, and other requirements. Once authorized, a provider is assigned a PIN and must decide whether to participate.

Participating Providers

Providers who participate agree to accept the TRICARE allowable charge as payment in full for services. Individual providers may decide whether to participate on a case-by-case basis. Participating providers are required to file claims on behalf of patients. The regional TRICARE contractor sends payment directly to the provider, and the provider collects the patient's share of the charges. Only participating providers may appeal claim decisions.

Nonparticipating Providers

A provider who chooses not to participate may not charge more than 115 percent of the allowable charge. If a provider bills more than 115 percent, the patient may refuse to pay the excess amount. For example, if the allowed charge for a procedure is $50.00, a nonparticipating provider may not charge more than $57.50 (115 percent of $50.00). If a nonparticipating provider were to charge $75.00 for the same procedure, the patient is not responsible for the amount that exceeded 115 percent of the allowed amount. The difference of $17.50 would have to be written off by the provider. The patient would pay the **cost-share** (either 20 or 25 percent)—a TRICARE term for the coinsurance, the amount that is the responsibility of the patient. Once the nonPAR provider submits the claim, TRICARE pays its portion of the allowable charges, but instead of going directly to the provider, the payment is mailed to the patient. The patient is responsible for paying the provider. Payment should be collected at the time of the visit.

cost-share Coinsurance for a TRICARE or CHAMPVA beneficiary.

Reimbursement

Providers who participate in the basic TRICARE plan are paid the amount specified in the Medicare Physician Fee Schedule for most procedures. Medical supplies, durable medical equipment, and ambulance services are not subject to Medicare limits. The maximum amount TRICARE will pay for a procedure is known as the TRICARE Maximum Allowable Charge (TMAC). Providers are responsible for collecting the patients' deductibles and their cost-share portions of the charges.

TRICARE Maxiumum Allowable Charge Table

www.tricare.mil/ allowablecharges/

Network and Nonnetwork Providers

Providers who are authorized to treat TRICARE patients may also contract to become part of the TRICARE network. These providers serve patients in one of TRICARE's managed care plans. They agree to provide care to beneficiaries at contracted rates and to act as participating providers on all claims in TRICARE's managed care programs.

Providers who choose not to join the network may still provide care to managed care patients, but TRICARE will not pay for the services. The patient is 100 percent responsible for the charges.

COMPLIANCE GUIDELINE

Covered Services

For a service to be eligible for payment, it must be:
- Medically necessary
- Delivered at the appropriate level for the condition
- At a quality that meets professional medical standards

BILLING TIP

TRICARE Fiscal Year

Check the date when collecting TRICARE deductibles; TRICARE's fiscal year is from October 1 through September 30, so annual deductibles renew based on this cycle.

THINKING IT THROUGH 11.2

1. The Military Health System (MHS) and the TRICARE health plan are required to comply with HIPAA privacy policies and procedures for the use and disclosure of PHI. The TRICARE website has this information about release of information:

   Some states have restrictions on disclosure of health information to family members to protect the privacy of certain minors and dependent adult family members. These restrictions on disclosure of information may include accessing personal health and medical information through electronic or Internet-based services. If you have questions regarding this matter, we recommend that you contact your local Military Treatment Facility (MTF) for more information about disclosure of health information and applicable privacy laws within the state or jurisdiction that you and your family receive care.

   What steps should medical assistants take to ensure compliance with this information?

11.3 TRICARE Plans

TRICARE offers beneficiaries access to a variety of health care plans.

TRICARE Standard

TRICARE Standard Fee-for-service health plan.

Military Treatment Facility (MTF) Provides medical services for members and dependents of the uniformed services.

TRICARE Standard is a fee-for-service program that replaces the CHAMPUS program, which was also fee-for-service. The program covers medical services provided by a civilian physician or by a **Military Treatment Facility (MTF).** Military families may receive services at an MTF, but available services vary by facility, and first priority is given to service members on active duty. When service is not available, the individual seeks treatment from a civilian provider, and TRICARE Standard benefits go into effect.

Under TRICARE Standard, medical expenses are shared between TRICARE and the beneficiary. Most enrollees pay annual deductibles. In addition, families of active-duty members pay 20 percent of outpatient charges. Retirees and their families, former spouses, and families of deceased personnel pay a 25 percent cost-share for outpatient services. A beneficiary who is treated by a provider who does not accept assignment, is also responsible for the provider's additional charges, up to 115 percent of the allowable charge, at the time of service unless other arrangements are in place.

catastrophic cap Maximum annual amount a TRICARE beneficiary must pay for deductible and cost-share.

Patient cost-share payments are subject to an annual **catastrophic cap,** a limit on the total medical expenses that beneficiaries are required to pay in one year. For active-duty families, the annual cap is $1,000, while for all other beneficiaries the limit is $3,000. Once these caps have been met, TRICARE pays 100 percent of additional charges for covered services for that coverage year.

catchment area Geographic area served by a hospital, clinic, or dental clinic.

TRICARE Standard covers care such as in- and outpatient services, diagnostic testing, and many preventive benefits. It does not cover cosmetic, custodial, or experimental procedures. A beneficiary who needs hospital care is encouraged by TRICARE to first seek care at a military treatment facility (MTF) if living in a **catchment area,** defined as a geographic area served by a hospital, clinic, or dental clinic and usually based on Zip codes to set an approximate 40-mile radius of military inpatient treatment facilities. Formerly, a person living in a catchment area had to get a nonavailability statement before being treated for inpatient non-emergency care at a civilian hospital. A **nonavailability statement (NAS)** is an electronic document stating that the required service is not available at the nearby military treatment facility. The form is electronically transmitted to the DEERS database. Currently, under the 2002 National Defense Authorization Act the requirement to obtain a NAS is eliminated, except for nonemergency inpatient mental health care services. However, some MTFs have been given an exemption and may still require a NAS. Best practice is to advise TRICARE standard beneficiaries to check with the Beneficiary Counseling and Assistance Coordinator at the nearest MTF.

nonavailability statement (NAS) Form required when a TRICARE member seeks medical services outside an MTF.

BILLING TIP

Preauthorization

Most high-cost procedures need preauthorization. Medical assistants should contact the TRICARE contractor for specific information.

TRICARE Prime

TRICARE Prime Basic managed care health plan.

Primary Care Manager (PCM) Provider who coordinates and manages the care of TRICARE beneficiaries.

TRICARE Prime is a managed care plan similar to an HMO. Note that all active-duty service members are limited in their choices and must enroll in one of the TRICARE Prime programs, rather than the additional TRICARE options.

After enrolling in the plan, individuals are assigned a **Primary Care Manager (PCM)** who coordinates and manages their medical care. The PCM may be a single military or civilian provider or a group of providers. In addition to most of the benefits offered by TRICARE Standard, TRICARE Prime offers preventive care, including routine physical examinations. Active-duty service members are automatically enrolled in TRICARE Prime. TRICARE Prime enrollees receive the majority of their health care services from military treatment facilities and receive priority at these facilities.

To join the TRICARE Prime program, individuals who are not active-duty family members must pay annual enrollment fees of $260 for an individual or $520 for a family. TRICARE Prime has no deductible, and no payment is required for outpatient treatment at a military facility. For active-duty family members, no payment is required for visits to civilian network providers, but different copayments apply for other beneficiaries. For example, for retirees and their family members, outpatient visits with civilian providers require $12 copayments.

Note that TRICARE Prime also has a point-of-service (POS) option that patients may select. The POS option has a deductible and coinsurance requirements.

TRICARE Prime Remote

TRICARE Prime Remote provides no-cost health care through civilian providers for service members and their families who are on remote assignment. Participants must live and work more than 50 miles (approximately one hour's drive time) from the nearest Military Treatment Facility. Their residence address must be registered with DEERS for eligibility, which is based on their Zip code.

TRICARE Prime Remote No-cost health care through civilian providers for service members and their families on remote assignment.

TRICARE Extra

TRICARE Extra is an alternative managed care plan for individuals who want to receive services primarily from civilian facilities and physicians rather than from military facilities. Since it is a managed care plan, individuals must receive health care services from a network of health care professionals. They may also seek treatment at military facilities, but active-duty personnel and other TRICARE Prime enrollees receive priority at those facilities, so care may not always be available.

TRICARE Extra is more expensive than TRICARE Prime, but less costly than TRICARE Standard. There is no enrollment fee, but there is an annual deductible of $150 for an individual and $300 for a family. TRICARE Extra beneficiaries pay 15 percent (5 percent less than TRICARE Standard enrollees) for civilian outpatient charges. Beneficiaries are not subject to additional charges of up to 115 percent of the allowable charge, since participating physicians agree to accept TRICARE's fee schedule.

TRICARE Extra Managed care health plan that offers a network of civilian providers.

TRICARE Reserve Select

Due to the large number of military reservists who have been called up for active duty, the Department of Defense implemented **TRICARE Reserve Select (TRS).** This program is a premium-based health plan available for purchase by certain members of the National Guard and Reserve activated on or after September 11, 2001. TRS provides comprehensive health care coverage similar to TRICARE Standard/Extra for TRS members and covered family members.

TRICARE Reserve Select (TRS) Coverage for reservists.

THINKING IT THROUGH 11.3

1. TRICARE claim forms are available from the program's website: www.tricare.mil/claims. Locate the website and review the information required for the TRICARE paper claim form DD 2642.

11.4 TRICARE and Other Insurance Plans

If the individual has other health insurance coverage that is primary to TRICARE, that insurance carrier must be billed first. TRICARE is a secondary payer in almost all circumstances; among the few exceptions is Medicaid.

Supplementary Plans

Many TRICARE beneficiaries purchase supplemental insurance policies to help pay deductible and cost-share or copayment fees. Most military associations offer supplementary plans, and so do private insurers. Supplemental plans are not regulated by TRICARE, so coverage varies. TRICARE is the primary payer; the purpose of a supplemental policy is simply to pick up the costs not paid by TRICARE.

TRICARE for Life

The Department of Defense offers a program for Medicare-eligible military retirees and Medicare-eligible family members called **TRICARE for Life (TFL)** that offers the opportunity to receive health care at a military treatment facility to individuals age sixty-five and over who are eligible for both Medicare and TRICARE. TRICARE beneficiaries entitled to Medicare Part A based on age, disability, or end stage renal disease are required by law to enroll in Medicare Part B to retain their TRICARE benefits. TRICARE for Life acts as a secondary payer to Medicare; Medicare pays first, and TRICARE pays the remaining out-of-pocket expenses. These claims are filed automatically. Enrollees do not need to submit a paper claim. Medicare pays its portion for Medicare covered services and automatically forwards the claim to WPS/TFL for processing. However, if the patient has other health insurance (OHI), the claim does not automatically cross over to TRICARE. Instead, the patient must submit a claim to WPS/TFL. The patient's Medicare Summary Notice along with a TRICARE paper claim (DD Form 2642) and the OHI's Explanation of Benefits (EOB) statement should be mailed by the patient to:

BILLING TIP

WPS

WPS stands for Wisconsin Physicians Service, the TFL contractor.

WPS/TFL

P.O. Box 7890

Madison, WI 53707-7890

BILLING TIP

Payers of Last Resort

TRICARE and TRICARE for Life are payers of the last resort, except when the patient also has Medicaid. In that case, TRICARE pays before Medicaid.

Benefits are similar to those of a Medicare HMO, with an emphasis on preventive and wellness services. Prescription drug benefits are also included. Other than Medicare costs, TRICARE for Life beneficiaries pay no enrollment fees and no cost-share fees for inpatient or outpatient care at a military facility. Treatment at a civilian network facility requires a copay.

THINKING IT THROUGH 11.4

1. If these three payers were involved with one claim, in what order would they pay?

   Medicaid

   TRICARE for Life

   Aetna BCBS

11.5 CHAMPVA

The **Civilian Health and Medical Program of the Department of Veterans Affairs (CHAMPVA)** is the government's health insurance program for the families of veterans with 100 percent service-related disabilities. Under the program, health care expenses are shared between the Department of Veterans Affairs (VA) and the beneficiary.

The Veterans Health Care Eligibility Reform Act of 1996 requires a veteran with a 100 percent disability to be enrolled in the program in order to receive benefits. Prior to this legislation, enrollment was not required.

Eligibility

The VA is responsible for determining eligibility for the CHAMPVA program. Eligible beneficiaries include:

▶ Dependents of a veteran who is totally and permanently disabled due to a service-connected injury.
▶ Dependents of a veteran who was totally and permanently disabled due to a service-connected condition at the time of death.
▶ Survivors of a veteran who died as a result of a service-related disability.
▶ Survivors of a veteran who died in the line of duty.

CHAMPVA Authorization Card

Each eligible beneficiary possesses a CHAMPVA Authorization Card, known as an A-Card. The provider's office checks this card to determine eligibility and photocopies or scans the front and back for inclusion in the patient record.

Services

Most persons enrolled in CHAMPVA pay an annual deductible and a portion of their health care charges. Some services are exempt from the deductible and cost-share requirement. A patient's out-of-pocket costs are subject to a catastrophic cap of $3,000 per calendar year. Once the beneficiary has paid $3,000 in medical bills for the year, CHAMPVA pays claims for covered services at 100 percent for the rest of that year.

CHAMPVA provides coverage for most medically necessary in- and outpatient services. Some procedures must be approved in advance; if they are not, CHAMPVA will not pay for them. It is the patient's responsibility, not the provider's, to obtain preauthorization.

Participating Providers

For most services, CHAMPVA does not contract with providers. Beneficiaries may receive care from providers of their choice, as long as those providers are properly licensed to perform the services being delivered and are not on the Medicare exclusion list. For mental health treatment, CHAMPVA maintains a list of approved providers. Providers who treat CHAMPVA patients are prohibited from charging more than the CHAMPVA allowable amounts. Providers agree to accept CHAMPVA payment and the patient's cost-share payment as payment in full for services.

In most cases, CHAMPVA pays equivalent to Medicare/TRICARE rates. The maximum amount CHAMPVA will pay for a procedure is known as the CHAMPVA Maximum Allowable Charge (CMAC). CHAMPVA has an outpatient deductible ($50 per person up to $100 per family per calendar year) and a cost-share of 25 percent. The cost-share percentages are 75 percent for CHAMPVA and 25 percent for the beneficiary. Beneficiaries are also responsible for the costs of health care services not covered by CHAMPVA.

CHAMPVA and Other Health Insurance Plans

When the individual has other health insurance benefits in addition to CHAMPVA, CHAMPVA is almost always the secondary payer. Two exceptions are Medicaid and supplemental policies purchased to cover deductibles, cost-shares, and other services.

Insurance claims are first filed with the primary payer. When the remittance advice from the primary plan arrives, a copy is attached to the claim that is then filed with CHAMPVA. Persons under age sixty-five who are eligible for Medicare benefits and who are enrolled in Parts A and B may also enroll in CHAMPVA.

CHAMPVA for Life

CHAMPVA for Life extends CHAMPVA benefits to spouses or dependents who are age sixty-five and over. Similar to TRICARE for Life, CHAMPVA for Life benefits are payable after payment by Medicare or other third-party payers. Eligible beneficiaries must be sixty-five or older and must be enrolled in Medicare Parts A and B. For services not covered by Medicare, CHAMPVA acts as the primary payer.

THINKING IT THROUGH 11.5

1. What is the difference between TRICARE and CHAMPVA?

11.6 Filing Claims

TRICARE Claims

TRICARE participating providers file claims on behalf of patients, following HIPAA regulations. Claims are filed with the regional contractor for their region, based on the patient's home address, not the location of the facility. Contact information for regional contractors is available on the TRICARE website. The three administration regions for TRICARE are TRICARE North, TRICARE South, and TRICARE West. A fourth region covers international claims.

Individuals file their own claims when services are received from nonparticipating providers, using DD Form 2642, Patient's Request for Medical Payment. A copy of the itemized bill from the provider must be attached to the form.

If a CMS-1500 paper claim is needed, follow the general guidelines shown in Table 7.3 (on pages 162–163) and Figure 11.2.

CHAMPVA Claims

The CHAMPVA program is covered by HIPAA regulations. Most CHAMPVA claims are filed by providers and are submitted to the centralized CHAMPVA claims processing center in Denver, Colorado. The information required on a claim is the same as the information required for TRICARE. In instances in which beneficiaries are filing their own claims, CHAMPVA Claim Form (VA Form 10-7959A) must be used. The claim must always be accompanied by an itemized bill from the provider. Claims must be filed within one year of the date of service or discharge.

THINKING IT THROUGH 11.6

1. If a TRICARE participating provider is filing a claim for a patient who visited a facility in another city, should they file the claim based on the patient's home address or the address of the facility?

Exercise 11.1 Completing a TRICARE Claim

Patient Elizabeth I. Wu has insurance coverage under a TRICARE plan. Create a claim for her recent visit with Dr. Clarke.

Follow the steps at www.mhhe.com/newbycarr to complete the exercise at connect.mcgraw-hill.com on your own once you have watched the demo and tried the steps with prompts in practice mode. Use the information provided in the scenario to complete the exercise.

connect™ plus+

DRAFT - NOT FOR OFFICIAL USE

HEALTH INSURANCE CLAIM FORM

APPROVED BY NATIONAL UNIFORM CLAIM COMMITTEE (NUCC) 02/12

☐☐ PICA   PICA ☐☐

1. MEDICARE	MEDICAID	TRICARE	CHAMPVA	GROUP HEALTH PLAN	FECA BLK LUNG	OTHER	1a. INSURED'S I.D. NUMBER (For Program in Item 1)
☐ (Medicare#)	☐ (Medicaid#)	☒ (ID#/DoD#)	☐ (Member ID#)	☐ (ID#)	☐ (ID#)	☐ (ID#)	301694218

2. PATIENT'S NAME (Last Name, First Name, Middle Initial)
RODRIGUEZ, MARIE, P

3. PATIENT'S BIRTH DATE MM 01 DD 14 YY 1975 SEX M ☐ F ☒

4. INSURED'S NAME (Last Name, First Name, Middle Initial)
RODRIGUEZ, JESUS, I

5. PATIENT'S ADDRESS (No., Street)
316 WASHINGTON AVE

6. PATIENT RELATIONSHIP TO INSURED
Self ☐ Spouse ☒ Child ☐ Other ☐

7. INSURED'S ADDRESS (No., Street)
SAME

CITY **CLEVELAND** STATE **OH**

8. RESERVED FOR NUCC USE

CITY   STATE

ZIP CODE **44101-3164** TELEPHONE (Include Area Code) ( )

ZIP CODE   TELEPHONE (Include Area Code) ( )

9. OTHER INSURED'S NAME (Last Name, First Name, Middle Initial)

10. IS PATIENT'S CONDITION RELATED TO:

11. INSURED'S POLICY GROUP OR FECA NUMBER

a. OTHER INSURED'S POLICY OR GROUP NUMBER

a. EMPLOYMENT? (Current or Previous) ☐ YES ☒ NO

a. INSURED'S DATE OF BIRTH MM DD YY SEX M ☐ F ☐

b. RESERVED FOR NUCC USE

b. AUTO ACCIDENT? ☐ YES ☒ NO PLACE (State)

b. OTHER CLAIM ID (Designated by NUCC)

c. RESERVED FOR NUCC USE

c. OTHER ACCIDENT? ☐ YES ☒ NO

c. INSURANCE PLAN NAME OR PROGRAM NAME

d. INSURANCE PLAN NAME OR PROGRAM NAME

10d. CLAIM CODES (Designated by NUCC)

d. IS THERE ANOTHER HEALTH BENEFIT PLAN?
☐ YES ☒ NO *If yes,* complete items 9, 9a, and 9d.

READ BACK OF FORM BEFORE COMPLETING & SIGNING THIS FORM.
12. PATIENT'S OR AUTHORIZED PERSON'S SIGNATURE I authorize the release of any medical or other information necessary to process this claim. I also request payment of government benefits either to myself or to the party who accepts assignment below.

SIGNED **SIGNATURE ON FILE** DATE _____

13. INSURED'S OR AUTHORIZED PERSON'S SIGNATURE I authorize payment of medical benefits to the undersigned physician or supplier for services described below.

SIGNED _____

14. DATE OF CURRENT ILLNESS, INJURY, or PREGNANCY (LMP) MM DD YY QUAL.

15. OTHER DATE QUAL. MM DD YY

16. DATES PATIENT UNABLE TO WORK IN CURRENT OCCUPATION FROM MM DD YY TO MM DD YY

17. NAME OF REFERRING PROVIDER OR OTHER SOURCE 17a. 17b. NPI

18. HOSPITALIZATION DATES RELATED TO CURRENT SERVICES FROM MM DD YY TO MM DD YY

19. ADDITIONAL CLAIM INFORMATION (Designated by NUCC)

20. OUTSIDE LAB? ☐ YES ☒ NO $ CHARGES

21. DIAGNOSIS OR NATURE OF ILLNESS OR INJURY Relate A-L to service line below (24E) ICD Ind. **0**

A. **I10** B. **I49.01** C. ____ D. ____
E. ____ F. ____ G. ____ H. ____
I. ____ J. ____ K. ____ L. ____

22. RESUBMISSION CODE _____ ORIGINAL REF. NO. _____

23. PRIOR AUTHORIZATION NUMBER

24. A. DATE(S) OF SERVICE					B. PLACE OF SERVICE	C. EMG	D. PROCEDURES, SERVICES, OR SUPPLIES (Explain Unusual Circumstances) CPT/HCPCS	MODIFIER	E. DIAGNOSIS POINTER	F. $ CHARGES	G. DAYS OR UNITS	H. EPSDT Family Plan	I. ID. QUAL.	J. RENDERING PROVIDER ID. #
From MM	DD	YY	To MM	DD	YY										
1 10	06	2016				11		99212		A	46 00	1		NPI	
2 10	06	2016				11		93000		AB	70 00	1		NPI	
3														NPI	
4														NPI	
5														NPI	
6														NPI	

25. FEDERAL TAX I.D. NUMBER **416246791** SSN ☐ EIN ☒

26. PATIENT'S ACCOUNT NO. **RODZIO**

27. ACCEPT ASSIGNMENT? (For govt. claims, see back) ☒ YES ☐ NO

28. TOTAL CHARGE $ **116 00**

29. AMOUNT PAID $

30. Rsvd for NUCC Use

31. SIGNATURE OF PHYSICIAN OR SUPPLIER INCLUDING DEGREES OR CREDENTIALS (I certify that the statements on the reverse apply to this bill and are made a part thereof.)

SIGNED _____ DATE _____

32. SERVICE FACILITY LOCATION INFORMATION

a. NPI b.

33. BILLING PROVIDER INFO & PH # (**614**) **3331212**
RUTH J. CLARKE, MD
841 ORCHARD HILL RD
COLUMBUS OH 43214 - 1234
a. **4675316922** b.

NUCC Instruction Manual available at: www.nucc.org *PLEASE PRINT OR TYPE* OMB APPROVAL PENDING

FIGURE 11.2 CMS-1500 (02/12) Claim Completion for TRICARE

Chapter Summary

Learning Outcomes	Key Concepts/Examples
11.1 Discuss the eligibility requirements for TRICARE. Pages 229–230	• Members of the Army, Navy, Air Force, Marine Corps, Coast Guard, Public Health Service, and National Oceanic and Atmospheric Administration and their families are eligible for TRICARE. • Reserve and National Guard personnel become eligible when on active duty for more than thirty consecutive days or on retirement from reserve status at age sixty.
11.2 Compare TRICARE participating and nonparticipating providers. Pages 230–231	Participating providers • Accept the TRICARE allowable charge as payment in full for services. • Are required to file claims on behalf of patients. • May appeal claim decisions. Nonparticipating providers • May not charge more than 115 percent of the allowable charge. • May not appeal a decision. • Are paid by the patient and TRICARE pays its portion of the allowable charges directly to the patient.
11.3 Differentiate among the various TRICARE plans. Pages 232–233	TRICARE Standard • Is a fee-for-service plan in which medical expenses are shared between TRICARE and the beneficiary. • Most enrollees pay annual deductibles and cost-share percentages. TRICARE Prime • Is a managed care plan. • Individuals are assigned a Primary Care Manager (PCM) who coordinates and manages that patient's medical care. • Enrollees receive most health care services from military treatment facilities. • In addition to most of the benefits offered by TRICARE Standard, TRICARE Prime offers additional preventive care, including routine physical examinations. TRICARE Extra • Is a managed care plan. • Services are primarily received from civilian facilities and physicians. • Individuals must receive health care services from a network of professionals.
11.4 Explain the TRICARE for Life program. Pages 233–234	• Under the TRICARE for Life program, individuals age sixty-five and over who are eligible for both Medicare and TRICARE may continue to receive health care at military treatment facilities.
11.5 Discuss the eligibility requirements for CHAMPVA. Pages 234–236	Individuals eligible for the CHAMPVA program include • Dependents of a veteran who is totally and permanently disabled due to service-connected injuries. • Dependents of a veteran who was totally and permanently disabled due to service-connected condition at the time of death. • Survivors of a veteran who died as a result of a service-related disability. • Survivors of a veteran who died in the line of duty.
11.6 Prepare accurate TRICARE and CHAMPVA claims. Pages 236–237	• Participating providers file TRICARE claims with the contractor for the region on behalf of patients. • Individuals file their own TRICARE claims when services are received from nonparticipating providers. • Most CHAMPVA claims are filed by providers and submitted to the centralized CHAMPVA claims processing center.

Using Terminology

Match the key terms in the left column with the definitions in the right column.

_____ 1. **[LO 11.1]** Civilian Health and Medical Program of the Uniformed Services (CHAMPUS)

_____ 2. **[LO 11.3]** Primary Care Manager (PCM)

_____ 3. **[LO 11.1]** Defense Enrollment Eligibility Reporting System (DEERS)

_____ 4. **[LO 11.3]** Nonavailability statement (NAS)

_____ 5. **[LO 11.4]** TRICARE for Life

_____ 6. **[LO 11.2]** Cost-share

_____ 7. **[LO 11.1]** Sponsor

_____ 8. **[LO 11.3]** Military Treatment Facility (MTF)

_____ 9. **[LO 11.3]** TRICARE Standard

_____ 10. **[LO 11.5]** Civilian Health and Medical Program of the Department of Veterans Affairs (CHAMPVA)

A. The government's health insurance program for veterans with 100 percent service-related disabilities and their families.

B. The Department of Defense's health insurance plan for military personnel and their families that was replaced by TRICARE.

C. TRICARE term for coinsurance.

D. A government database that contains information about patient eligibility for TRICARE.

E. A place where medical care is provided to members of the military service and their families.

F. An electronic document stating that the service the patient requires is not available at the local military treatment facility.

G. A provider who coordinates and manages a patient's medical care under a managed care plan.

H. The uniformed service member whose status makes it possible for other family members to be eligible for TRICARE coverage.

I. Program for beneficiaries who are both Medicare and TRICARE eligible.

J. A fee-for-service program that covers medical services provided by a civilian physician or a military treatment facility .

Checking Your Understanding

Write the letter of the choice that best completes the statement or answers the question.

1. **[LO 11.3]** The TRICARE plan that is an HMO and requires a PCM is _____.
   A. TRICARE Prime
   B. TRICARE for Life
   C. CHAMPVA
   D. TRICARE Standard

2. **[LO 11.4]** A TRICARE for Life beneficiary must be at least age _____.
   A. Seventy
   B. Twenty-one
   C. Sixty-five
   D. Thirty

3. **[LO 11.4]** TRICARE is secondary to all other health plans except _____.
   A. Medicare
   B. Group health insurance
   C. Medicaid
   D. Private health insurance

4. **[LO 11.3]** The TRICARE plan that has a POS option is _____.
   A. TRICARE Standard
   B. TRICARE for Life
   C. TRICARE Reserve Select
   D. TRICARE Prime

5. **[LO 11.2]** A nonparticipating provider may not charge more than what percentage of TRICARE's allowable charge? _____
   A. 80 percent
   B. 20 percent
   C. 115 percent
   D. 25 percent

connect plus+

Enhance your learning at mcgrawhillconnect.com!
- Practice Exercises
- Worksheets
- Activities
- Integrated eBook

6. **[LO 11.3]** In a military treatment facility first priority is given to members of _____.
   A. TRICARE Prime
   B. TRICARE Standard
   C. TRICARE Extra
   D. TRICARE for Life

7. **[LO 11.6]** TRICARE claims are filed based on _____.
   A. The military facility's address
   B. The patient's home address
   C. The physician's address
   D. The address of the regional contractor

8. **[LO 11.4]** For individuals enrolled in TRICARE for Life, the primary payer is _____.
   A. TRICARE   C. A supplementary plan
   B. CHAMPVA   D. Medicare

9. **[LO 11.1]** Decisions about an individual's eligibility for TRICARE are made by the _____.
   A. Military treatment facility
   B. Provider
   C. Defense Enrollment Eligibility Reporting System
   D. Branch of military service

10. **[LO 11.2]** The TRICARE health care program is a covered entity and subject to privacy rules under _____.
    A. NAS   C.   TCS
    B. HIPAA D.   CHAMPVA

Applying Your Knowledge

[LO 11.2]   Case 11.1

Fill in the blanks in the following payment situations:

Participating Provider

Physician's standard fee	$350.00
TRICARE fee	$265.00
TRICARE pays 80%	$ _____
Patient pays 20%	$ _____
Provider adjustment (write-off)	$ _____

Nonparticipating Provider (Accepts Assignment)

Physician's standard fee	$285.00
TRICARE fee	$165.00
TRICARE pays 80%	$ _____
Patient pays 20%	$ _____
Provider adjustment (write-off)	$ _____

Nonparticipating Provider (Does Not Accept Assignment)

Physician's standard fee	$130.00
TRICARE fee	$ 95.00
Limiting charge	$ _____
Total provider can collect	$ _____
TRICARE pays patient	$ _____
Patient out-of-pocket expense	$ _____
Provider adjustment (write-off)	$ _____

connect plus+

Enhance your learning at mcgrawhillconnect.com!
- Practice Exercises
- Worksheets
- Activities
- Integrated eBook

WORKERS' COMPENSATION AND AUTOMOBILE/ DISABILITY INSURANCE

12

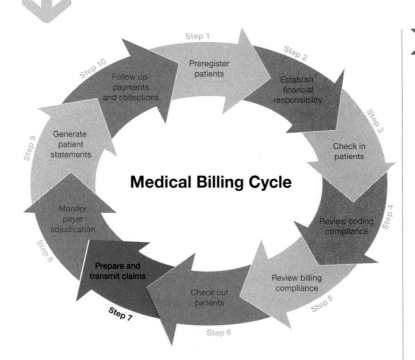

Medical Billing Cycle

- Step 1 — Preregister patients
- Step 2 — Establish financial responsibility
- Step 3 — Check in patients
- Step 4 — Review coding compliance
- Step 5 — Review billing compliance
- Step 6 — Check out patients
- Step 7 — Prepare and transmit claims
- Step 8 — Monitor payer adjudication
- Step 9 — Generate patient statements
- Step 10 — Follow up payments and collections

KEY TERMS

Admission of Liability
automobile insurance policy
disability compensation programs
Federal Employees' Compensation Act (FECA)
Federal Insurance Contribution Act (FICA)
final report
first report of injury
independent medical examination (IME)
lien
Notice of Contest
occupational diseases or illnesses
Occupational Safety and Health Administration (OSHA)
Office of Workers' Compensation Programs (OWCP)
personal injury protection (PIP)
physician of record
progress report
Social Security Disability Insurance (SSDI)
subrogation
Supplemental Security Income (SSI)
vocational rehabilitation

Learning Outcomes

After studying this chapter, you should be able to:

12.1 Explain the four federal workers' compensation plans.

12.2 Describe the two types of state workers' compensation benefits.

12.3 Classify work-related injuries.

12.4 Complete workers' compensation claims.

12.5 Compare automotive insurance and disability compensation programs.

*Workers' compensation was developed to benefit both the employer and the employee. It provides employees who are injured on the job with compensation for their injuries, and it protects employers from liability for employees' injuries. The **Occupational Safety and Health Administration (OSHA)** was created by Congress in 1970 to protect workers from health and safety risks on the job. OSHA sets standards to guard against known dangers in the workplace, such as toxic fumes, faulty machinery, and excess noise. Businesses must meet health and safety standards set by OSHA. If they do not, they are subject to significant fines. Other types of insurance—disability, automotive, and liability—are individual policies that protect against the financial risk of injury and loss of income in certain situations. All of these insurance plans may require the medical office to follow procedures and file claims on behalf of their patients.*

12.1 Federal Workers' Compensation Plans

Work-related illnesses or injuries suffered by civilian employees of federal agencies, including occupational diseases acquired by them, are covered under various programs administered by the **Office of Workers' Compensation Programs (OWCP)**. OWCP is part of the U.S. Department of Labor. The programs are:

▶ The Federal Employees' Compensation Program, which provides workers' compensation benefits to individuals employed by the federal government under the **Federal Employees' Compensation Act (FECA).**
▶ The Federal Black Lung Program, which provides benefits to individuals working in coal mines under the Black Lung Benefits Act.
▶ The Energy Employees Occupational Illness Compensation Program, which went into effect on July 31, 2001, and provides benefits under the Energy Employees Occupational Illness Compensation Program Act for workers who have developed cancer and other serious diseases because of exposure to radiation, beryllium, or silica at atomic weapons facilities or at certain federally owned facilities in which radioactive materials were used.
▶ The Longshore and Harbor Workers' Compensation Program, which provides coverage for individuals employed in the maritime field under the Longshore and Harbor Workers' Compensation Act and for certain other classes of workers covered by extensions of the act.

Each program provides medical treatment, cash benefits for lost wages, vocational rehabilitation, and other benefits to workers of the employee group or industry it represents who have sustained workplace injuries or acquired occupational diseases.

FECA Program Information
www.oig.dol.gov/
fecaprogram.htm

THINKING IT THROUGH 12.1

1. Workers' compensation coverage provides important medical insurance benefits to people who experience work-related injuries or illnesses. Unfortunately, many instances of abuse of workers' compensation have been uncovered. In a significant number of these situations, court cases have found workers' claims for temporary or permanent disability to be untruthful. Are medical office staff members responsible for questioning or reporting information they suspect to be fraudulent?

12.2 State Workers' Compensation Plans

Each state administers its own workers' compensation program and has its own statutes that govern workers' compensation, so coverage varies from state to state. However, all states provide two types of workers' compensation benefits. One pays the employee's medical expenses that result from the work-related injury, and the other compensates the employee for lost wages while he or she is unable to return to work. Workers' compensation pays for all reasonable and necessary medical expenses resulting from the work-related injury.

Employers obtain workers' compensation insurance from one of the following sources: (1) a state workers' compensation fund, (2) a private plan, or (3) directly with a self-insured fund (as described in the chapter about Medicare). Under a state fund, companies pay premiums into a central state insurance fund from which claims are paid. Many employers contract with private insurance carriers, which provide access to their networks of providers (primary care physicians, occupational medical centers, urgent care centers, physical therapy providers, chiropractors, radiology centers, orthopedists, and orthopedic surgeons and facilities). When a firm self-insures, it sets money aside in a fund that is to be used to pay workers' compensation claims. Most states require a company to obtain authorization before choosing to self-insure. Regardless of the source of workers' compensation insurance, the money that funds workers' compensation insurance is fully paid by the employer; no money is withdrawn from an employee's pay.

Employers or their insurance carriers must file proof of workers' compensation insurance with the state Workers' Compensation Board. In some states, this proof may be filed electronically through a web-based data-entry application. In addition, the employer must post a Notice of Workers' Compensation Coverage in a place accessible to all employees. This notice must list the name, address, and telephone number of the administrator of the company's workers' compensation program.

Links to States' Workers' Compensation Agencies
www.workerscompensation.com

Eligibility

Most states require public and private companies to provide workers' compensation coverage to all full-time and part-time employees, including minors. Companies that are required to carry workers' compensation insurance but fail to do so are subject to legal penalties.

Benefits

Workers' compensation insurance covers injuries, illnesses, and job-related deaths. Injuries are not limited to on-the-job occurrences. An injury may occur while performing an off-site service for the company, such as driving to the post office on its behalf. Accidents such as falls in the company parking lot are also covered under workers' compensation rules.

Occupational diseases or illnesses develop as a result of workplace conditions or activities. These include lung disorders caused by poor air quality, repetitive motion illnesses such as carpal tunnel syndrome, and occupational hearing loss, among others. Illnesses may develop rapidly or over the course of many years.

Medical benefits are payable from the first day of the injury. Cash benefits vary from state to state and are generally not paid for the first seven days of disability. In most states, a worker must be disabled for more than seven calendar days before benefits are payable. However, if the disability extends beyond fourteen days, a worker may become retrospectively eligible for cash benefits for the first seven days. Different states have different methods of determining wage-loss benefits. Usually, the benefits are a percentage of the worker's salary before the injury. For example, it is not uncommon for workers to be compensated at two-thirds of their average weekly wage, up to a weekly maximum. The weekly maximums differ among states, as do the formulas for determining workers' average weekly wages. When an individual is fatally injured on the job, workers' compensation pays death benefits to the employee's survivors. Funeral expenses may also be paid.

BILLING TIP

Workers' Compensation Fees

Some states have mandated the use of RVS unit values as the schedule of fees for workers' compensation services. These states have often also set a conversion factor. Many, however, do not use RVS or the CPT codes for their fee schedules. The office may have to crosswalk from the CPT code to the workers' compensation fee schedule.

occupational diseases or illnesses Caused by the work environment over a period longer than one workday or shift.

Covered Injuries and Illnesses

States determine the types of injuries that are covered under workers' compensation. Generally, an injury is covered if it meets all of the following criteria:

▶ It results in personal injury or death.
▶ It occurs by accident.
▶ It arises out of employment.
▶ It occurs during the course of employment.

An accident can be either an immediate event or the unexpected result of an occurrence over time. A worker who cuts a finger while using a box cutter is an example of an immediate accident. An employee who suffers a repetitive stress injury that developed over the course of several years is an example of an unexpected result over time. The following are examples of covered injuries:

▶ Back injuries due to heavy lifting or falls.
▶ Repetitive stress injuries such as carpal tunnel syndrome.
▶ Parking lot injuries such as falls.
▶ Heat-related injuries such as heat stroke or heat exhaustion if the job requires a lot of work time in the hot sun.
▶ Hernias if they are related to a work injury.
▶ Personal time injuries, such as injuries that occur in the cafeteria or restroom.

Some generally covered injuries may be excluded from workers' compensation, or benefits may be reduced if certain conditions were present at the time of the injury, such as employee intoxication by alcohol or failure to follow safety procedures.

THINKING IT THROUGH 12.2

1. Joe Marino works in the mailroom of a large telecommunications company. His job requires lifting packages in excess of eighty pounds. Over the course of his employment with the company, Joe has been out on temporary disability several times because of back pain. On his way home from work last Friday, Joe stopped by the post office to drop off some personal mail. As he was walking into the post office, he slipped on an icy patch on the sidewalk and injured his back. After an examination by his physician, Joe was ordered to stay out of work for a minimum of two weeks. Would this injury be covered under workers' compensation insurance? Provide an argument to support your position.

12.3 Workers' Compensation Terminology

Classification of Injuries

Work-related injuries are grouped into five categories.

Injury without Disability

A worker is injured on the job and requires treatment, but is able to resume working within several days. All medical expenses are paid by workers' compensation insurance.

Injury with Temporary Disability

A worker is injured on the job, requires treatment, and is unable to return to work within several days. All medical expenses are paid by workers' compensation insurance, and the employee receives compensation for lost wages. Compensation varies from state to state and is usually a percentage of the worker's salary before injury. Before an injured employee can return to work, the physician must file a doctor's **final report** indicating that he or she is fit to return to work and resume normal job activities.

Injury with Permanent Disability

A worker is injured on the job, requires treatment, is unable to return to work, and is not expected to be able to return to his or her regular job in the future. Usually this employee has been on temporary disability for an extended period of time and is still unable to resume work. When that is the case, the physician of record files a report stating that the individual is permanently disabled. The state workers' compensation office or the insurance carrier may request an additional medical opinion before a final determination is made. An impartial physician is called in to provide an **independent medical examination (IME)**. Once the IME report is submitted, a final determination of disability is made, and a settlement is reached. The length of coverage varies from state to state.

Injury Requiring Vocational Rehabilitation

A worker is injured on the job, requires treatment, and is unable to return to work without vocational rehabilitation. All medical expenses are paid by workers' compensation insurance, as are the costs of the vocational rehabilitation program. **Vocational rehabilitation** is the process of retraining an employee to return to the workforce, although not necessarily in the same position as before the injury. For example, an employee who injured his or her back working in a job that required heavy lifting may be trained for work that does not involve lifting.

Injury Resulting in Death

A worker dies as a result of an injury on the job. Death benefits are paid to survivors based on the worker's earning capacity at the time of the injury.

Pain and Disability

Physicians who examine patients under workers' compensation coverage use a set of standardized terms to describe the effects of work-related injuries and illnesses. These widely accepted terms are used by most states and insurance carriers. Different terminology is used to describe levels of pain and the effects of injuries or illnesses. Pain is classified as minimal, slight, moderate, or severe. Disabilities due to spinal injuries, heart disease, pulmonary disease, or abdominal weakness are classified on a scale from limitation to light work to precluding very heavy lifting. Those due to lower extremity injuries can be classified as limited to sedentary or semi-sedentary work.

Workers' Compensation and HIPAA

Workers' compensation cases are one of the few situations in which a health care provider may disclose a patient's protected health information (PHI) to an employer without the patient's authorization. Workers' compensation claim information is not subject to the same confidentiality rules as other medical records.

Most states allow claims adjusters and employers unrestricted access to the workers' compensation files. Likewise, at the federal level the HIPAA Privacy Rule permits disclosures of PHI for workers' compensation purposes without the patient's authorization. Likewise, workers' compensation claims do not have to adhere to the HIPAA Transactions and Code Sets regulations.

final report Filed by the physician in a state workers' compensation case when the patient is discharged.

independent medical examination (IME) Examination conducted by a physician to confirm that an individual is permanently disabled.

vocational rehabilitation Program to prepare a patient for reentry into the workforce.

12.4 Claim Process

When an employee is injured on the job, the injury must be reported to the employer within a certain time period. Most states require notification in writing. Once notified, the employer must notify the state workers' compensation office and the insurance carrier, also within a certain period of time. In some cases, the employee is given a medical service order to take to the physician who provides treatment.

In most instances, the injured employee must be treated by a provider selected by the employer or insurance carrier. Some employers contract with a managed care organization for services. In these cases, the patient must be examined and treated by a physician in the managed care plan's network. If the employee refuses to comply with the request, benefits may not be granted.

Responsibilities of the Physician of Record

physician of record Provider who first treats a patient and assesses the level of disability.

progress report Filed by the physician in state workers' compensation cases when a patient's medical condition or disability changes.

The physician who first treats the injured or ill employee is known as the **physician of record.** This physician is responsible for treating the patient's condition and for determining the percentage of disability and the possible return-to-work date, if applicable. The physician of record also files a **progress report** with the insurance carrier every time there is a substantial change in the patient's condition that affects disability status or when required by state rules. Providers submit their charges to the workers' compensation insurance carrier and are paid directly by the carrier. Charges are limited to an established fee schedule. Patients may not be billed for any medical expenses related to the case's E/M and treatment. In addition, the employer may not be billed for any amount that exceeds the established fee for the service provided.

Responsibilities of the Employer and Insurance Carrier

first report of injury Filed in state workers' compensation cases, containing employer and accident information, and patient's description of the accident.

The **first report of injury** form must be filed by either the employer or the physician (under state law) within a certain time period. The amount of time varies among states; the range is normally from twenty-four hours to ten days. The form contains information about the patient, the employer, and the injury or illness. Depending on the insurance carrier, the report may be filed electronically or mailed to the carrier.

Admission of Liability Determination that an employer is responsible for an employee's claim under workers' compensation.

Notice of Contest Determination to deny liability for an employee's workers' compensation claim.

The insurance carrier assigns a claim number to the case, determines whether the claim is eligible for workers' compensation, and notifies the employer. This determination is either an **Admission of Liability,** stating that the employer is responsible for the injury, or a **Notice of Contest,** which is a denial of liability. The worker must be informed of the outcome within a given number of days.

If the employee is eligible for compensation for lost wages, checks are sent directly to him or her, and no income taxes are withheld from the payments. If the claim is denied, the employee must pay all medical bills associated with the accident. These charges may be submitted to the individual's own health insurance carrier for payment.

Billing and Claim Management

Workers' compensation claims require special handling. The first medical treatment report on the case must be exact. If it is not, future treatments may appear unrelated to the original injury and may be denied.

When a patient makes an appointment for an injury that could have occurred on the job, the scheduler asks whether the visit is work-related. If the answer is yes, pertinent information should be collected before the office visit:

▶ Date of injury
▶ Workers' compensation carrier
▶ Employer at time of injury
▶ Patient's other insurance

The medical assistant contacts the workers' compensation carrier for authorization to treat the patient before the initial visit. Note that the practice management program (PMP) captures workers' compensation and injury-related information when the patient's injury case record is created and updated.

There are no universal rules for completing a claim form. Some plans use the HIPAA 837 or the CMS-1500, while other plans have their own claim forms. Although the specific procedures vary depending on the state and the insurance carrier, the following are some general guidelines:

▶ Payment from the insurance carrier must be accepted as payment in full. Patients or employers may not be billed for any of the medical expenses.
▶ A separate file must be established when a provider treats an individual who is already a patient of the practice. Information in the patient's regular medical record (non-workers' compensation) must not be released to the insurance carrier.
▶ The patient's signature is not required on any billing forms.
▶ The workers' compensation claim number should be included on all forms and correspondence.
▶ Use the eight-digit format when reporting dates such as the date last worked.

The NUCC has recommended the following information for completing a CMS-1500 workers' compensation claim:

Item Number	Data
1a	Enter the Employee ID
4	Enter the name of the employer
7	Enter the address of the employer
10d	The following is a list of Condition Codes for workers' compensation claims that are valid for use on the CMS-1500. They are required when the bill is a duplicate or an appeal. The Original reference Number must be entered for Item Number 22 for these conditions. Note that these are not used for submitting a revised or corrected claim. W2 Duplicate of original bill W3 Level 1 appeal W4 Level 2 appeal W5 Level 3 appeal
11	Enter the Workers' Compensation claim number assigned by the payer.
19	Required based on Jurisdictional Workers' Compensation Guidelines.
23	Required when a prior authorization, referral, concurrent review, or voluntary certification was received.

THINKING IT THROUGH 12.4

1. Anna Ferraro has an accident at work when the arm of her office chair gives way. She is covered by her employer's insurance. She is also a Medicare beneficiary. Should the claim connected with the accident be filed with her employer's workers' compensation carrier or with Medicare?

Exercise 12.1 Completing a Workers' Compensation Claim

Patient Shih-Chi Yang has a workers' compensation case being handled by Dr. Clarke. Create a claim for the recent visit with Dr. Clarke for this situation.

Follow the steps at www.mhhe.com/newbycarr to complete the exercise at connect.mcgraw-hill.com on your own once you have watched the demo and tried the steps with prompts in practice mode. Use the information provided in the scenario to complete the exercise.

12.5 Automobile Insurance and Disability Compensation Programs

Automobile Insurance

automobile insurance policy
Insurance contract for coverage of specified car-related financial losses.

When the medical office treats patients injured in a motor vehicle accident (MVA), the patient's **automobile insurance policy** often covers the cost of the treatment. An automobile insurance policy is a contract between an insurance company and an individual, under which the individual pays a premium in exchange for coverage of specified car-related financial losses. These policies provide several basic types of coverage:

personal injury protection (PIP)
Coverage for expenses related to a motor vehicle accident.

▶ **Personal injury protection (PIP)** or medical payments (MedPay)—covers the driver and passengers of a policyholder's car. PIP, sometimes referred to as "no-fault" coverage, is insurance coverage for medical expenses and other expenses related to an MVA.
▶ Liability—covers damages the policyholder causes to someone else's body or property.
▶ Collision—covers damages to the policyholder's car resulting from a collision.
▶ Comprehensive—covers damages to the policyholder's vehicle that do not involve a collision with another car.
▶ Additional types of coverage—includes coverage for uninsured motorists, emergency road services, rental reimbursement, and property damage.

Treating patients covered under an automobile insurance policy may require the medical assistant to perform specific actions to receive the maximum appropriate payment, including:

▶ Coordinating claims with the insurance company that provides the patient's automobile insurance policy, including verifying their benefits and obtaining preauthorization prior to treatment when possible.
▶ Ruling out coverage under workers' compensation by asking if the patient's MVA was work-related.

- Handling **liens**—which are written, legal claims on property to secure the payment of a debt—properly to help ensure payment.
- Filling out boxes 10b and 14 on the CMS-1500 to indicate that the patient's condition is related to an MVA and the date of the MVA, and including the accident claim number.
- Talking with a patient's attorney to stay informed and prepare for the possible settlement of a claim.
- Making a copy of the patient's health insurance card to provide the practice with an alternative source of reimbursement in the event the automobile insurance carrier does not pay for a claim, or does not fully cover a claim.

The laws and guidelines surrounding automobile insurance policies vary by state. Therefore, medical assistants learn and follow the policies of the state under which the patient is covered. Policies also vary by the type of insurance plan, including fee-for-service and capitation plans, among other types. All of these factors, including the appropriate coordination of benefits, are taken into account in filing claims for the treatment of a patient injured in a motor vehicle accident.

lien Legal claim on property to secure payment of debt.

Subrogation

When working with workers' compensation or liability/automotive claims, medical insurance specialists should be aware of the payers' subrogation rights. **Subrogation** refers to actions an insurance company takes to recoup expenses for a claim it paid out, when another party should have been responsible for paying at least a portion of that claim.

Primary payment responsibility on the part of workers' compensation, liability insurance (including self-insurance), and no-fault insurance is generally set according to settlements, judgments, awards, or other payments. These programs "settle" with the patient, sometimes long after the accident or situation that caused the injury. In these cases, the payer that made payments before the case was settled takes action to get their payments back.

subrogation Action by payer to recoup expenses for a claim it paid when another party should have been responsible for paying at least a portion of that claim.

Disability Compensation Programs

Disability compensation programs do not provide policyholders with reimbursement for health care charges. Instead, they provide partial reimbursement for lost income when a disability—whether work-related or not—prevents the individual from working. Benefits are paid in the form of regular cash payments. Workers' compensation coverage is a type of disability insurance, but most disability programs do not require an injury or illness to be work-related in order to pay benefits.

To receive compensation under a disability program, an individual's medical condition must be documented in his or her medical record. The medical record often serves as substantiation for the disability benefits, and an inadequate or incomplete medical record may result in a denial of disability benefits. The more severe the disability, the greater the standard of medical documentation required. For this reason, an accurate and thorough medical record is of primary significance in disability cases.

disability compensation programs Provide partial reimbursement for lost income when a disability prevents an individual from working.

Private Programs

Employers are not required to provide disability insurance. Many companies provide employees with disability coverage and pay a substantial amount of the premiums, but others do not. Federal or state government employees are eligible for a public disability program. Individuals not covered by employer- or government-sponsored plans may purchase disability policies from private insurance carriers.

Government Programs

The federal government provides disability benefits to individuals through several different programs. The major government disability programs are:

- ► Workers' compensation (covered earlier in the chapter)
- ► Social Security Disability Insurance (SSDI)
- ► Supplemental Security Income (SSI)
- ► Federal Employees Retirement System (FERS) or Civil Service Retirement System (CSRS)
- ► Department of Veterans Affairs disability programs

People who become disabled may qualify for **Social Security Disability Insurance (SSDI)** benefits if one of the following applies:

- ► They are salaried or hourly wage employees whose payroll deductions included those for the **Federal Insurance Contribution Act (FICA).**
- ► They are self-employed and paid Social Security taxes for the required minimum number of quarters.
- ► They are widows, widowers, or minor children of deceased workers who would be qualified for Social Security benefits if they were still alive.

Disability under the SSDI program is defined as a condition that prevents the worker from doing any work and that is expected to last at least twelve consecutive months or can be expected to result in the worker's death. Part of the review process includes an assessment of whether the worker can perform a different job or learn new skills that the condition will allow him or her to use.

The **Supplemental Security Income (SSI)** program is a welfare program, not an entitlement program. SSI provides payments to individuals in need, including aged, blind, and disabled individuals. Eligibility is determined using nationwide standards.

The Federal Employees Retirement System (FERS) provides disability coverage to federal workers hired after 1984. Employees hired before 1984 enrolled in the Civil Service Retirement System (CSRS). The FERS program consists of a federal disability program and the Social Security disability program. The two parts of the program have different eligibility rules, and some workers qualify for FERS benefits but not for SSDI benefits. If a worker is eligible for both, the amount of the SSDI payment is reduced based on the amount of the FERS payment.

Veterans of the uniformed services are covered by two federal plans, the Veteran's Compensation Program and the Veteran's Pension Program. Certain veterans may qualify to receive benefits from both VA programs. The Veteran's Compensation Program provides coverage for individuals with permanent and total disabilities that resulted from service-related illnesses or injuries. In order for a veteran to be eligible for benefits, the disability must affect his or her earning capacity. The Veteran's Pension Program provides benefits for service-related permanent disabilities to those who are unable to obtain gainful employment.

In states with disability programs, State Disability Insurance (SDI) covers most workers in the state, although in some states employees of the state and federal government, school district employees, and employees of churches are ineligible. As with Social Security Disability Insurance, SDI is usually paid for through payroll deductions.

Preparing Disability Reports

When a request is made for a medical report to support a disability claim, the physician or a member of the staff prepares the report by abstracting information from the patient's medical record. It is important to thoroughly document each

Social Security Disability Insurance (SSDI) Federal disability compensation program for some qualified people.

Federal Insurance Contribution Act (FICA) Authorizes payroll deductions for the Social Security Disability Program.

Supplemental Security Income (SSI) Helps pay living expenses for low-income older people and those who are blind or have disabilities.

examination by the physician. In many cases, an incomplete or inadequate medical report leads to denial of a disability claim.

The report for a disability claim should include the following medical information:

► Medical history
► Subjective complaints
► Objective findings
► Diagnostic test results
► Diagnosis
► Treatment
► Description of patient's ability to perform work-related activities and limitations, if any

Supporting documents, such as X-rays, pulmonary function tests, range of motion tests, and ECGs, should also be included when appropriate.

THINKING IT THROUGH 12.5

1. Explain the difference between SSI and SSDI.

Chapter Summary

Learning Outcomes	Key Concepts/Examples
12.1 Explain the four federal workers' compensation plans. Page 242	The four workers' compensation plans that provide coverage to federal government employees are: • The Federal Employees' Compensation Program • The Federal Black Lung Program • The Energy Employees Occupational Illness Compensation Program • The Longshore and Harbor Workers' Compensation Program
12.2 Describe the two types of state workers' compensation benefits. Pages 242–244	• States provide two types of workers' compensation benefits. • One pays the worker's medical expenses that result from work-related illness or injury. • The other pays for lost wages while the worker is unable to return to work.
12.3 Classify work-related injuries. Pages 244–246	Work-related injuries are classified as: • Injury without disability • Injury with temporary disability • Injury with permanent disability • Injury requiring vocational rehabilitation • Injury resulting in death
12.4 Complete workers' compensation claims. Pages 246–248	• Payment from the insurance carrier must be accepted as payment in full. • A separate file must be maintained when a provider treats an established patient for a work-related injury. • The patient's signature is not required on any billing forms. • The workers' compensation claim number should be included on all forms and correspondence. • Use the eight-digit format when reporting dates such as the date last worked.

Learning Outcomes	Key Concepts/Examples
12.5 Compare automotive insurance and disability compensation programs. Pages 248–251	Automobile insurance policies provide several basic types of coverage: • Personal Injury Protection (PIP) • Liability • Collision • Comprehensive • Automobile insurance may also include coverage for uninsured motorist, emergency road services, rental reimbursement, and property damage. Disability compensation programs provide partial reimbursement for lost income. The major government disability programs are: • Workers' Compensation • Social Security Disability Insurance (SSDI) • Supplemental Security Income (SSI) • Federal Employees Retirement System (FERS) or Civil Service Retirement System (CSRS)

Using Terminology

Match the key terms in the left column with the definitions in the right column.

_____ 1. **[LO 12.5]** Personal Injury Protection (PIP)

_____ 2. **[LO 12.3]** Final report

_____ 3. **[LO 12.2]** Occupational diseases or illnesses

_____ 4. **[LO 12.5]** Supplemental Security Income (SSI)

_____ 5. **[LO 12.4]** First report of injury

_____ 6. **[LO 12.1]** Office of Worker's Compensation Program (OWCP)

_____ 7. **[LO 12.4]** Admission of Liability

_____ 8. **[LO 12.1]** Occupational Safety and Health Administration (OSHA)

_____ 9. **[LO 12.1]** Federal Employees' Compensation Act (FECA)

_____ 10. **[LO 12.5]** Social Security Disability Insurance (SSDI)

A. Determination that the employer is responsible for the worker's injury or illness.

B. Legislation that provides workers' compensation benefits to individuals employed by the federal government.

C. Conditions caused by the work environment over a period longer than one workday or shift.

D. A document that contains information about the patient, the employer, and the injury or illness that must be filed by the employer, often within twenty-four hours of the incident.

E. A document indicating that an individual is fit to return to work and resume normal job activities.

F. Agency set up by congress in 1970 to protect workers from health and safety risks on the job.

G. The government agency that administers workers' compensation programs for civilian employees of federal agencies.

H. Insurance coverage for medical expenses and other expenses related to a motor vehicle accident.

I. Program funded by workers' payroll deductions and matching employer contributions that provides compensation for lost wages due to disability.

J. A welfare program that provides financial assistance to individuals in need, including those who are aged, blind, and disabled.

connect plus+

Enhance your learning at mcgrawhillconnect.com!
• Practice Exercises   • Worksheets
• Activities   • Integrated eBook

Checking Your Understanding

Write the letter of the choice that best completes the statement or answers the question.

1. **[LO 12.4]** If an employer denies liability, the workers' compensation insurance carrier issues a _____.
   A. First Report of Liability
   B. Notice of Contest
   C. No Fault Notice
   D. Denial of Finding

2. **[LO 12.4]** When a patient with a work-related injury has a significant change in her or his condition, the treating physician files _____.
   A. A progress report
   B. A doctor's final report
   C. An admission of liability report
   D. A final report of injury

3. **[LO 12.1]** Workers' compensation insurance coverage is provided to employees of the federal government through the _____.
   A. Office of Workers' Compensation Programs (OWCP)
   B. Federal Insurance Contribution Act (FICA)
   C. Supplemental Security Income (SSI)
   D. Federal Employees' Compensation Act (FECA)

4. **[LO 12.5]** Legislation that authorizes payroll deductions for the Social Security Disability Programs is known as _____.
   A. Federal Employees' Compensation Act (FECA)
   B. Federal Insurance Contribution Act (FICA)
   C. Employment Retirement Income Security Act (ERISA)
   D. Payroll Deduction Act (PDA)

5. **[LO 12.1]** An employee who believes the work environment to be dangerous may file a complaint with the _____.
   A. Office of Workers' Compensation Programs (OWCP)
   B. Local Social Security office
   C. Occupational Safety and Health Administration (OSHA)
   D. Workers' Compensation Board in the state in which the company is headquartered

6. **[LO 12.2]** Identify the source from which employers cannot obtain workers' compensation insurance. _____
   A. Private plan
   B. State workers' compensation fund
   C. Directly with a self-insured fund
   D. Physician of record

7. **[LO 12.2]** Which of the following is an example of an immediate accident? _____
   A. Employee develops chronic back pain after years of heavy lifting.
   B. Employee is diagnosed with carpal tunnel syndrome from too much typing.
   C. Employee begins to have lung problems as a result of working in a dusty factory.
   D. Employee slips on a wet surface at work and breaks her arm.

8. **[LO 12.3]** For individuals with job-related injuries vocational rehabilitation programs provide _____.
   A. Physical therapy
   B. Compensation for lost wages
   C. Training in a different job
   D. Payment for medical expenses

connect plus+

Enhance your learning at mcgrawhillconnect.com!
- Practice Exercises
- Worksheets
- Activities
- Integrated eBook

9. **[LO 12.3]** Workers' compensation claim information _____.
   A. Is confidential and must be authorized for release
   B. Can only be accessed by the provider
   C. Must contain HIPAA codes
   D. Can be accessed by employers

10. **[LO 12.5]** Which type of coverage in an automobile insurance policy compensates for damages caused by the policyholder to someone else's body or property? _____
   A. Personal Injury Protection (PIP)
   B. Liability
   C. Collision
   D. Comprehensive

Applying Your Knowledge

[LO 12.4]   Case Study 12.1   Workers' Compensation

Evelyn Wakefield hurt her shoulder while at work. Assume that the first report of injury has been filed and claim number CG465637 has been issued.

Physician Information
Name: Nicole Gary, MD
Employer ID Number: 23-8591473
National Provider Identifier: 5398742311

Patient Information
Name: Evelyn Wakefield (New Patient)
Sex: Female
Birth Date: 02-20-66
Address: 2517 Atlee Rd
     Butler, Maryland 21023
Social Security Number: 164-58-7412
Employer: Cupcakes Galore Bakery
     7401 Broad St
     Butler, Maryland 21023
Phone: 443-574-2828

Workers' Compensation Information
Workers Compensation Carrier: CGB Insurance Group
Carrier Address: 404 Main St
     Butler, Maryland 21023
Insurance Group Number: B642
Claim Number: CG465637

connect plus+
Enhance your learning at mcgrawhillconnect.com!
• Practice Exercises   • Worksheets
• Activities   • Integrated eBook

Patient's Encounter Form

Date: June 16, 2016

CC: Patient stated that on Wednesday June 16, 2016 a container of butter crème frosting fell from the shelf as she entered the pantry and hit her right shoulder.

Dx: Right shoulder dislocation

List of Fees for the Service:

Charges: Office visit, Level II $85

   Shoulder X Ray 1 View $68

Supply the following data elements:

Billing Provider _____

Billing Provider's Primary Identifier _____

Patient _____

Relationship _____

WC Claim Number _____

WC Plan _____

WC Group Number _____

Claim Information:

Accident Cause (check One)

Auto Accident ___ Another Responsible Party ___

Employment Related ___ Other Accident ___

Date of Accident _____

Service Line Information:

Date of Service _____

Procedure Code(s) _____

Diagnosis Code(s) _____

Total Charges _____

13

CLAIM PROCESSING, PAYMENTS, AND COLLECTIONS

KEY TERMS

adjudication
adjustment code
aging
appeal
autoposting
bad debt
collections
cycle billing
day sheet
determination
development
downcoding
electronic funds transfer (EFT)
electronic remittance advice (ERA)
Equal Credit Opportunity Act (ECOA)
explanation of benefits (EOB)
Fair Debt Collection Practices Act (FDCPA)
    of 1977
guarantor billing
insurance aging report
NSF checks
overpayment
patient aging report
patient ledger
patient statement
patient refund
reconciliation
Telephone Consumer Protection Act of 1991
Truth in Lending Act
uncollectible account
upcoding

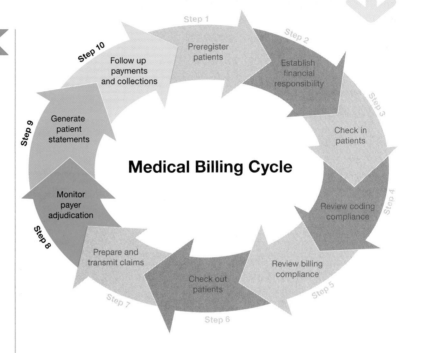

Medical Billing Cycle

Step 1 — Preregister patients
Step 2 — Establish financial responsibility
Step 3 — Check in patients
Step 4 — Review coding compliance
Step 5 — Review billing compliance
Step 6 — Check out patients
Step 7 — Prepare and transmit claims
Step 8 — Monitor payer adjudication
Step 9 — Generate patient statements
Step 10 — Follow up payments and collections

Learning Outcomes

After studying this chapter, you should be able to:

13.1 Outline the steps of claim adjudication, explaining the effect of upcoding and downcoding on the process.

13.2 Process RAs.

13.3 Discuss the purpose and general steps of the appeal process.

13.4 Describe the purpose and content of patient statements.

13.5 Apply regulations and guidelines to the collection process.

13.6 Explain the procedures for writing off uncollectible accounts.

13.7 Describe the physician's responsibilities when terminating the provider–patient relationship.

Clean claims increase the probability of being paid in full and on time. Claims that payers pay late, decide not to pay, or pay at a reduced level have a negative effect on accounts receivable (AR). Likewise, patient balances that fail to be collected affect revenue. To follow up on claims and patient balances, medical assistants need to understand the process that payers follow to determine payments and the subsequent collection process involving patients.

13.1 Health Plan Claim Processing by Payers

When the payer receives claims, it issues an electronic response to the sender showing that the transmission has been successful. Each claim then undergoes a process known as **adjudication,** made up of five steps designed to judge how it should be paid:

adjudication Health plan process of examining claims and determining benefits.

1. Initial processing
2. Automated review
3. Manual review
4. Determination
5. Payment

Initial Processing

Each claim's data elements are checked by the payer's front-end claims processing system. Paper claims and any paper attachments are date-stamped and entered into the payer's computer system, either by data-entry personnel or by the use of a scanning system. Initial processing might find such problems as the following:

▶ The patient's name, plan identification number, or place of service code is wrong.
▶ The diagnosis code is missing or is not valid for the date of service.
▶ The patient is not the correct sex for a reported gender-specific procedure code.

Claims with errors or simple mistakes are rejected, and the payer transmits instructions to the provider to correct errors and/or omissions and to rebill the service. The medical insurance specialist should respond to such a request as quickly as possible by supplying the correct information and, if necessary, submitting a clean claim (see the chapter covering health care claim preparation and transmission) that is accepted by the payer for processing.

Automated Review

Payers' computer systems then apply edits that reflect their payment policies. For example, a Medicare claim is subject to the Correct Coding Initiative (CCI) edits (see the chapter on Medicare). The automated review checks for the following:

1. *Patient eligibility for benefits*: Is the patient eligible for the services that are billed?
2. *Time limits for filing claims:* Has the claim been sent within the payer's time limits for filing claims?
3. *Preauthorization and referral:* Are valid preauthorization or referral numbers present as required under the payer's policies? Some authorizations are for specific dates or number of service, so these data will be checked, too.
4. *Duplicate dates of service:* Is the claim billing for a service on the same date that has already been adjudicated?
5. *Noncovered services:* Are the billed services covered under the patient's policy?
6. *Valid code linkages:* Are the diagnosis and procedure codes properly linked for medical necessity?
7. *Bundled codes:* Have surgical code bundling rules and global periods been followed?
8. *Medical review:* Are there charges for services that are not medically necessary or that are over the frequency limits of the plan? The payer's medical director and other professional medical staff have a medical review program to ensure that providers give patients the most appropriate care in the most cost-effective

manner. The basic medical review edits that are done at this stage are based on its guidelines.

9. *Utilization review:* Are the hospital-based health care services appropriate? Are days and services authorized consistent with services and dates billed?

10. *Concurrent care:* If concurrent care (medical situations in which a patient receives extensive care from two or more providers on the same date of service) is being billed, was it medically necessary?

Manual Review

development Process of gathering information to adjudicate a claim.

If problems result from the automated review, the claim is suspended and set aside for **development**—the term used by payers to indicate that more information is needed for claim processing. These claims are sent to the medical review department, where a claims examiner reviews the claim. The examiner may ask the provider for clinical documentation to check:

▶ Where the service took place.
▶ Whether the treatments were appropriate and a logical outcome of the facts and conditions shown in the medical record.
▶ That services provided were accurately reported.

Claims examiners are trained in the payer's payment policies, but they usually have little or no clinical medical background. When there is insufficient guidance on the point in question, examiners may have it reviewed by staff medical professionals—nurses or physicians—in the medical review department. This step is usually followed, for example, to review the medical necessity of an unlisted procedure.

Determination

determination Payer's decision about the benefits due for a claim.

For each service line on a claim, the payer makes a payment **determination**—a decision whether to (1) pay it, (2) deny it, or (3) pay it at a reduced level. If the service falls within normal guidelines, it will be paid. If it is not reimbursable, the item on the claim is denied. Or, the examiner may decide that the procedure code assigned is at too high a level for the diagnosis, and assign a lower-level code, called **downcoding.**

downcoding Payer's review and reduction of a procedure code.

Downcoding may occur because the procedure's place of service is an emergency department, but the patient's problem is not considered an emergency. Claims may also be downcoded because the documentation fails to support the level of service claimed. For example, if the physician has coded a high-level evaluation and management service for a patient who presents with an apparently straightforward problem, this is considered **upcoding,** and the claims examiner is likely to request the encounter documentation. The medical record should contain information about the type of medical history and examination done as well as the complexity of the medical decision making that was performed. If the documentation does not support the service, the examiner downcodes the E/M code to a level considered appropriate.

upcoding Use of a procedure code that provides a higher payment.

Payment

If payment is due, the payer sends it to the provider along with a remittance advice (RA) (see the first chapter), also known as an **electronic remittance advice (ERA),** a transaction that explains the payment decisions to the provider.

electronic remittance advice (ERA) Transaction that explains payment decisions to the provider.

Overdue Claims

Just as medical offices are required to file claims within a certain period of time, health plans have contractual or legal agreements to pay claims within a period of time from receipt. Claims must be monitored until payments are received. Monitoring claims during adjudication requires two types of information. The first is the amount of time the payer is allowed to take to respond to the claim, and the second is how long the claim has been in process.

Valley Associates, P.C.
Primary Insurance Aging
As of November 30, 2016

Date of Service	Procedure	Current 0 - 30	Past 31 - 60	Past 61 - 90	Past 91 - 120	Past 121 ---->	Total Balance

Aetna Choice (AET00) (555)777-1000

WILLIWA0   Walter Williams

Claim: 65   Initial Billing Date: 9/2/2016   Last Billing Date: 9/2/2016   Policy: ABC103562239 Group: BDC1001

9/2/2016	99212			31.00			31.00
9/2/2016	93000			70.00			70.00
	Claim Totals:	0.00	0.00	101.00	0.00	0.00	101.00
	Insurance Totals:	0.00	0.00	101.00	0.00	0.00	101.00

Oxford Freedom (OXF00) (555)666-1111

PORCEJE0 Jennifer Porcelli

Claim: 63   Initial Billing Date: 10/3/2016   Last Billing Date: 10/3/2016   Policy: 712340808X   Group: G0119

10/3/2016	99211		15.00				15.00
	Claim Totals:	0.00	15.00	0.00	0.00	0.00	15.00

SMITHJO0 Josephine Smith

Claim: 64   Initial Billing Date: 10/6/2016   Last Billing Date: 10/6/2016   Policy: 610327842X   Group: G0119

10/6/2016	99212		36.00				36.00
	Claim Totals:	0.00	36.00	0.00	0.00	0.00	36.00
	Insurance Totals:	0.00	51.00	0.00	0.00	0.00	51.00

Report Aging Totals		$0.00	$51.00	$101.00	$0.00	$0.00	$152.00
Percent of Aging Total		0.0 %	12.9 %	87.1 %	0.0 %	0.0 %	100.0 %

FIGURE 13.1 Example of an Insurance Aging Report

COMPLIANCE GUIDELINE

Claim Status

Medical offices use a HIPAA transaction called the "claim status inquiry" to electronically follow up with payers. The payer responds with the status of the claim.

Payers also have to process clean claims within the claim turnaround time as specified by the participation contract or governed by state or federal rules. The other factor in claim follow-up is **aging**—how long a payer has had the claim. The practice management program is used to generate an **insurance aging report** that lists the claims transmitted on each day and shows how long they have been in process with the payer. A typical report, shown in Figure 13.1, lists claims that were sent fewer than thirty days ago, between thirty and sixty days ago, and so on.

aging Classification of accounts receivable by length of time.

insurance aging report Report grouping unpaid claims transmitted to payers by the length of time they remain due.

THINKING IT THROUGH 13.1

1. In Figure 13.1, are any of the accounts past due thirty-one to sixty days?

FIGURE 13.2 Medicare RA

13.2 Processing the Remittance Advice

explanation of benefits (EOB)
Document showing how the amount of a benefit was determined.

The RA sent by the payer to the medical office summarizes the determinations for a number of claims. See Figure 13.2 for an example of a Medicare RA received by a medical office. (The document the patient receives, called the **explanation of benefits** or **EOB,** covers just the patient's determination.) The RA shows the claim control number, patient name, dates of service, types of service, and charges, along with an explanation of the way the amount of the benefit payment was determined.

RAs cover claims for a number of patients, and payments may not be made for every service line on a particular claim. Payers use standard types of HIPAA administrative codes to explain their adjustments—situations where the payment is different than the amount billed. For example, the **adjustment code** PR indicates that the amount can be billed to the patient/insured, and code PI means payer-initiated reduction, which might result from the payer's downcoding an E/M code.

adjustment code Explains an adjustment on the insured's account.

Review Procedure

COMPLIANCE GUIDELINE

RA Codes

Access the website www. wpc-edi.com/codes for updated lists of the HIPAA administrative codes reported on RAs.

An RA repeats the unique claim control number that the provider assigned to the claim when sending it. This number is the resource needed to match the payment to a claim. To process the RA, each claim is located in the practice management program—either manually or automatically by the computer system. The remittance data are reviewed and then posted to the practice management program (PMP).

This procedure is followed to double-check the remittance data:

1. Check the patient's name, account number, insurance number, and date of service against the claim.
2. Verify that all billed CPT codes are listed.
3. Check the payment for each CPT against the expected amount, which may be an allowed amount or a percentage of the usual fee. Many practice management programs build records of the amount each payer has paid for each CPT code as the data are entered. When another RA payment for the same CPT is posted, the program highlights any discrepancy for review.
4. Analyze the payer's adjustment codes to locate all unpaid, downcoded, or denied claims for closer review.

5. Pay special attention to the RA for claims submitted with modifiers. Some payers' claim processing systems automatically ignore modifiers, so that E/M visits billed on the same date of service as a procedure are always unpaid and should be appealed.

6. Decide whether any items on the RA need clarifying with the payer, and follow up as necessary.

Posting Procedure

Many practices that receive RAs authorize the payer to provide an **electronic funds transfer (EFT)** of the payment. Payments are deposited directly into the practice's bank account. Otherwise, the payer sends a check to the practice, and the check is taken to the practice's bank for deposit. Regulations mandated under the Affordable Care Act (ACA) as of January 1, 2014, require a trace number to appear on both the EFT and its ERA, so the documents are easy to match up electronically.

electronic funds transfer (EFT) Electronic routing of funds between banks.

Applying Payments

Payment and adjustment transactions are entered in the practice management program. The data entry includes

▶ Date of deposit.
▶ Payer name and type.
▶ Check or EFT number.
▶ Total payment amount.
▶ Amount to be applied to each patient's account, including type of payment. Codes are used for payments, adjustments, deductibles, and other specific types.

Some PMPs have an **autoposting** feature. Instead of posting payments manually, this feature automatically posts the payment data in the RA to the correct account. The software allows the user to establish posting rules, such as "post a payment automatically only if the claim is paid at 100 percent," so that the medical assistant can examine claims that are not paid as expected.

autoposting Software feature enabling automatic entry of payments on a remittance advice.

Reconciling Payments

The process of **reconciliation** means making sure that the totals on the RA EOB check out mathematically. The total amount billed minus the adjustments (such as for allowed amounts and patient responsibility to pay) should equal the total amount paid. For example, study this report for an assigned claim:

reconciliation Comparison of two numbers.

POS	PROC	BILLED	ALLOWED	DEDUCT	COINS	UNALLOWED	PROV PD
11	99213	85.00	57.87	0.00	11.57	27.13	46.30

RECONCILIATION
Amount Billed	$85.00
(Coinsurance)	−11.57
(Unallowed)	−27.13
Payment	$46.30

In this case, the allowed amount (ALLOWED) of $57.87 is made up of the coinsurance (COINS) to be collected from the patient of $11.57 plus the amount the payer pays to the provider (PROV PD) of $46.30. The difference between the billed amount (BILLED) of $85.00 and the allowed amount of $57.87 is $27.13.

This amount is written off unless it can be billed to the patient under the payer's rules.

Handling Overpayments

overpayment Improper or excessive payment resulting from billing errors.

From the payer's point of view, **overpayments** (also called credit balances) are improper or excessive payments resulting from billing errors for which the provider owes refunds. Examples are:

▶ A payer may mistakenly overpay a claim.
▶ A payer's postpayment audit may find that a claim that has been paid should be denied or downcoded because the documentation does not support it.
▶ A provider may collect a primary payment from Medicare when another payer is primary.

In such cases, reimbursement that the provider has received is considered an overpayment, and the payer will ask for a refund (with the addition of interest for Medicare). If the audit shows that the claim was for a service that was not medically necessary, the provider also must refund any payment collected from the patient. Most often, the procedure is to promptly refund the overpayment.

COMPLIANCE GUIDELINE

Overpayments

Part of the compliance plan is a regular process to self-audit and discover any overbilling situations—and then to send the payer a refund.

Denial Management

Typical problems and solutions are:

▶ *Rejected claims:* A claim that is not paid due to incorrect information must be corrected and sent to the payer according to its procedures.
▶ *Procedures not paid:* If a procedure that should have been paid on a claim was overlooked, another claim is sent for that procedure.
▶ *Partially paid, denied, or downcoded claims:* If the payer has denied payment, the first step is to study the adjustment codes to determine why. If a procedure is not a covered benefit or if the patient was not eligible for that benefit, typically the next step will be to bill the patient for the noncovered amount. If the claim is denied or downcoded for lack of medical necessity, a decision about the next action must be made. The options are to bill the patient, write off the amount, or challenge the determination with an appeal, as discussed on pages 263–264. Some provider contracts prohibit billing the patient if an appeal or necessary documentation has not been submitted to the payer.

To improve the rate of paid claims over time, medical assistants track and analyze each payer's reasons for denying claims. This record may be kept in a denial log or by assigning specific denial-reason codes for the practice management program to store and report on. Denials should be grouped into categories, such as:

▶ Coding errors (incorrect unbundling, procedure codes not payable by plan with the reported diagnosis codes).
▶ Registration mistakes, such as incorrect patient ID numbers.
▶ Billing errors, such as failure to get required preauthorizations or referral numbers.
▶ Payer requests for more information or general delays in claims processing.

The types of denials should be analyzed to find out what procedures can be implemented to fix the problems. For example, educating the staff members responsible for getting preauthorizations about each payer's requirements may be necessary.

Exercise 13.1 Posting an Insurance Payment

Post the payment that has been transmitted to Dr. Clarke's bank account from Ann Ingram's insurance carrier.

Follow the steps at www.mhhe.com/newbycarr to complete the exercise at connect.mcgraw-hill.com on your own once you have watched the demo and tried the steps with prompts in practice mode. Use the information provided in the scenario to complete the exercise.

connect (plus+)

THINKING IT THROUGH 13.2

1. Based on the RA below:

   A. What is the total amount paid by check? (Fill in the "Amt paid provider" column before calculating the total.)

   B. Were any procedures paid at a rate lower than the claim charge? If so, which?

   C. What might be the reason that there is no insurance payment for services for Gloria Vanderhilt?

   D. Was payment denied for any claim? For what reason?

Date prepared: 6/22/2016   **Claim number: 0347914**

Patient's name	Dates of service from - thru	POS	Proc	Qty	Charge amount	Eligible amount	Patient liability	Amt paid provider
Kavan, Gregory	04/15/16 - 04/15/16	11	99213	1	$48.00	$48.00	$4.80	_____
Ferrara, Grace	05/11/16 - 05/11/16	11	99212	1	$35.00	$35.00	$3.50	_____
Cornprost, Harry	05/12/16 - 05/12/16	11	99214	1	$64.00	$54.00	-0-	_____
Vanderhilt, Gloria	05/12/16 - 05/12/16	11	99212	1	$35.00	$35.00	$35.00	-0-
Dallez, Juan	05/13/16 - 05/13/16	11	99212	1	$35.00	*	*	-0-

* * * * * * * *   Check #1039242 is attached in the amount of _____   * * * * * * * *

* Procedure not covered under Medicaid

13.3 Appeals

When a claim has been denied or payment reduced, an appeal may be filed with the payer for reconsideration.

The General Appeal Process

An **appeal** is a process that can be used to challenge a payer's decision to deny, reduce, or otherwise downcode a claim. A provider or a patient may begin the appeal process by asking for a review of the payer's decision.

Each payer has consistent procedures for handling appeals. These procedures are based on the nature of the appeal. The practice staff reviews the appropriate guidelines for the particular insurance carrier before starting an appeal and plans its actions according to the rules. Appeals must be filed within a specified time after the

appeal Request for reconsideration of a claim adjudication.

claim determination. Most payers have an escalating structure of appeals, such as (1) a complaint, (2) an appeal, and (3) a grievance. The claimant must move through the three levels in pursuing an appeal, starting at the lowest and continuing to the highest, final level. Some payers also set a minimum amount that must be involved in an appeal process, so that a lot of time is not spent on a small dispute.

A claimant can take another step if the payer has rejected all the appeal levels on a claim. Because they license most types of payers, state insurance commissions have the authority to review appeals that payers reject. If a claimant decides to pursue an appeal with the state insurance commission, copies of the complete case file—all documents that relate to the initial claim determination and the appeal process—are sent, along with a letter of explanation.

Medicare Appeals

Medicare participating providers have appeal rights. Note, though, that there is no need to appeal a claim if it has been denied for minor errors or omissions. The provider can instead ask the MAC to reopen the claim so the error can be fixed, rather than going through the appeals process.

The Medicare appeal process involves five steps:

1. *Redetermination:* The first step, called *redetermination*, is a claim review by an employee of the Medicare carrier who was not involved in the initial claim determination. The request, which must be made within 120 days of receiving the initial claim determination, is made by completing a form or writing a letter and attaching supporting medical documentation. If the decision is favorable, payment is sent. If the redetermination is either partially favorable or unfavorable, the answer comes as a letter called the Medicare Redetermination Notice (MRN). The decision must be made within 60 days; and the letter is sent to both the provider and the patient.

2. *Reconsideration:* The next step is a reconsideration request. This request must be made within 180 days of receiving the redetermination notice. At this level, the claim is reviewed by qualified independent contractors (QICs).

3. *Administrative law judge:* The third level is a hearing by an administrative law judge. The amount in question must be over $130, and the hearing must be requested within 60 days of receiving the reconsideration notice.

4. *Medicare Appeals Council:* The fourth level must be requested within 60 days of receiving the response from the hearing by the administrative law judge. No monetary amount is specified.

5. *Federal court (judicial) review:* The fifth and final Medicare appeal level is a hearing in federal court. The amount in dispute must be at least $1,350, and the hearing must be requested within 60 days of receiving the department appeals board decision.

THINKING IT THROUGH 13.3

1. Create a flowchart based on the five steps in the Medicare appeals process.

13.4 Patient Billing and Adjustments

Effective patient billing begins with sound financial policies that are clearly communicated to patients so that they understand their responsibilities for payment. The process continues throughout the medical billing cycle, as patients' eligibility and benefits are verified, charges are carefully posted to the practice management program, clean claims are submitted, and RAs are received. At this point, the PMP is updated as follows:

1. The payer's payment for each reported procedure is entered.
2. The amount the patient owes for each reported procedure is calculated.
3. If any part of a charge must be written off due to a payer's required adjustment, this amount is also entered. The PMP uses this information to update the **day sheet,** which is a summary of the financial transactions that occur each day. The **patient ledger**—the patient's account—is also updated. These data are used to generate **patient statements,** bills that show the amount each patient owes. Patient statements are called patient ledger cards when billing is done manually rather than by computer. Patients may owe coinsurance, deductibles, and fees for noncovered services.

day sheet Report summarizing the business day's charges and payments.

patient ledger Record of a patient's financial transactions.

patient statement Shows services provided to a patient, total payments made, total charges, adjustments, and balance due.

Working with Statements

Statements are mailed (or in some offices e-mailed) to patients for payment. They must be easy for the patient to read, and they must be accurate. They contain all necessary information so that there is no confusion about the amount owed:

▶ The name of the practice and the patient's name, address, and account number.
▶ A cost breakdown of all services provided.
▶ An explanation of the costs covered by the patient's payer(s).
▶ The date of the statement (and sometimes the due date for the payment).
▶ The balance due (if a previous balance was due on the account, the sum of the old balance and the new charges).
▶ In some cases, the payment methods the practice accepts.

For example, review the following section taken from a patient statement. This patient's policy is a high-deductible PPO that does not cover preventive services.

DATE	CODE	DESCRIPTION				CHARGES	CREDITS
09/10/16	99396	Prev Check up, Est. 40–64 Yr				169.00	
09/10/16	85018	Hemoglobin Count, Colorimetric				6.10	
09/10/16	81002	Urinalysis, Non-automated, w/o s				4.20	
09/11/16		Golden Rule Ins. Co. #31478				Filed	
10/17/16		Denied Golden Rule Ins. Co. #31478					00.00
10/17/16		Repriced Golden Rule Inc. Co. #31478					51.80—
10/17/16		$127.50 = deductible for 9/10/16 visit					
CURRENT	**30–60**	**60–90**	**>90**	**TOTAL**	**INS PENDING**	**TOTAL DUE FROM PATIENT**	
127.50	0.00	0.00	0.00	127.50	0.00	127.50	

This section summarizes the following encounter and transaction information for the patient:

▶ The patient had a preventive checkup with a hemoglobin level check and urinalysis on September 10, for which the provider's usual charges are shown.
▶ On the next day, the claim for the visit was sent to the payer, Golden Rule Insurance Company.
▶ On October 17, the RA/EOB for the claim was posted. The payer did not pay the claim ("denied it") because the patient's plan does not cover these preventive

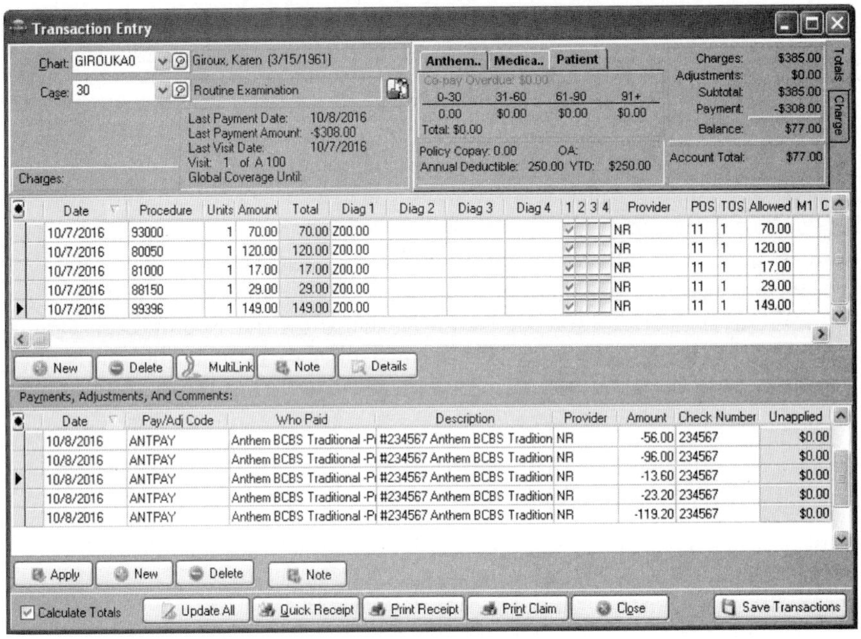

FIGURE 13.3a Patient Transaction Data Entry Screen

Patient Account Ledger

As of October 31, 2016

Show all data where the Chart Number is between GIROUKA0,GIROUKA0

Entry	Date	POS	Description	Procedure	Document	Provider	Amount
GIROUKA0	**Karen Giroux**			(555)683-5364			
	Last Payment: -308.00		On: 10/8/2016				
76	10/07/2016	11		93000	1610070000	NR	70.00
77	10/07/2016	11		80050	1610070000	NR	120.00
78	10/07/2016	11		81000	1610070000	NR	17.00
79	10/07/2016	11		88150	1610070000	NR	29.00
80	10/07/2016	11		99396	1610070000	NR	149.00
81	10/08/2016		#234567 Anthem BCBS Traditiona	ANTPAY	1610070000	NR	-56.00
82	10/08/2016		#234567 Anthem BCBS Traditiona	ANTPAY	1610070000	NR	-96.00
83	10/08/2016		#234567 Anthem BCBS Traditiona	ANTPAY	1610070000	NR	-13.60
84	10/08/2016		#234567 Anthem BCBS Traditiona	ANTPAY	1610070000	NR	-23.20
85	10/08/2016		#234567 Anthem BCBS Traditiona	ANTPAY	1610070000	NR	-119.20
						Patient Total:	77.00
						Ledger Total:	$77.00

FIGURE 13.3b Patient Account Ledger

services. The payer repriced the charges according to the PPO's in-network allowed amount for the service. The PPO total allowed amount for the visit is $127.50.

- The patient has not met the annual deductible, so the repriced charge of $127.50 is being billed to the patient.

Study parts a, b, and c of Figure 13.3 to observe the connections among the practice management program's data entry screen, the patient ledger, and the patient statement.

Example

Patient: Karen Giroux

Date of Service: 10/7/16

Date of RA: 10/8/16

Orchard Hill Medical Center
Ruth J. Clarke, MD
841 Orchard Hill Rd.
Columbus, OH 43214-1234

Statement Date	Chart Number	Page
10/31/2016	GIROUKA0	1

Make Checks Payable To:

Orchard Hill Medical Center
Ruth J. Clarke, MD
841 Orchard Hill Rd.
Columbus, OH 43214-1234

Karen Giroux
14A West Front St
Brooklyn, OH 44144-1234

Date of Last Payment: 10/8/2016   Amount: -308.00   Previous Balance: 0.00

Patient: Karen Giroux   Chart Number: GIROUKA0   Case: Routine Examination

Dates	Procedure	Charge	Paid by Primary	Paid by Secondary	Paid By Guarantor	Adjustments	Remainder
10/07/16	93000	70.00	-56.00	0.00		0.00	14.00
10/07/16	80050	120.00	-96.00	0.00		0.00	24.00
10/07/16	81000	17.00	-13.60	0.00		0.00	3.40
10/07/16	88150	29.00	-23.20	0.00		0.00	5.80
10/07/16	99396	149.00	-119.20	0.00		0.00	29.80

Amount Due
77.00

FIGURE 13.3c Patient Statement

The screen in Figure 13.3a illustrates the entry of the charges for Karen Giroux's office visit on October 7, 2016, and a payment received from the health plan on October 8, 2016. The patient ledger in Figure 13.3b shows each charge and each payment. The patient statement in Figure 13.3c is sent to the patient or guarantor and shows the balance that is owed. Compare the statement to the ledger to check the amounts charged and paid. ◄

Cycle versus Guarantor Billing

Instead of generating all statements at the end of a month, practices follow some kind of billing cycle to spread out the workload. **Cycle billing** is used to assign patient accounts to a specific time of the month and to standardize the times when statements will be mailed and payments will be due. If the billing cycle is weekly, for example, the patient accounts are divided into four groups—usually alphabetically—so that 25 percent of the bills go out each week.

Practices may send statements to each individual patient, as shown in Figure 13.3c, or they may send one statement to the guarantor of a number of different accounts, called **guarantor billing**. For example, if a patient is responsible for his own bill as well as the bills of his wife and children, all of the family's recent charges can be categorized and sent together on one statement.

cycle billing Type of billing which divides patients with current balances into groups to even out monthly statement printing and mailing.

guarantor billing Grouping patient billing under the insurance policyholder.

Patient Advocacy

Patients often have complaints and problems with their health plans that they become aware of when they receive their bills. The medical assistant may serve as a go-between to contact the carrier and get questions answered. Handling these situations with expertise and objectivity can build good will for the physician's office by using problem-solving and communication skills to fulfill this role. The first step in answering patients' inquiries about claims is to find out exactly what the problem is. Ask the patient whether he or she has:

► Contacted the health plan.
► Talked to the service representative.
► Reviewed and understands the policy.

Often, the answer is no. The patient may not understand the insurance policy or may be confused about the rules, such as in- and out-of-network billing. On other occasions, the payer has made an error, and the patient is correct.

Understandably, patients get upset when they receive unexpected large bills or incorrect payments or when payments are delayed. The medical assistant is the patients' advocate with the health plan. Sometimes the problem is just a misunderstanding because the patient does not know the right questions to ask, does not understand the answers, or is unaware that benefits have changed. In other situations, the patient may accuse the office staff of billing incorrectly. In these cases, try to listen carefully for the facts without letting feelings interfere.

If the patient has already called the health plan but is still upset or confused, the medical assistant should call again and listen carefully to the explanation. The patient may have been too stressed to understand it. Explaining the solution again to the patient may help clear up misunderstandings.

Following are some techniques to use when explaining insurance issues to patients:

▶ Volunteer to explain. Speak slowly and calmly.
▶ Use simple language. Try to avoid insurance jargon.
▶ Explain more than once when necessary.
▶ Ask the patient "Do you understand?" or say "Perhaps I can explain that better."
▶ Remember, patients are under stress. Use respect and care.

Credit Balances, Refunds, and NSF Fee Posting

Some situations require adjustments to the *patient's* account using the practice management program. (Handling overpayments from payers is covered on page 262.) The medical office focuses on accounts receivable, but at times the practice may need to issue **patient refunds.** Refunds are made when the practice has overcharged a patient for a service and the patient has a credit balance, so the extra amount needs to be repaid. Note that the balance due must be refunded promptly if the practice has completed the patient's care. However, if the practice is still treating the patient, the credit balance may be carried forward—that is, noted on the patient's statement and account to be applied toward the copayment or other charges for the next visit.

Another adjustment to patient accounts occurs when a patient makes a payment by check, does not have adequate funds in his or her checking account to cover the check, and it is not honored by the bank. These checks are referred to as **NSF checks,** for "nonsufficient funds." They are also commonly called "bounced" and "returned" checks. A bank may also not honor a check if the account has been closed. When a practice receives an NSF notice from a bank, an adjustment is made in the patient's account, since the patient now owes the practice the amount of the returned check. In addition, most practices charge a fee for a returned check. The maximum amount of the fee is governed by state laws.

patient refund Money owed to a patient.

NSF check Check written from an account that does not have adequate funds to cover the check.

Exercise 13.2 Generating a Patient Statement

The insurance payment for Ann Ingram's visit has been posted and subtracted from her balance. Generate a current statement that shows her balance due.

Follow the steps at www.mhhe.com/newbycarr to complete the exercise at connect.mcgraw-hill.com on your own once you have watched the demo and tried the steps with prompts in practice mode. Use the information provided in the scenario to complete the exercise.

connect™ plus+

THINKING IT THROUGH 13.4

1. Examine the patient statement in Figure 13.3c. Based on the procedure code 99396, what is Karen's age range? Is she a new patient of the practice? What percentage of the charges does her insurance pay?

13.5 Collecting Outstanding Patient Accounts

The term **collections** refers to all the activities that are related to patient accounts and follow-up. Collection activities should achieve a suitable balance between maintaining patient satisfaction and generating cash flow. While most patients pay their bills on time, every medical practice has patients who do not pay their monthly statements when they receive them. Many simply forget to pay the bills and need a reminder, but others require more attention and effort. A patient may not pay a bill for several reasons:

▶ The patient thinks the bill is too high.
▶ The patient thinks that the care rendered was not appropriate or not effective.
▶ The patient has personal financial problems or just does not plan to pay the bill.
▶ The bill was sent to an inaccurate address.
▶ There is a misunderstanding about the amount the patient's insurance pays on the bill.

A great deal of accounts receivable can be tied up in unpaid bills, and these funds can mean the difference between a successful and an unsuccessful practice.

collections All activities related to patient accounts and follow-up.

Regulations

Collection Activities

Collections from patients are classified as consumer collections and are regulated by federal and state laws. The Federal Trade Commission enforces the **Fair Debt Collection Practices Act (FDCPA) of 1977** and the **Telephone Consumer Protection Act of 1991** that regulate collections to ensure fair and ethical treatment of debtors. The following guidelines apply:

▶ Contact patients once daily only, and leave no more than three messages per week.
▶ Do not call a patient before 8 A.M. or after 9 P.M.
▶ Do not threaten the patient or use profane language.
▶ Identify the caller, the practice, and the purpose of the call; do not mislead the patient.
▶ Do not discuss the patient's debt with another person, such as a neighbor.
▶ Do not leave a message on an answering machine that indicates that the call is about a debt or send an e-mail message stating that the topic is debt.
▶ If a patient requests that all phone calls cease and desist, do not call the patient again, but instead contact the patient via mail.
▶ If a patient wants calls to be made to an attorney, do not contact the patient directly again unless the attorney says to or cannot be reached.

State law may not permit contacting debtors at their place of employment, so this aspect needs to be checked. In addition to state and federal laws, the practice's policies for dealing with patients need to be followed. If the practice chooses to add late fees or finance charges to patient's accounts, it must do so in accordance with these laws. Often, it is required to disclose these at the time services are rendered.

Fair Debt Collection Practices Act (FDCPA) of 1977 Laws regulating collection practices.

Telephone Consumer Protection Act of 1991 Law regulating consumer collections to ensure fair and ethical treatment of debtors.

Credit Arrangements and Payment Plans

A practice may decide to extend credit to patients through a payment plan that lets patients pay bills over time, rather than in a single payment. The Federal Trade Commission (FTC) enforces the **Equal Credit Opportunity Act (ECOA),** which prohibits credit discrimination on the basis of race, color, religion, national origin, sex, marital status, age, or because a person receives public assistance. If the practice decides not to extend credit to a particular patient, while extending it to others, under the ECOA the patient has a right to know why. Factors like income, expenses, debts, and credit history are among the considerations lenders use to determine creditworthiness. The practice must be specific in answering such questions.

Both the patient and the practice must agree to all the terms before the arrangement is finalized. Patients agree to make set monthly payments; if no finance charges are applied to the account, the arrangement is not regulated by law. However, if the practice applies finance charges or late fees, or if payments are scheduled for more than four installments, the payment plan is governed by the **Truth in Lending Act,** which is part of the Consumer Credit Protection Act. Patients must sign off on the terms on a truth-in-lending form that the practice negotiates with the patient.

Practices have guidelines for appropriate time frames and minimum payment amounts for payment plans. For example, the following schedule might be followed:

- ▶ $50 balance or less: Entire balance due the first month
- ▶ $51–$500 balance due: $50 minimum monthly payment
- ▶ $501–$1,000 balance due: $100 minimum monthly payment
- ▶ $1,001–$2,500 balance due: $200 minimum monthly payment
- ▶ Over $2,500 balance due: 10 percent of the balance due each month

The practice works out payment plans using patient information such as the amount of the bill, the date of the payday, the amount of disposable income the patient has, and any other contributing factors.

Procedures

The medical office tracks overdue bills by reviewing the **patient aging report.** Like the insurance aging report, it is analyzed to determine which patients are overdue on their bills and to group them into categories for efficient collection efforts (see Figure 13.4). Aging begins on the date of the bill. The patient aging report includes the patient's name, the most recent payment, and the remaining balance.

Equal Credit Opportunity Act (ECOA) Prohibits credit discrimination on the basis of race, color, religion, national origin, sex, marital status, age, or because a person receives public assistance.

Truth in Lending Act Law requiring disclosure of finance charges and late fees for payment plans.

patient aging report Report grouping unpaid patients' bills by the length of time they remain due.

Valley Associates, P.C.
Patient Aging by Date of Service
As of November 30, 2016

Chart	Name		Current 0 - 30	Past 31 - 60	Past 61 - 90	Past 91 ---->	Total Balance
GIROUKA0	Karen Giroux		9.20	77.00			86.20
Last Pmt: -36.80	On: 11/25/2016	(555)683-5364					
PORCEJE0	Jennifer Porcelli			15.00			15.00
Last Pmt: -15.00	On: 10/3/2016	(555)709-0388					
SHAHKAL0	Kalpesh Shah		48.00		63.00		111.00
Last Pmt: -15.00	On: 11/8/2016	(555)608-9772					
SMITHJO0	Josephine Smith			36.00			36.00
Last Pmt: -10.00	On: 10/6/2016	(555)214-3349					
WILLIWA0	Walter Williams				101.00		101.00
Last Pmt: -15.00	On: 9/2/2016	(555)936-0216					
	Report Aging Totals		$57.20	$128.00	$164.00	$0.00	$349.20
	Percent of Aging Total		16.4%	36.7%	47.0%	0.0%	100.0%

FIGURE 13.4 Example of a Patient Aging Report

It divides the information into these categories based on each statement's beginning date:

1. Current or up-to-date: Thirty days
2. Past due: Thirty-one to sixty days
3. Past due: Sixty-one to ninety days
4. Past due: More than ninety days

For example, Figure 13.4 shows that Karen Giroux owes two charges. The $9.20 charge is current, and the $77.00 charge is thirty-one to sixty days past due.

Each practice sets its own procedures for the collections process. Large bills have priority over smaller ones. Usually, an automatic reminder notice and a second statement are mailed when a bill has not been paid thirty days after it was issued. Some practices phone a patient with a thirty-day overdue account. If the bill is not then paid, a series of collection letters is generated at intervals, each more stringent in its tone and more direct in its approach. Some practices use small claims court or outside collection agencies to pursue significant unpaid bills.

Posting Collection Agency Payments

A collection agency that is hired by a practice transmits monies it has collected according to the terms of its business associate (BA) contract. The payment is made up of amounts collected from various patients with various account ages. The agency includes a statement showing which patient accounts have been paid.

Payments are processed and posted in a manner similar to that used for RAs covered earlier in this chapter. Each patient account is located and the payment posted to the correct charge. The PMP then subtracts the amount due from the account. Often an amount less than that which is due is accepted as payment in full, and the uncollected difference will be written off, as explained in the next section.

THINKING IT THROUGH 13.5

1. Patient statements may be prepared using a spreadsheet format. The AMT DUE column is a running total; that is, the charge for each service line is added to the previous AMT DUE figure. The total due on the statement can be cross-checked by comparing the AMT DUE in the last box with the total of all CHARGES. These amounts should be the same. For example:

SERVICE DATE	PT NAME	PROC CODE	DIAG. CODE	SERVICE DESCRIPTION	CHARGES	INS. PAID	ADJ.	PT PAID	AMT DUE
10/14/2016	Lund, Alan.	99384	Z02.89	NP preventive visit	182.00	-0-	-0-	-0-	182.00
		81001		UA	10.00	-0-	-0-	-0-	192.00
					192.00				**192.00**

A. If for the 10/14/2016 charges, the patient made a payment of $50 and the third-party payer paid $20, what balance would be due?

B. What balance would be due if the patient and payer made these payments but the previous statement showed a $235 balance?

▶13.6 Writing Off Uncollectible Accounts

uncollectible account Money that cannot be collected and must be written off.

After the practice has exhausted all of its collection efforts and a patient's balance is still unpaid, the account may be labeled as an **uncollectible account,** also known as a write-off account. Uncollectible accounts are those with unpaid balances that the practice does not expect to be able to collect and that are not worth the time and cost to pursue. Also, accounts over a year old have little chance of collection.

The practice must determine which debts to write off in the practice management program and whether to continue to treat the patients. Practice management programs can be set to automatically write off small balances, such as less than $5.00. After an account is determined to be uncollectible, it is removed from the practice's expected accounts receivable and classified as **bad debt.**

bad debt Account deemed uncollectible.

Common Types

The most common reason an account becomes uncollectible is that a patient cannot pay the bill. Under federal and state laws, there are means tests that help a practice decide whether patients are indigent. The patient completes a form that is used to evaluate ability to pay. A combination of factors, such as income level (verified by recent federal tax returns) as compared to the federal poverty level, other expenses, and the practice's policies, are used to determine what percentage of the bill will be forgiven and written off.

Another reason that an account is uncollectible is that the patient cannot be located, so the account must be written off. Accounts of patients who have died are often marked as uncollectible. Large unpaid balances of deceased patients may be pursued by filing an estate claim or by working—considerately—with the deceased patient's family members.

Another reason for a write-off is a patient's bankruptcy. Debtors may choose to file for bankruptcy when they determine that they will not be able to repay the money they owe. When a patient files for bankruptcy, the practice, which is considered to be an unsecured creditor, must file a claim in order to join the group of creditors that may receive some compensation for unpaid bills. Claims must be filed by the date specified by the bankruptcy court so as not to forfeit the right to any money.

Practices only rarely sue individuals to collect money they are owed. Usually, unpaid balances are deemed uncollectible to avoid going through the expense of a court case with uncertain results.

Avoiding Fraudulently Writing Off Accounts

Practices must follow strict guidelines and the established office policy for write-offs. Both Medicare and Medicaid require a practice to follow a specific series of steps before an account can be written off. Writing off some accounts and not others could be considered fraud if there are discrepancies between charges for the same services.

Exercise 13.3 Write Off an Uncollectable Account

Small or uncollectible account balances are often written off. Follow the instructions to clear the small balance from Orchard Hill Medical Center's accounts receivable.

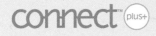

Follow the steps at www.mhhe.com/newbycarr to complete the exercise at connect.mcgraw-hill.com on your own once you have watched the demo and tried the steps with prompts in practice mode. Use the information provided in the scenario to complete the exercise.

THINKING IT THROUGH 13.6

1. The following patient bill has been in collections and is going to be written off:

DATE	CODE	DESCRIPTION	CHARGES	CREDITS
09/10/16	99396	Prev Check up, Est. 40–64 Yr	169.00	
09/10/16	85018	Hemoglobin Count, Colorimetric	6.10	
09/10/16	81002	Urinalysis, Non-automated, w/o s	4.20	
09/11/16		Golden Rule Ins. Co. #31478 Filed		
10/17/16		Denied Golden Rule Ins. Co. #31478		00.00
10/17/16		Repriced Golden Rule Ins. Co. #31478		51.80—
10/17/16		$127.50 = deductible for 9/10/16 visit		

CURRENT	30–60	60–90	>90	TOTAL	INS PENDING	TOTAL DUE FROM PT
0.00	0.00	0.00	127.50	127.50	0.00	127.50

A. What amount has previously been written off as an adjustment due to the payer's allowed charge?

B. What amount must now be deemed bad debt?

13.7 Terminating the Provider–Patient Relationship

A physician has the right to terminate the provider–patient relationship for any reason under the regulations of each state. The doctor also has the right to be paid for care provided. The physician may decide to dismiss a patient who does not pay medical bills. If the patient is to be dismissed, this action should be documented in a letter to the patient that:

▶ Offers to continue care for a specific period of time after the date of the dismissal letter, so that the patient is never endangered.

▶ Provides suggestions of services that provide referrals to other physicians and offers to send copies of the medical record.

▶ Does not state a specific reason for the dismissal; the letter must be tactful and carefully worded.

The letter should be signed by the physician and mailed certified, return receipt requested, so there will be proof that the patient received it.

BILLING TIP

Locating State Regulations

Each state's insurance commission has regulations on handling terminating the provider's relationship with the patient that must be observed.

THINKING IT THROUGH 13.7

1. Generally speaking, is it sufficient for a physician to inform a patient face-to-face that he is ending the provider–patient relationship?

Chapter Summary

Learning Outcomes	Key Concepts/Examples
13.1 Outline the steps of claim adjudication, explaining the effect of upcoding and downcoding on the process. Pages 257–259	The adjudication process is made up of 5 steps: • Initial processing • Automated review • Manual review • Determination • Payment Upcoding by the practice may lead to requests for additional documentation and delay payment. Downcoding by the payer may result when the coding or medical necessity are called into question, reducing the payment.
13.2 Process RAs. Pages 260–263	• The unique claim control number reported on the RA is used to match up claims sent and payments received. • Then basic data are checked against the claim, billed procedures are verified, the payment for each CPT is checked against the expected amount, adjustment codes are reviewed to locate all unpaid, downcoded, or denied claims, and items are identified for follow up.
13.3 Discuss the purpose and general steps of the appeal process. Pages 263–264	• An appeal process is used to challenge a payer's decision to deny, reduce, or otherwise downcode a claim. • Each payer has a graduated level of appeals, deadlines for requesting them, and medical review programs to answer them. • In some cases, appeals may be taken beyond the payer to an outside authority, such as a state insurance commission.
13.4 Describe the purpose and content of patient statements. Pages 264–269	• Updated patient ledgers reflecting all charges, adjustments, and previous payments to patients' accounts are used to generate patient statements, printed bills that show the amount each patient owes. • Patients may owe coinsurance, deductibles, and fees for noncovered services. • Statements are designed to be direct and easy to read, clearly stating the services provided, balances owed, due dates, and accepted methods of payment.
13.5 Apply regulations and guidelines to the collection process. Pages 269–271	• Collections from patients are regulated by federal and state laws. • The Fair Debt Collection Act (FDCPA) of 1977 is such a law.
13.6 Explain the procedures for writing off uncollectible accounts. Pages 272–273	• The practice reviews unpaid balances to determine which accounts are uncollectible. • Practice management programs can be set to automatically write off small balances. • Balances can be forgiven and a percentage of a bill can be written off if patients' financial status classifies them as indigent based upon federal and state laws. • Account balances can be written off if a patient dies, files for bankruptcy, or can't be located. • Practices must follow strict guidelines and use caution when writing off account balances to avoid activity that could be considered fraudulent.
13.7 Describe the physician's responsibilities when terminating the provider–patient relationship. Page 273	• To inform the patient tactfully in a carefully worded letter of the dismissal. • To continue care for a specified period of time after the date of dismissal. • To suggest services that the patient could use that would provide a referral to another physician.

Using Terminology

Match the key terms in the left column with the definitions in the right column.

_____ 1. **[LO 13.6]** Uncollectible account

_____ 2. **[LO 13.5]** Fair Debt Collection Practices Act (FDCPA) of 1977

_____ 3. **[LO 13.2]** Electronic funds transfer (EFT)

_____ 4. **[LO 13.5]** Patient aging report

_____ 5. **[LO 13.1]** Adjudication

_____ 6. **[LO 13.4]** Cycle billing

_____ 7. **[LO 13.2]** Autoposting

_____ 8. **[LO 13.2]** Overpayment

_____ 9. **[LO 13.1]** Insurance aging report

_____ 10. **[LO 13.3]** Appeal

A. Process followed by health plans to determine claim payment.

B. Software feature enabling automatic entry of payments on an RA.

C. Request sent to a payer for reconsideration of a claim.

D. A banking service for directly transmitting funds from one bank to another.

E. Law that regulates collection practices.

F. Analysis of how long a payer has held submitted claims.

G. Assigns patient accounts to a specific time of the month and standardizes the times when statements will be mailed and payments will be due.

H. Improper or excessive payments resulting from billing errors for which the provider owes refunds.

I. Shows which patients are overdue on their bills and groups them into distinct categories for efficient collection efforts.

J. Patient balance that the practice has not collected and does not expect to be able to collect.

Checking Your Understanding

Write the letter of the choice that best completes the statement or answers the question.

1. **[LO 13.1]** A payer's initial processing of claims screens for _____.
   A. Utilization guidelines
   B. Medical edits
   C. Basic errors in claim data or missing information
   D. Claims attachments

2. **[LO 13.1]** A claim may be downcoded because _____.
   A. The claim does not list a charge for every procedure
   B. The claim is for noncovered services
   C. The documentation does not justify the level of service
   D. The procedure code applies to a patient of the other gender

3. **[LO 13.1]** Payers should comply with the required _____.
   A. Insurance aging report
   B. Claim turnaround time
   C. Remittance advice
   D. Retention schedule

4. **[LO 13.2]** If a postpayment audit determines that a paid claim should have been denied or reduced, _____.
   A. The provider is subject to civil penalties
   B. The provider must refund the incorrect payment
   C. The provider bills the patient for the denied claim
   D. The provider does not need to take any action

connect (plus+)
Enhance your learning at mcgrawhillconnect.com!
• Practice Exercises   • Worksheets
• Activities   • Integrated eBook

5. **[LO 13.4]** The day sheet produced by the practice management program shows _____.
   A. What each patient owes the practice as of that date
   B. What each payer owes the practice as of that date
   C. The payment and charges that occurred on that date
   D. The overdue accounts on that date

6. **[LO 13.5]** Collection calls are regulated by the guidelines set by _____.
   A. FCRA
   B. FACTA
   C. HIPAA
   D. FDCPA

7. **[LO 13.6]** Accounts might be considered uncollectible when a patient _____.
   A. Files for bankruptcy
   B. Directs phone calls to an attorney
   C. Needs a payment plan
   D. Has not responded to the first bill

8. **[LO 13.5]** The patient aging report is used to _____.
   A. Enter payments in the patient billing system
   B. Enter write-offs to a patient's account
   C. Track overdue claims from payers
   D. Collect overdue accounts from patients

9. **[LO 13.6]** Bad debt is defined as
   A. Payer refunds
   B. Patient refunds
   C. Uncollectible A/R
   D. Collectible A/R

10. **[LO 13.7]** What must occur for a physician to cancel a provider–patient relationship? _____
   A. The patient must be past due on his medical bills.
   B. The patient must be proven to have not followed the physician's treatment instructions.
   C. The physician must be able to legally prove that she is no long er capable of providing health care services to the patient.
   D. The physician may cancel the provider–patient relationship for any reason under state regulations.

Applying Your Knowledge

[LO 13.2]   Case 13.1

Determine the amount due from the patient of a PAR physician based on the following information from the RA/EOB, explaining your reasoning.

Charges:	$25.00
Disallowed:	$ 3.42
Allowed Charge:	$21.58
Deductible:	0
Coinsurance:	$10.00
Amount Due from Carrier:	$11.58
Additional Amount Due from Patient: $ _____	

HOSPITAL INSURANCE

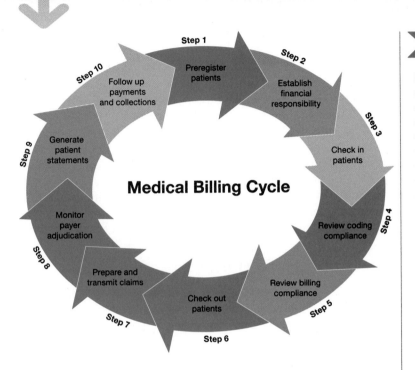

Medical Billing Cycle

Step 1 Preregister patients
Step 2 Establish financial responsibility
Step 3 Check in patients
Step 4 Review coding compliance
Step 5 Review billing compliance
Step 6 Check out patients
Step 7 Prepare and transmit claims
Step 8 Monitor payer adjudication
Step 9 Generate patient statements
Step 10 Follow up payments and collections

Learning Outcomes

After studying this chapter, you should be able to:

14.1 Compare inpatient and outpatient hospital services.

14.2 List the major steps relating to the hospital billing cycle.

14.3 Contrast coding diagnoses and procedures for hospital inpatient cases and physician office services.

14.4 Compare the Medicare Inpatient and Outpatient Payment Systems.

14.5 Prepare an accurate UB-04 claim.

Although this text focuses on billing and reimbursement in medical practices, medical assistants should be aware of the coding systems and billing cycle used in hospitals. There are many financial agreements between physicians and hospitals; for example, physicians in practices may have staff privileges at hospitals. Medical office staff members also must bill for the procedures physicians perform in the hospital environment. It is important to distinguish between hospital and physician services for accurate billing.

14.1 Health Care Facilities: Inpatient versus Outpatient

Inpatient Care

inpatient Person admitted for services that require an overnight stay.

Inpatient facilities are equipped for patients to stay overnight. In addition to hospital admission, inpatient care may be provided in:

▶ *Skilled Nursing Facilities (SNF)*—Facilities that provide skilled nursing or rehabilitation services to help with recovery after a hospital stay. Skilled nursing care includes care given by licensed nurses under the direction of a physician, such as intravenous injections, tube feeding, and changing sterile dressings on a wound.
▶ *Long-Term Care Facilities*—This term describes facilities such as nursing homes that provide care for patients with chronic disabilities and prolonged illnesses.
▶ *Hospital Emergency Rooms or Departments*—*Emergency care* involves a situation in which a delay in the treatment of the patient would lead to a significant increase in the threat to life or a body part. Emergency care differs from urgently needed care, in which the condition must be treated right away but is not life-threatening.

Outpatient or Ambulatory Care

Within the hospital environment, emergency rooms (ERs) or departments (EDs) are the most familiar type of outpatient service. *Emergency care* involves a situation in which a delay in treatment would lead to a significant increase in the threat to a patient's life or body part. (Emergency care differs from urgently needed care, in which the condition must be treated right away but is not life-threatening.) Patients treated in an emergency room are either discharged or admitted as inpatients to the hospital after treatment or observation.

ambulatory care Outpatient care.

Many hospitals have expanded beyond inpatient and ER services to offer a variety of outpatient services. Outpatient care, often called **ambulatory care,** covers all types of health services that do not require an overnight hospital stay. Most hospitals, for example, have outpatient departments that provide same-day surgery.

Different types of outpatient services are also provided in patients' home settings. Home health care services include care given at home, such as physical therapy or skilled nursing care. Home health care is provided by a home health agency (HHA), an organization that provides home care services, including skilled nursing, physical therapy, occupational therapy, speech therapy, and care by home health aides. At-home recovery care is a different category; it includes help with the activities of daily living (ADLs), such as bathing and eating. Hospice care is a special approach to caring for people with terminal illnesses—that is, people who are not expected to live longer than six months—in a familiar and comfortable place, either a special hospice facility or the patient's home.

THINKING IT THROUGH 14.1

1. When a patient of the practice is admitted to the hospital, and the admitting physician first visits the patient there, what CPT code range is used to report that service? What code range is used for subsequent hospital care by this physician? Would the hospital use these same codes?

14.2 Hospital Billing Cycle

Hospitals generally have large departments that are responsible for major business functions. The admissions department records the patient's personal and financial information. As in medical offices, hospital admissions staff must be sure patients give written consent for the work to be done and for the claim reporting that follows. The patient accounting department handles billing, and there is often a separate collections department. Organizing and maintaining patient medical records in hospitals are the duties of the *health information management (HIM)* department. Hospitals are also structured into departments for patient care. For example, there are professional services departments, such as laboratory, radiology, and surgery, as well as support services departments, such as food service and housekeeping.

From the insurance perspective, the three major steps in a patient's hospital stay are:

1. Admission, for creating or updating the patient's medical record, verifying patient insurance coverage, securing consent for release of information to payers, and collecting advance payments as appropriate.
2. Treatment, during which the various departments' services are provided and charges generated.
3. Discharge from the hospital or transfer to another facility, at which point the patient's record is compiled, claims or bills are created, and payment is followed up on.

Admission

Patients are admitted to hospitals in a process called **registration.** Like physician practices, hospitals must keep clear, accurate records of their patients' diagnoses and treatments. The record begins at a patient's first admission to the facility. More information is gathered for a hospital admission than is required for a visit to a physician practice. Special points about the patient's care, such as language requirements, religion, or disabilities, are also entered in the record.

The HIM department keeps a health record system that permits storage and retrieval of clinical information by patient name or number, by **attending physician** (the physician who is primarily responsible for the care of the patient during the hospital stay), and by diagnosis and procedure. At almost every facility, a part or all of the records are stored in a computer system. Each patient is listed in a patient register under a unique number. These numbers make up the **master patient index (MPI)**—the main database that identifies patients.

Outpatient department and emergency room insurance claims are often delayed because it is difficult to verify insurance coverage in these settings. The emergency department has its own registration system because people who come for emergency and urgent treatment must receive care immediately. Both outpatient and emergency room procedures must be established so as to collect the maximum amount of information available at that time. Many admissions departments as well as emergency departments join online insurance verification systems so that payers can be contacted during the registration process and verification can be received in seconds.

Records of Treatments and Charges During the Hospital Stay

The patient's hospital medical record contains (1) notes of the attending physician and of other treating physicians; (2) ancillary documents like nurses' notes, medication administration records, and pathology, radiology, and laboratory reports; (3) patient data, including insurance information for patients who have been in the hospital before; and (4) a correspondence section that contains signed consent forms

COMPLIANCE GUIDELINE

Notice of Privacy Practices

Under the HIPAA Privacy Rule, hospitals must give patients a copy of their privacy practices at registration and ask them to sign an acknowledgment that they have received this notice. Patients have many privacy rights, such as choosing whether they wish their names to appear in the hospital's registry.

registration Process of gathering information about a patient during admission to a hospital.

attending physician Clinician primarily responsible for a patient's care from the beginning of a hospitalization.

master patient index (MPI) Hospital's main patient database.

and other documents. In line with HIPAA security requirements, the confidentiality and security of patients' medical records are guarded by all hospital staff members. Both technical means, such as passwords and encryption, and legal protections, such as requiring staff members to sign confidentiality pledges, are used to ensure privacy.

Inpatients are usually charged by hospitals for the following services (the *technical component* of procedures):

▶ Room and board.
▶ Medications.
▶ Ancillary tests and procedures, such as laboratory workups.
▶ Equipment used during surgery or therapy.
▶ The amount of time spent in an operating room, recovery room, or intensive care unit.

Patients are charged according to the type of accommodations and services they receive. For example, the rate for a private room is higher than for a semiprivate room, and intensive care unit or recovery room charges are higher than charges for standard rooms. When patients are transferred to these various services, this activity is tracked. In an outpatient or an emergency department encounter, there is no room and board charge; instead, there is a visit charge.

Discharge and Billing

By the time patients are discharged from the hospital, their accounts have usually been totaled and insurance claims or bills created. The goal in most cases is to file a claim or bill within seven days after discharge. The items to be billed are recorded on the hospital's charge description master file, usually called the **charge master** or **charge ticket,** which is similar to a computerized medical office encounter form but with many more entries. This master list contains the following information for each billable item:

▶ The hospital's code for the service and a brief description of it.
▶ The charge for the service.
▶ The hospital department (such as laboratory).
▶ The hospital's cost to provide the service.
▶ A procedure code for the service.

The hospital's computer system tracks the patient's services. For example, if the patient is sent to the intensive care unit after surgery, the intensive care department's billing group reports the specific items performed for the patient, and these charges are entered on the patient's account.

THINKING IT THROUGH 14.2

1. What are some of the differences between working for a hospital facility and for a physician practice? Which employment setting is more likely to have specialized job functions?

14.3 Inpatient (Hospital) Coding

The HIM department is also responsible for diagnostic and procedural coding of the patients' medical records, based on the discharge summary signed by the attending physician. Coding is done by inpatient medical coders as soon as the patient is discharged. Some inpatient coders are generalists; others may have special skills in a certain area, like surgical coding or Medicare. ICD-10-CM is used to code inpatient diagnoses, as of October 1, 2014 (dates of discharge earlier than this use

ICD-9-CM), and **ICD-10-PCS** (procedural coding system) Volume 3 is used to code procedures performed during hospitalization.

Hospital Diagnostic Coding

Different rules apply for assigning inpatient codes than for physician office diagnoses. The rules are extensive; three of them are described briefly below to illustrate some of the major differences in inpatient versus outpatient coding.

Rule 1—Principal Diagnosis

For ICD-10-CM diagnostic coding in medical practices, the first code listed is the primary diagnosis, defined as the main reason for the patient's encounter with the provider. Under hospital inpatient rules, the **principal diagnosis (PDX)** is listed first. The principal diagnosis is the condition established *after study* to be chiefly responsible for the admission. This diagnosis is listed even if the patient has other, more severe diagnoses. In some cases, the **admitting diagnosis (ADX)**—the condition identified by the physician at admission to the hospital—is also reported.

Rule 2—Suspected or Unconfirmed Diagnoses

When the patient is admitted for workups to uncover the cause of a problem, inpatient medical coders can also use a suspected or unconfirmed condition (rule out) if it is listed as the admitting diagnosis. The admitting diagnosis may not match the principal diagnosis once a final determination is made.

Rule 3—Comorbidities and Complications

The inpatient coder also lists all the other conditions that have an effect on the patient's hospital stay or course of treatment. Other conditions at admission that affect care during the hospitalization are called **comorbidities,** meaning coexisting conditions. Conditions that develop as complications of surgery or other treatments are coded as **complications.**

Comorbidities and complications are shown in the patient medical record with the initials *CC.* Coding CCs is important because their presence may increase the hospital's reimbursement level for the care. The hospital insurance claim form discussed later in this chapter allows for up to 18 additional conditions to be reported.

CMS has also put into place the requirement for a **present on admission (POA)** indicator for every reported diagnosis code for a patient upon discharge. *Present on admission* means that a condition existed at the time the order for inpatient admission occurs. This requirement is based on a federal mandate to Medicare to stop paying for conditions that hospitals cause or allow to develop during inpatient stays. Such conditions are now referred to as "never events," meaning that payers will not ever pay for them. Medicare will not assign an inpatient hospital discharge to a higher-paying category if a selected hospital-acquired condition was not POA. The case will be paid as though the secondary diagnosis was not present.

Hospital Procedural Coding

In inpatient coding, ICD-10-PCS is used to assign procedure codes. Reporting the correct ICD-10-PCS codes when appropriately documented may increase the hospital's reimbursement level for a patient's care because some procedures require more hospital time for recovery.

ICD-10-PCS has a multiaxial code structure. This term means that a table format is used to present options for building a code. An axis is a column or row in a table; columns are vertical, while rows are horizontal. The coder picks the correct values from one of the rows in a table to build a seven-character code for each procedure. This approach provides a unique code for every substantially different procedure and allows new procedures to be easily incorporated as new codes. A finished code looks like this: 02103D4.

The code set is contained both online and in a printed reference. It is updated annually. The Code Tables, the main part of the code set, begin with an index to assist in locating common procedures. Then procedures are divided into 16 sections that identify the general type of procedure, such as medical and surgical, obstetrics, or imaging.

The **principal procedure** assigned by the inpatient medical coder is the procedure that is most closely related to the treatment of the principal diagnosis. It is usually a surgical procedure. If no surgery is performed, the principal procedure may be a therapeutic procedure.

principal procedure Procedure most closely related to treatment of the principal diagnosis.

THINKING IT THROUGH 14.3

1. A patient is admitted for gastrointestinal bleeding due to diverticulitis. The initial treatment plan is for the patient to undergo a sigmoid resection, but the patient decides to postpone the surgery for personal reasons.

   A. What is the principal diagnosis in this case?

   B. What kind of additional diagnosis code is reported to show that the patient decided not to proceed?

14.4 Payers and Payment Methods

Medicare and Medicaid both provide coverage for eligible patients' hospital services. Medicare Part A, known as hospital insurance, helps pay for inpatient hospital care, skilled nursing facilities (SNF), hospice care, and home health care. Private payers also offer hospitalization insurance. Most employees have coverage for hospital services through employers' programs.

Medicare Inpatient Payment System

DRGs

diagnosis-related groups (DRGs) System of analyzing conditions and treatments for similar groups of patients.

Medicare's actions to control the cost of hospital services began in 1983 with **diagnosis-related groups (DRGs).** Under the DRG classification system, the hospital stays of patients who had similar diagnoses were studied. Groupings were created based on the relative value of the resources that physicians and hospitals nationally used for patients with similar conditions. The calculations combine data about the patient's diagnosis and procedures with factors that affect the outcome of treatment, such as age, gender, comorbidities, and complications. At the same time the DRG system was created, Medicare changed the way hospitals were paid. Payment changed from a fee-for-service approach to the Medicare **Inpatient Prospective Payment System (IPPS).** In the IPPS, the payment for each type of service is set ahead of time based on the DRG.

Inpatient Prospective Payment System (IPPS) Medicare payment system for hospital services.

When DRGs were established, Medicare also set up Peer Review Organizations (PROs), which were later renamed Quality Improvement Organizations (QIOs). Made up of practicing physicians and other health care experts, these organizations are contracted by CMS in each state to review Medicare and Medicaid claims for the appropriateness of hospitalization and clinical care. QIOs aim to ensure that payment is made only for medically necessary services. QIOs are also resources for investigating patients' complaints regarding the quality of care at a given facility or through a managed care plan.

MS-DRGs

In 2008 Medicare adopted a new type of DRG called **Medicare-Severity DRGs (MS-DRGs)** to better reflect the different severity of illness among patients who have the same basic diagnosis. The system recognizes the higher cost of treating patients with more complex conditions. Hospital admissions are grouped according to their expected use of hospital resources. The groups are based on:

▶ Principal diagnosis
▶ Surgical procedure(s)
▶ Age
▶ Sex
▶ Complications
▶ Comorbidities
▶ Signs and symptoms (if the diagnosis is not yet known)
▶ Discharge disposition (routine, transferred, deceased)

Medicare Outpatient Payment System

The use of DRGs under an IPPS system proved to be very effective in controlling costs. In 2000, this approach was implemented for outpatient hospital services, which previously were paid on a fee-for-service basis. For example, the Hospital **Outpatient Prospective Payment System (OPPS)** is used to pay for hospital outpatient services. In place of DRGs, patients are grouped under an ambulatory patient classification (APC) system. Reimbursement is made according to preset amounts based on the value of each APC.

Private Insurance Companies

Because of the expense involved with hospitalization, private payers encourage providers to minimize the number of days patients stay in the hospital. Most private payers establish the standard number of days allowed for various conditions and compare this number to the patient's actual stay. Many private payers have also adopted the DRG method of setting prospective payments for hospital services. Hospitals and the payers, which may include Blue Cross and Blue Shield or other managed care plans, negotiate the rates for each DRG.

THINKING IT THROUGH 14.4

1. What is the purpose of a QIO?

14.5 Claims and Follow-Up

Hospitals must submit claims for Medicare Part A reimbursement to Medicare fiscal intermediaries using the HIPAA health care claim called **837I.** This electronic data interchange (EDI) format, similar to the 837 claim, is called I for Institutional; the physicians' claim is called 837P (Professional). In some situations, a paper claim form called the **UB-04** (uniform billing 2004), also known as the **CMS-1450,** is also accepted. The UB-04 is maintained by the National Uniform Billing Committee. This form was previously called the UB-92.

837I Health Care Claim Completion

The 837I, like the 837P, has sections requiring data elements for the billing and the pay-to provider, the subscriber and patient, and the payer, plus claim and service level details. Most of the data elements report the same information as summarized in Table 14.1 for the paper claim.

Table 14.1 UB-04 Form Completion

Form Locator	Description	Medicare Required?
1 (Unlabeled Field) (Provider Name, Address, and Telephone Number)	The name, address (service location), and telephone number of the provider submitting the bill.	Yes
2 (Unlabeled Field) (Pay-to Name and Address)	To be used only if the provider would like payments mailed to a different address from that listed in FL 1; for example, a central processing office or a PO box.	Situational
3a Patient Control Number	Patient's unique number assigned by the facility and used to locate the patient's financial record. For example, the patient control number is used to identify payments on RAs.	Yes
3b Medical Record Number	Number assigned by the facility to the patient's medical record and used to locate the patient's treatment history.	Yes
4 Type of Bill	Four-digit alphanumeric code: First digit is a leading 0 (*Note:* The leading 0 is not included on electronic claims.) Second digit identifies the facility type (e.g., 1 = hospital, 2 = SNF). Third digit identifies the care type (e.g., 1 = inpatient Part A, 2 = inpatient Part B, 3 = outpatient). Fourth digit identifies the billing sequence in this episode of care (e.g., 1 = this bill encompasses entire inpatient confinement or course of outpatient treatment for which provider expects payment from the payer; 2 = this bill is the first bill in an expected series of bills).	Yes
5 Federal Tax Number	Also known as the TIN or EIN; a ten-digit alphanumeric number (XX-XXXXXXXX) reported in the bottom line of FL 5. (*Note:* The hyphen in the number is not used on electronic claims.) The top line of FL 5 may be used as necessary to report a federal tax sub-ID for an affiliated subsidiary of the hospital, such as a hospital psychiatric pavilion.	Yes
6 Statement Covers Period (From–Through)	The beginning and ending dates (MMDDYY) of the period included on the bill; dates before patient's entitlement are not shown. From date is used to determine timely filing.	Yes
7 (Unlabeled Field)	Reserved for national assignment.	
8a Patient Identifier	May be used if the patient and the insured are not the same; the patient identifier is the number assigned to the patient by the patient's insurance carrier (this number would be different from the Insured's Unique Identifier in FL 60).	Situational
8b Patient Name	Patient's last name, first name, and middle initial. A comma (or space) is used to separate last and first names on the paper claim.	Yes
9 a, b, c, d, e Patient's Address	Patient's full mailing address: (a) street number and name, PO Box or RFD; (b) city; (c) state; (d) ZIP Code; and (e) country code (if other than USA).	Yes
10 Patient Birth Date	Patient's birth date (MMDDYYYY); for paper claims, if birth date is unavailable, report eight zeroes.	Yes
11 Patient Sex	For Medicare claims, report M for male; F for female. Other payers may also accept U for Unknown.	Yes
12 Admission, Start of Care Date	Date of admission for inpatient care, or start of care date for home health services (MMDDYY).	Yes
13 Admission Hour	The hour during which the patient was admitted for inpatient care. A two-digit hour code, based on military time, is used to indicate hour (e.g., 3:15 a.m. = 03; 1:40 p.m. = 13).	No

Table 14.1 UB-04 Form Completion *(continued)*

Form Locator	Description	Medicare Required?
14 Type of Admission/Visit	Required for inpatient bills: 1 = emergency 2 = urgent 3 = elective 4 = newborn 5 = trauma 9 = information not available (rarely used)	Yes
15 Point of Origin for Admission or Visit	Point of origin for IP admission or OP visit: 1 = non-health care facility (e.g., home, a physician's office, or workplace) 2 = clinic 3 = reserved 4 = transfer from a hospital (different facility) 5 = transfer from an SNF or ICF 6 = transfer from another health care facility 7 = emergency room 8 = court/law enforcement 9 = information not available A = reserved B = transfer from another home health agency C = readmission to same home health agency D = transfer from one distinct unit of the hospital to another distinct unit of the same hospital resulting in a separate claim to the payer E = transfer from ambulatory surgery center F = transfer from hospice and is under a hospice plan of care or enrolled in a hospice program G-Z = reserved Code structure for newborns 1-4 = reserved 5 = born inside this hospital 6 = born outside of this hospital 7-9 = reserved	Yes
16 Discharge Hour	Code indicating the hour patient was discharged from inpatient care. Hour codes are based on military time (see FL 13, Admission Hour).	No
17 Patient Discharge Status	For Part A inpatient, SNF, hospice, home health, and outpatient hospital services: 01 = discharge to home or self-care (routine discharge) 02 = discharge to another short-term general hospital 03 = discharge to SNF 04 = discharge to ICF 05 = discharge to a designated cancer center or children's hospital 06 = discharge to home under care of a home health service organization 07 = left against medical advice or discontinued care 09 = admitted as inpatient (after outpatient services) 20 = expired 30 = still patient or expected to return for outpatient services 40 = expired at home (hospice claims only) 41 = expired in a medical facility (hospice claims only) 42 = expired, place unknown (hospice claims only) 50 = hospice—home 51 = hospice—medical facility 70 = discharge to another type of health care institution not defined elsewhere in this code list	Yes

(continued)

Table 14.1 UB-04 Form Completion *(continued)*

Form Locator	Description	Medicare Required?
18–28 Condition Codes	Codes relating to bill that affect processing; examples include: 02 = condition is employment-related 04 = information only bill 05 = lien has been filed 06 = ESRD-patient in first eighteen months of entitlement covered by employer group health insurance 07 = treatment of nonterminal condition for hospice patient 08 = beneficiary would not provide information concerning other insurance coverage 09 = neither patient nor spouse is employed 10 = patient and/or spouse employed, but no employer group health plan coverage exists 31 = patient is student (full-time, day) 40 = same day transfer 50 = product replacement for known recall of a product 67 = beneficiary elects not to use lifetime reserve days A9 = second opinion surgery C3 = partial approval (after review by the QIO or intermediary)	Situational
29 Accident State	State where an accident occurred on claims containing services related to an auto accident; two-digit state abbreviation is reported.	No
30 (Unlabeled Field)	Reserved for national assignment.	
31–34 Occurrence Codes and Dates	Codes and date data (MMDDYY) relating to bill that affect processing; examples include: 01 = accident/medical coverage 04 = accident/employment related 05 = accident/no medical or liability coverage 11 = onset of symptoms/illness 17 = date occupational therapy plan established or reviewed 18 = date of patient/beneficiary retirement 19 = date of spouse retirement 21 = utilization notice received 24 = date insurance denied by primary payer 25 = date benefits terminated by primary payer 31 = date beneficiary notified of intent to bill for inpatient care accommodations 32 = date beneficiary notified of intent to bill for Medicare medically unnecessary procedures or treatments 45 = date treatment started for speech therapy A1 = birthdate—insured A A2 = effective date—insured A policy A3 = benefits for insured A exhausted A4 = split bill date (date patient became Medicaid-eligible)	Situational
35, 36 Occurrence Span Codes and Dates	Codes and beginning/ending dates (MMDDYY) for specific events relating to the billing period that affect processing, such as: 72 = first/last visit dates (actual dates of first and last visits in this billing period when different from FL 6, Statement Covers Period) 77 = provider liability period (from and through dates of a period of noncovered care for which provider is liable; utilization is charged)	Situational

Table 14.1 UB-04 Form Completion *(continued)*

Form Locator	Description	Medicare Required?
37 (Unlabeled Field)	Reserved for national assignment.	
38 (Unlabeled Field) (Responsible Party Name and Address)	May be used on commercial claims if a window envelope is used for mailing the claim. For Medicare as secondary payer, the address of the primary payer may be shown here.	No
39, 40, 41 Value Codes and Amounts	Codes and related dollar amounts required to process the claim; examples include: 08 = Medicare lifetime reserve amount for first calendar year in billing period 09 = Medicare coinsurance amount for first calendar year in billing period 14 = no-fault, including auto/other, when primary payer payments are being applied to covered Medicare charges on this bill 31 = patient liability amount; the amount approved by hospital or the QIO to charge the beneficiary for noncovered services 50 = physical therapy visits; number of visits provided from onset of treatment through this billing period 80 = number of days covered by the primary payer (as qualified by the payer) (*Note:* For paper claims only.) 81 = number of days not covered by the primary payer (*Note:* For paper claims only.) A1, B1, C1 = amounts assumed by provider to be applied to the patient's deductible amount for payer A, B, or C (*Note:* For paper claims only.) A2, B2, C2 = amounts assumed by provider to be applied to the patient's coinsurance amount involving payer A, B, or C (*Note:* For paper claims only.) A3, B3, C3 = amount estimated by provider to be paid by payer A, B, or C D3 = amount estimated by the provider to be paid by the indicated patient	Situational
42 (lines 1-23) Revenue Code	Lines 1-22: For reporting the appropriate four-digit code(s) to identify a specific-accommodation and/or ancillary service. The corresponding narrative description is reported next to the code in FL 43 (Revenue Description). Up to 22 codes (lines 1-22) can be listed on each page. Line 23: On paper claims, code 0001 (total charges) is placed before the total charge amount and reported on line 23 of the final claim page.	Yes
43 (lines 1-22) Revenue Description	Line 1-22: Narrative description for each revenue code used in FL42. (*Note:* Not used on electronic claims.) Line 23: Incrementing page count and total number of pages (Page __ of __) is reporting on line 23 on each page.	No
44 (lines 1-22) HCPCS/ (Accommodation) Rates/HIPPS Rate Codes	HCPCS codes for applicable procedures (ancillary and outpatient services); accommodation rates for inpatient bills; or HIPPS rate codes for determining payment for service line item under certain prospective payment systems.	Yes
45 (lines 1-23) Service Date	Lines 1-22: For outpatient claims, the date (MMDDYY) the outpatient service was provided. A single line item date is required for every revenue code. Line 23: The creation date is required in line 23 of this field for all pages of the claim.	Yes
46 (lines 1-22) Service Units	Number of units for each applicable service provided, such as number of accommodation days, pints of blood, or number of lab tests.	Yes
47 (lines 1-23) Total Charges	Lines 1-22: Total line item charges. Line 23: On paper claims, the sum total of charges for the billing period is reported in line 23 on final page of bill, using revenue code 0001.	Yes
48 (lines 1-23) Noncovered Charges	Lines 1-22: Total of noncovered charges of those listed in FL 42. Line 23: On paper claims, the sum total of noncovered charges is reported in line 23 on final page of bill, using revenue code 0001.	Yes

(continued)

Table 14.1 UB-04 Form Completion *(continued)*

Form Locator	Description	Medicare Required?
49 (Unlabeled Field)	Reserved for national assignment.	
50 (lines A, B, C) Payer Name (payers A, B, C)	The name of the payer organization from which the provider is expecting payment; lines A, B, and C are used to report the primary, secondary, and tertiary payer. Information in FLs 51-55 on the same line all pertains to this payer. If Medicare is primary payer, Medicare is entered on line A. If Medicare is secondary or tertiary payer, the primary payer is entered on line A, and Medicare information on lines B or C.	Yes
51 (lines A, B, C) Health Plan Identification Number (payers A, B, C)	For reporting the HIPAA national health plan identifier when one is established; otherwise, the provider's six-digit Medicare-assigned number, or legacy number assigned by other payer, is entered on the line corresponding to payer A in FL 50. If other payers are involved, their ID numbers are reported in lines B and C.	Yes
52 (lines A, B, C) Release of Information Certification Indicator (payers A, B, C)	A code indicating whether the provider has obtained release of information authorization from the patient. Codes include: Y = provider has on file a signed statement permitting data release to other organizations in order to adjudicate the claim. *(Note:* The back of the UB-04 contains this certification.) I = provider has informed consent to release medical information for conditions or diagnoses regulated by federal statues (to be used when the provider has not collected a signature and state and federal laws do not supersede the HIPAA Privacy Rule).	Yes
53 (lines A, B, C) Assignment of Benefits Certification Indicator (payers A, B, C)	A code indicating whether the provider has obtained a signed form from the patient authorizing the third-party payer to send payments directly to the provider. Codes include: N = no W = not applicable (when patient refuses to assign benefits; for paper claims only) Y = yes *(Note:* Not required for Medicare claims.)	No
54 (lines A, B, C) Prior Payments—Payer (payers A, B, C)	The amount provider has received to date (from payer A, B, or C) toward payment of this bill.	Situational
55 (lines A, B, C) Estimated Amount Due—Payer (payers A, B, C)	The amount the provider estimates is due from the indicated payer (A, B, or C) toward payment of this bill.	Situational
56 National Provider Identifier—Billing Provider	The billing provider's ten-digit National Provider Identifier (NPI); HIPAA mandated use of NPIs as of May 23, 2007.	Yes
57 (lines A, B, C) Other (Billing) Provider Identifier	For reporting health plan legacy number assigned to provider by the indicated payer in FL 50 (payer A, B, C). No longer a required field on Medicare claims after HIPAA's mandated use of NPIs in FL 56. For non-Medicare claims, required only when there is no NPI in FL 56 and an identification number other than the NPI is necessary for the receiver to identify the provider.	No
58 (lines A, B, C) Insured's Name	The name of the insured individual in whose name the insurance, as reported in FL 50 A, B, or C, is listed. The information in FLs 59–62 on the same line all pertains to this person. This name (last name, first name, and middle initial) must correspond to the name on the insured's health insurance card.	Yes

Table 14.1 UB-04 Form Completion *(continued)*

Form Locator	Description	Medicare Required?
59 (lines A, B, C) Patient's Relationship to Insured	Code for patient's relationship to insured: 01 = spouse 18 = self 19 = child 20 = employee 21 = unknown 39 = organ donor 40 = cadaver donor 53 = life partner G8 = other relationship	Yes
60 (lines A, B, C) Insured's Unique Identifier	The identification number assigned to the insured by the payer organization; for example, in the case of Medicare, the patient's Medicare number.	Yes
61 (lines A, B, C) Insured's Group Name	The name of the group or plan under which the individual is insured; used when available and the group number (FL 62) is not used. For Medicare secondary, the primary payer's insurance group or plan name, if known, is reported in line A.	Situational
62 (lines A, B, C) Insured's Group Number	The number assigned by the insurance company to identify the group or plan under which the individual is insured. For Medicare secondary, the primary payer's insurance group number, if known, is reported in line A.	Situational
63 (lines A, B, C) Treatment Authorization Codes	Number or other indicator that designates that the treatment covered by this bill has been authorized by the payer indicated in FL 50 (lines A, B, C). On Medicare claims, whenever the QIO review is performed for outpatient preadmission, preprocedure, or inpatient preadmission, authorization number is shown.	Situational
64 (lines A, B, C) Document Control Number (DCN)	The internal control number assigned to the original bill by the indicated health plan (FL 50 A, B, C); reported when filing a replacement or cancellation to a previously processed claim.	Situational
65 (lines A, B, C) Employer Name of the Insured	The name of the employer that is providing health care coverage for the insured indicated in FL 58 A, B, or C. (*Note:* Not used on electronic claims.)	Situational
66 Diagnosis and Procedure Code Qualifier (ICD Version Indicator)	ICD version indicator. Codes include: 9 = ICD-9-CM 0 = ICD-10-CM (not yet accepted on claims; for future use when ICD-10-CM codes are implemented)	Yes
67 Principal Diagnosis Code and POA Indicator *As of 2011, CMS accepted 24 secondary ICD-9-CM codes and related POA indicators, up from 8.	ICD-9-CM diagnosis codes reported to highest level of specificity available. A POA (present on admission) code indicator is required in the eighth position of this FL (shaded area) to indicate whether the diagnosis was present at the time of admission. POA indicators include: Y = yes N = no U = no information in the record W = clinically undetermined 1 or Blank = exempt from POA reporting (1 on electronic claims)	Yes
67 A-Q Other Diagnoses Codes with POA Indicators *As of 2011, CMS accepted 24 secondary ICD-9-CM codes and related POA indicators, up from 8.	Codes for additional conditions that coexisted at admission or developed and that had an effect on the treatment or the length of stay. A POA indicator is required in the eighth position of this field (shaded area). See list of POA code indicators in FL 67 above (*Note:* The UB-04 form provides fields A-Q for up to eighteen additional codes. Medicare allows for up to eight additional codes, reported in the top line in fields A-H.)	Yes

(continued)

Table 14.1 UB-04 Form Completion *(continued)*

Form Locator	Description	Medicare Required?
68 (Unlabeled Field)	Reserved for national assignment.	
69 Admitting Diagnosis Code	For inpatient claims only. The patient's admitting diagnosis is required if the claim is subject to QIO review.	Yes
70 a, b, c Patient's Reason for Visit	For outpatient claims only. The patient's reason for visit is required for all unscheduled outpatient visits. Up to three diagnosis codes can be reported (a, b, c). *(Note:* May be reported for scheduled outpatient visits, such as for ancillary tests, when this information provides additional support for medical necessity.)	Situational
71 Prospective Payment System (PPS) Code	Used to identify the DRG. Required on IP claims if the hospital's DRG contract with the payer stipulates that this information be provided. *(Note:* Not used for Medicare claims; workers' compensation programs often require this information.)	No
72 a, b, c External Cause of Injury (ECI) Code	The ICD-9-CM code(s) for an external cause of injury, poisoning, or other adverse effect. *(Note:* Not used for Medicare claims.) POA: FLs 72 a, b, c contain a shaded area for reporting a POA indicator code. *(Note:* Medicare only requires POA codes for ECI codes when they are being reported in FLs 67 A-Q as other diagnosis codes.)	No
73 (Unlabeled Field)	Reserved for national assignment.	
74 Principal Procedure Code and Date	For reporting the ICD-9-CM procedure code most closely related to principal diagnosis code, along with corresponding date of procedure (MMDDYY). Required on inpatient claims only. Not to be used on outpatient claims.	Situational
74 a-e Other Procedure Codes and Dates	For reporting up to five additional ICD-9-CM procedure codes and dates. Required oninpatient claims only. Not to be used on outpatient claims.	Situational
75 (Unlabeled Field)	Reserved for national assignment.	
76 Attending Provider Name and Identifiers	*Line 1:* NPI (primary identifier) of the attending provider. Required for any services received other than nonscheduled transportation services. On non-Medicare claims, a secondary identifier may be reported in line 1 when an NPI has not been obtained and an identification number other than the NPI is necessary for the receiver to identify the provider. Report secondary identifier qualifier followed by ID number. Secondary identifier qualifiers include: OB = state license number. 1G = provider UPIN number. G2 = provider commercial number. *(Note:* For Medicare claims after May 23, 2008, the NPI alone is required in this form locator.) *Line 2:* Last name and first name of attending provider.	Situational
77 Operating Physician Name and Identifiers	*Line 1:* NPI (primary identifier) of physician who also performed principal or surgical procedures; required when a surgical procedure code is reported on the claim. On non-Medicare claims, a secondary identifier may be reported in line 1 when an NPI is not used. See FL 76 above. *(Note:* For Medicare claims after May 23, 2008, the NPI alone is required in this form locator.) *Line 2:* Last name and first name of operating physician.	Situational

Table 14.1   UB-04 Form Completion *(continued)*

Form Locator	Description	Medicare Required?
78, 79 Other Provider Name and Identifiers	*Line 1:* Provider type qualifier code and NPI of other provider such as a referring or assisting provider. Provider type qualifier codes include: DN = referring provider. ZZ = other operating physician. 82 = rendering provider. On non-Medicare claims, a secondary identifier may be reported in line 1 when an NPI is not used. See FL 76 above. (*Note:* For Medicare claims after May 23, 2008, the NPI alone is required in this form locator.) *Line 2:* Last name and first name of other provider.	Situational
80 Remarks	For providing information that is not shown elsewhere on the claim and that is necessary for proper payment; for example, DME and Medicare Secondary Payer information.	Situational
81 a, b, c, d Code-Code Field	For reporting FL overflow codes or to report externally maintained codes approved by the NUBC, such as taxonomy codes or public health reporting codes, not used in current form. Report code qualifier followed by code. Code qualifiers for overflow codes (not used on Medicare claims) include: A1 = condition codes A2 = occurrence codes and dates A3 = occurrence span codes and dates A4 = value codes and amounts Other example of code qualifiers: B3 = health care provider taxonomy code (billing provider only). (*Note:* Taxonomy code is required for institutional providers submitting Medicare claims; used to identify subparts of facility when provider has chosen not to apply for individual subpart NPIs.)	Situational

UB-04 Claim Form Completion

The UB-04 claim form has eighty-one data fields, some of which require multiple entries (see Figure 14.1). The information for the form locators often requires choosing from a list of codes. Figure 14.1 shows required information and possible choices for a Medicare claim. (In some cases, because the list of code choices is extensive, selected entries are shown as examples.) Private-payer-required fields may be slightly different, and other condition codes or options are often available.

Remittance Advice Processing

Hospitals receive a remittance advice (RA) when payments are transmitted by payers to their accounts. The patient accounting department and HIM check that appropriate payment has been received. Unless the software used for billing automatically reports that the billed code is not the same as the paid code, procedures to find and follow up on these exceptions must be set up between the two departments.

Similar to medical practices, hospitals set up schedules when accounts receivable are due and follow up on late payments. The turnaround time for electronic claims is usually from ten to fifteen days faster than for manual paper claims, so the follow-up procedures are organized according to each payer's submission method and usual turnaround time. Payers' requests for attachments such as emergency department reports may delay payment.

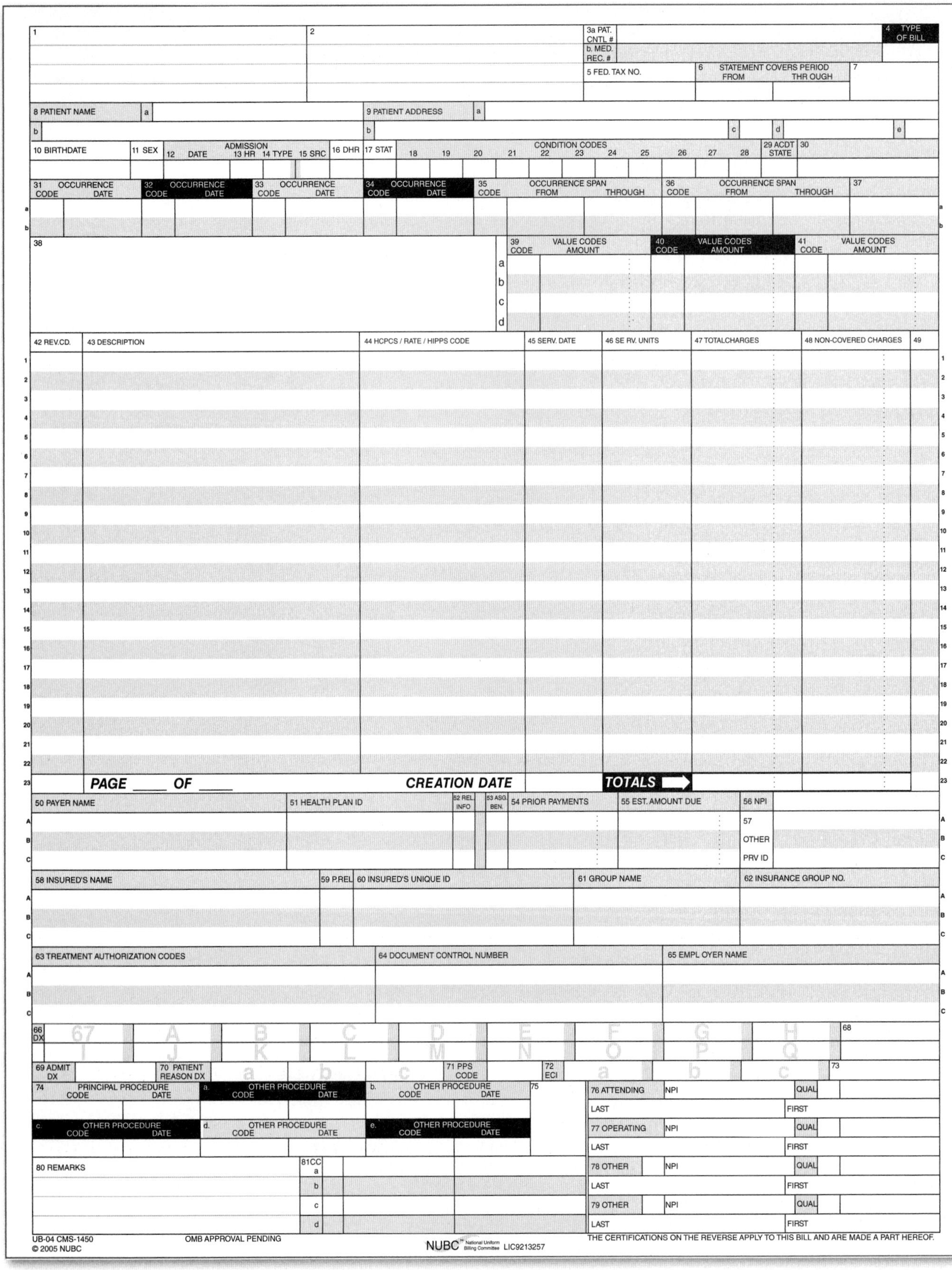

FIGURE 14.1 UB-04 Form

THINKING IT THROUGH 14.5

1. Based on the guidelines in Table 14.1, assign a form locator to each of the following data items. The first has been completed for you.

Form Locator   Data Item

__1__   **A.** Facility name and address

_____   **B.** Federal tax number

_____   **C.** Statement covers period (from—through)

_____   **D.** Patient's name

_____   **E.** Patient's address

_____   **F.** Patient birth date

_____   **G.** Patient's health plan ID

_____   **H.** Patient control number

_____   **I.** Patient's sex

_____   **J.** Patient's medical record number

_____   **K.** Admission hour

_____   **L.** Type of admission

_____   **M.** Discharge hour

_____   **N.** Insured's name

_____   **O.** Patient's relationship to insured

_____   **P.** Insured's payer ID number

_____   **Q.** Payer name

_____   **R.** Revenue code(s)

_____   **S.** Revenue description

_____   **T.** Units

_____   **U.** Charges

_____   **V.** Principal diagnosis code and POA indicator

_____   **W.** Attending provider name and ID

Chapter Summary

Learning Outcomes	Key Concepts/Examples
14.1 Compare inpatient and outpatient hospital services. Page 278	Inpatient services: • Involve an overnight stay. • Are provided by general and specialized hospitals, skilled nursing facilities, and long-term care facilities. Outpatient services: • Are provided by ambulatory surgical centers or units, by home health agencies, and by hospice staff.
14.2 List the major steps relating to the hospital billing cycle. Pages 279–280	• Admitting (registering) the patient. • Entering personal and financial information in the hospital's health record system. • Verifying insurance coverage. • Signing consent forms by the patient.

Learning Outcomes	Key Concepts/Examples
	• Presenting a notice of the hospital's privacy policy to the patient. • Collecting some pretreatment payments. • Tracking and recording the patient's treatments and transfers among the various departments in the hospital. • Discharging and billing. • Following the discharge of the patient from the facility and the completion of the patient's record.
14.3 Contrast coding diagnoses and procedures for hospital inpatient cases and physician office services. Pages 280–282	• The main diagnosis, called the principal rather than the primary diagnosis, is established after study in the hospital setting. • Coding an unconfirmed (rule-out) as the admitting diagnosis is permitted in the hospital setting. • Comorbidities and complications are also reported and may increase the hospital's reimbursement for level of care. • In the hospital setting ICD-10-PCS is used to assign procedure codes.
14.4 Compare the Medicare Inpatient and Outpatient Payment Systems. Pages 282–283	• Medicare pays for inpatient services under its Inpatient Prospective Payment System (IPPS), which uses diagnosis-related groups (DRGs) to classify patients into similar treatment and length-of-hospital-stay units and sets prices for each classification group. • Medicare pays for outpatient hospital services under its Outpatient Prospective Payment System (PPS), which groups patients under an ambulatory patient classification (APC) system that reimburses preset amounts based on the value of each APC.
14.5 Prepare an accurate UB-04 claim. Pages 283–293	• The 837I—the HIPAA standard transaction for the facility claim—or, in some cases, the UB-04 form (CMS-1450), is used to report facility charges. • Some of the information that is reported on the form includes patient data, insured information, facility and patient type, admission source, principal and admitting diagnosis, principal procedure code, attending and other key physicians, and charges.

Using Terminology

Match the key terms in the left column with the definitions in the right column.

_____ **1.** [LO 14.2] Attending physician

_____ **2.** [LO 14.3] Principal diagnosis (PDX)

_____ **3.** [LO 14.2] Charge master

_____ **4.** [LO 14.1] Inpatient

_____ **5.** [LO 14.4] Diagnosis-related groups (DRGs)

A. A person admitted to a hospital for services that require an overnight stay.

B. The main service performed for the condition listed as the principal diagnosis for a hospital inpatient.

C. The clinician primarily responsible for the care of the patient from the beginning of the hospital episode.

D. Outpatient care.

E. HIPAA standard transaction for the facility claim.

connect plus+

Enhance your learning at mcgrawhillconnect.com!
• Practice Exercises • Worksheets
• Activities • Integrated eBook

_____ **6.** [LO 14.3] Comorbidities

_____ **7.** [LO 14.3] Admitting diagnosis (ADX)

_____ **8.** [LO 14.3] Principal procedure

_____ **9.** [LO 14.1] Ambulatory care

_____ **10.** [LO 14.5] 837I

F. A hospital's list of the codes and charges for its services.

G. The patient's condition identified by the physician at admission to the hospital.

H. A system of analyzing conditions and treatments for similar groups of patients used to establish Medicare fees for hospital inpatient services.

I. Conditions in addition to the principal diagnosis that the patient had at hospital admission which affect the length of the hospital stay or the course of treatment.

J. The condition that after study is established as chiefly responsible for a patient's admission to a hospital.

Checking Your Understanding

Write the letter of the choice that best completes the statement or answers the question.

1. [LO 14.2] When the hospital staff collects data on a patient who is being admitted for services, the process is called _____.
   A. Health information management
   B. Registration
   C. MSP
   D. Precertification

2. [LO 14.5] Name the paper claim form used by hospitals to submit claims for Medicare Part A reimbursement. _____
   A. CMS-1500
   B. 837I
   C. UB-92
   D. UB-04

3. [LO 14.2] Patient charges in hospitals vary according to _____.
   A. Their accommodations only
   B. Their services only
   C. Their accommodations and services
   D. Their age and gender

4. [LO 14.2] In the HIM department the master patient index contains _____.
   A. The main database that identifies patients
   B. The list of patients waiting to be admitted
   C. The total hospital patient count for each day
   D. Patient satisfaction survey data

5. [LO 14.3] Conditions that arise during the patient's hospital stay as a result of surgery or treatments are called _____.
   A. Comorbidities
   B. Admitting diagnoses
   C. Complications
   D. Correlates

6. [LO 14.3] In inpatient coding, the initials *CC* mean _____.
   A. Chief complaint
   B. Comorbidities and complications
   C. Cubic centimeters
   D. Convalescent center

connect plus+
Enhance your learning at mcgrawhillconnect.com!
• Practice Exercises   • Worksheets
• Activities   • Integrated eBook

7. **[LO 14.3]** Upon discharge, CMS requires that every reported diagnosis be submitted with _____.
   A. A progress report
   B. A procedure code
   C. The initials CC
   D. A present on admission indicator

8. **[LO 14.4]** Under an Inpatient Prospective Payment System (IPPS), payments for services are _____.
   A. Set in advance
   B. Based on the provider's fees
   C. Discounts to the provider's usual fees
   D. Negotiable depending upon the case

9. **[LO 14.3]** Which of the following codes are used to assign procedure codes in an inpatient setting? _____
   A. CPT
   B. ICD-10-CM
   C. Revenue Codes
   D. ICD-10-PCS

10. **[LO 14.2]** Which of the following hospital departments has different procedures for collecting patients' personal and insurance information? _____
    A. Accounting department
    B. Surgery department
    C. Emergency department
    D. Collections department

Copyright © 2014 The McGraw-Hill Companies

connect plus+

Enhance your learning at mcgrawhillconnect.com!
• Practice Exercises   • Worksheets
• Activities   • Integrated eBook

Guide to Medisoft®

This Guide contains an introduction to the Medisoft Advanced Patient Accounting program, including an introduction to the program's databases, an explanation of how claims are created in Medisoft, and illustrations of the major dialog boxes that are used for data entry. If directed by your instructor, you will be completing exercises from the book using the simulated Medisoft exercises available through **Connect Plus.** Connect Plus provides simulated Medisoft exercises in four modes: Demo, Practice, Test, and Assessment. Using the scenario provided in the book, along with the steps available at www.mhhe.com/newbycarr, you will complete the exercises at connect.mcgraw-hill.com. Before getting started, please read through this Guide to get a better understanding of what Medisoft is and the essential tasks that you will be completing in Connect Plus.

Before a medical office begins to create claims using Medisoft, basic information about the practice and its patients must be entered into the program. The medical practice with which you will work is called Orchard Hill Medical Center.

Overview

Medisoft, a computerized patient billing system, is used in this textbook as an example of the type of program with which Medical Assistants often work. Processing information to complete insurance claim forms is one of the main functions of the Medisoft program.

Medisoft's Database Design

The Medisoft program is designed to collect information and store it in databases.

A database is a collection of related facts. For example, a provider database contains information about a practice's physicians while a patient database contains each patient's unique chart number and personal information, including address, phone, employer, assigned provider, and so on. The major databases in the Medisoft program are:

- *Provider:* The provider database has information about the physician(s) as well as the practice, such as the practice's name, address, phone number, and tax and provider identifier numbers.
- *Patient/Guarantor:* Each patient information form is stored in the computer system's patient/guarantor database. The database includes the patient's unique chart number and personal information: name, address, phone number, birth date, Social Security number, gender, marital status, employer, and guarantor (the insured person if other than the patient).
- *Insurance Carriers:* The insurance carrier database contains the names, addresses, plan types, and other data about all insurance carriers used by the practice's

patients. This database also stores information about each carrier's electronic claim submission.

- *Diagnosis Codes:* The diagnosis code database contains the most frequently used ICD codes that indicate the reason a service is provided. The practice's encounter form serves as a source document in setting up this database.
- *Procedure Codes:* The procedure code database contains the data needed to create charges. The CPT codes most often used by the practice are selected for this database. The practice's encounter form is a good source document for these codes also. Other claim data, such as place of service (POS) codes and the charge for each procedure, are stored in this database as well.
- *Transactions:* The transaction database stores information about each patient's visits, diagnoses, and procedures, as well as received and outstanding payments.

How Insurance Claims Are Created in Medisoft

Three major steps are followed to create insurance claims using Medisoft: (1) setting up the practice, (2) entering patient and transaction information, and (3) creating insurance claims.

Setting Up the Practice

Before Medisoft can be used to store information about patients and their visits, basic facts about the practice itself are entered into several of the databases mentioned above. Information about the providers in the practice is recorded in the provider database, including each provider's National Provider Identifier (NPI), tax identification numbers, or other provider IDs as needed. In addition, frequently used diagnosis and procedure codes are entered in their own databases with code descriptions. Finally, insurance carrier data are entered. The insurance carrier database contains information about the carriers that most patients use, as well as options for electronic claim submission and paper claim printing. These databases are created once during the setup of the practice. However, they may be updated as often as necessary.

Entering Patient and Transaction Information

Entering patient and transaction information in the database is an ongoing process. After a patient visits a physician in the practice, the medical insurance specialist organizes the information gathered on the patient information form and the encounter form.

After analyzing and checking the data, each element is entered in Medisoft.

A new record must be created for a new patient, and information on established patients may need to be updated. Next, the appropriate insurance carrier for the visit is selected. Usually, this is the patient's primary insurance carrier, but in workers' compensation cases, for example, the carrier will be different. After that, the purposes of the visit, the diagnosis codes, and the procedure codes are entered, with the appropriate charges.

Creating Insurance Claims

When all patient and transaction information has been entered and checked, the medical insurance specialist issues the command to Medisoft to create an insurance claim form. Medisoft then organizes the necessary databases. Within Medisoft, each database is linked, or related, to each of the others by having at least one fact in common. For example, the patient's chart number appears in both the patient/guarantor database and the transaction database, thereby linking the two. Medisoft selects data from each database as needed. The program follows the instructions for printing the form or transmitting the information electronically to the designated receiver, which is often a clearinghouse.

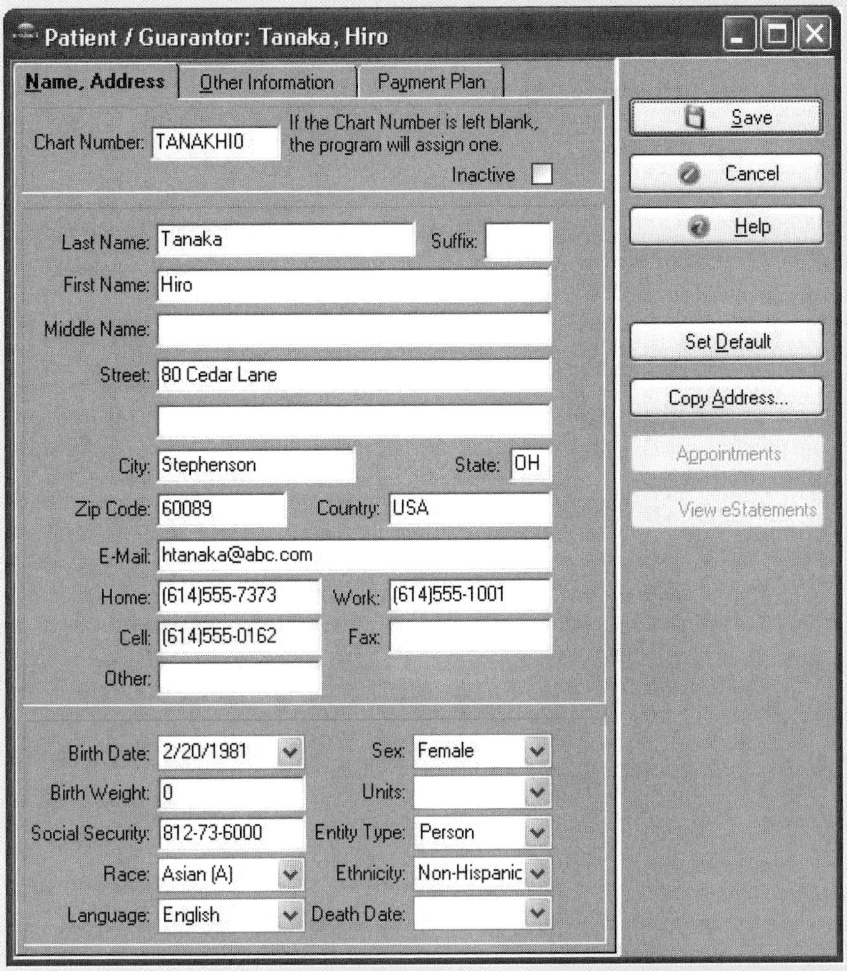

FIGURE 1 Name, Address Tab in the Patient/Guarantor Dialog Box

Data Entry in Medisoft

The following section provides illustrations and descriptions of the main areas in which data are entered in Medisoft.

Patient/Guarantor Information

The Patient/Guarantor dialog box is where basic information about patients is entered. The dialog box has three "pages," or tabs, used to enter information about patients. Tabs are so named because they resemble the tab on a file folder. When a tab name is clicked, the entire contents of that tab are displayed. Each tab contains fields in which data is keyed. The patient's unique chart number, which can be created by the user or assigned by Medisoft, is entered in the first field in the Name, Address tab of the Patient/Guarantor dialog box (see Figure 1). Then, the patient's personal information (name, address, contact numbers, birth date, Social Security number, and so on) is entered.

Many Medisoft dialog boxes include default entries to save time when various types of data are entered. For example, in the Country field in the Name, Address tab, the entry "USA" automatically appears. If this entry is correct, the user moves on to the next entry, accepting the default. This information is stored when the user clicks the Save button. If the default entry is not correct, other data may be entered and stored in its place.

The second tab in the Patient/Guarantor dialog box, called the Other Information tab, contains information about the patient's employment and other miscellaneous data. The third tab, Payment Plan, is used to enter the terms for the patient's payment plan, provided the practice offers a payment plan and the patient requests one. For the Medisoft work in this text, patient information has already been entered in the tabs of the Patient/Guarantor dialog box for you.

Case Information

Once a patient's personal information is entered, then a new case can be created each time the patient visits the medical office with a different complaint. A new case is also set up if the insurance carrier differs from the patient's primary carrier, such as in a workers' compensation case, in order to keep the information separate from other office visits. A patient's case information is stored in the Case dialog box (see Figure 2).

The Case dialog box contains eleven tabs for entering a patient's case information: Personal, Account, Diagnosis, Policy 1, Policy 2, Policy 3, Condition, Miscellaneous, Medicaid and TRICARE, Comment, and EDI. These tabs contain information about the patients' billing account, insurance coverage, medical condition, and other miscellaneous information that may be required to create an insurance claim.

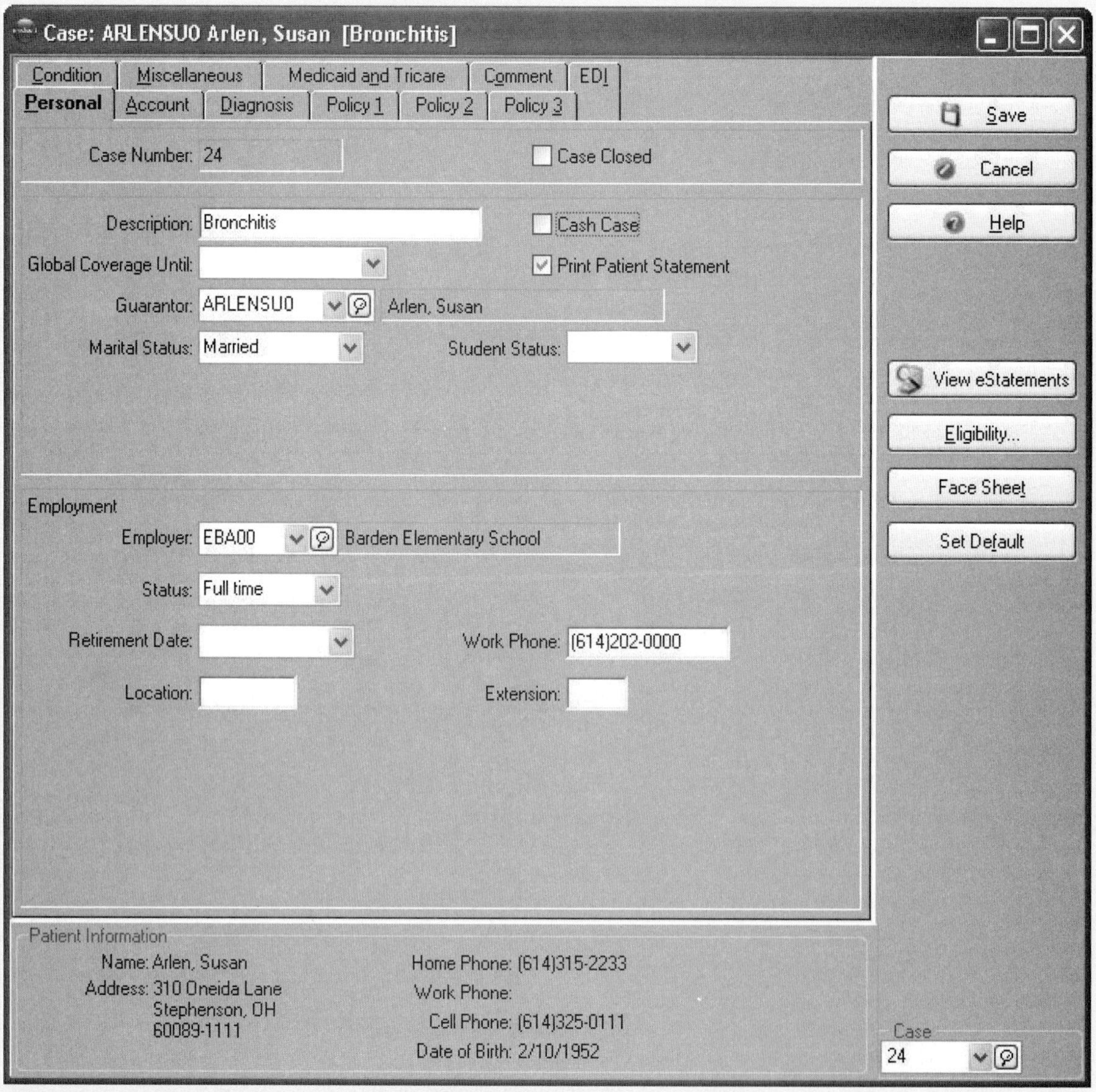

FIGURE 2 Case Dialog Box with the Personal Tab Active

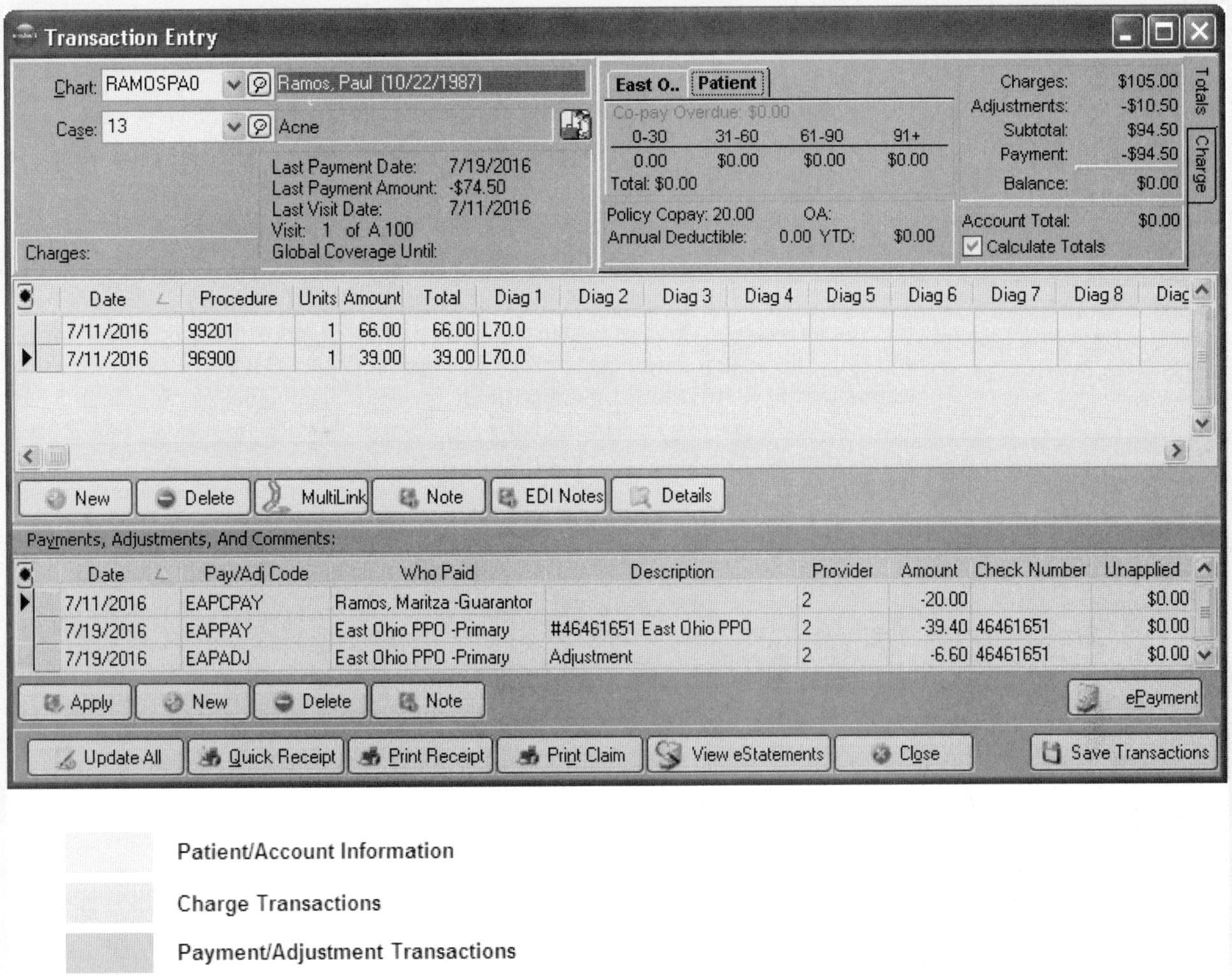

FIGURE 3 Transaction Entry Dialog Box with Three Sections Highlighted

Transaction Entry

Transactions—patients' visits and charges, as well as payments and adjustments—are entered in the Transaction Entry dialog box (see Figure 3). When the patient's chart number and case number are selected in the Transaction Entry dialog box, Medisoft displays information previously entered in other dialog boxes, such as the patient's name and birth date, case name, and insurance carrier information, in the top portion of the Transaction Entry dialog box for easy reference.

Charge transactions are created by clicking the New button in the middle portion of the Transaction Entry dialog box, labeled the Charges section. This section is used for entering procedure codes and charges. Procedures are selected in the Procedure field from a drop-down list of procedure codes. The list shows the CPT codes and descriptions that are frequently used by the practice. If the correct procedure has not already been included in Medisoft, a dialog box can be accessed to add it.

Patient copayments are entered by clicking the New button in the lower third of the Transaction Entry dialog box, the Payments, Adjustments, and Comments section. This section is used for recording payments received from patients and insurance carriers. The type of payment is selected in the Pay/Adj Code field from a drop-down list of codes (see Figure 3). Transaction entries must be saved by clicking the Save Transactions button in the bottom right corner of the dialog box. Any transaction can be edited by clicking in the field to be edited and making the change.

When the transaction entry is complete, a receipt, called a walkout receipt, can be printed for the patient by clicking the Print Receipt button at the bottom of the Transaction Entry dialog box. The walkout receipt is a printed statement showing what the patient paid that day and what is owed. Patients who file their own insurance claims use this information to complete the claim form.

Claim Management

Once a patient's transaction entries have been completed for a visit, a claim can be created. The Claim Management dialog box is used to (1) create batches of claims for transmission, (2) transmit claims electronically or print them on paper forms, and (3), if necessary, make corrections to existing claims. Medisoft creates a list of claims that have been sent by either mode (print or electronic) in the Claim Management dialog box so that each claim can be marked with its status when RA reports arrive from carriers (see Figure 4).

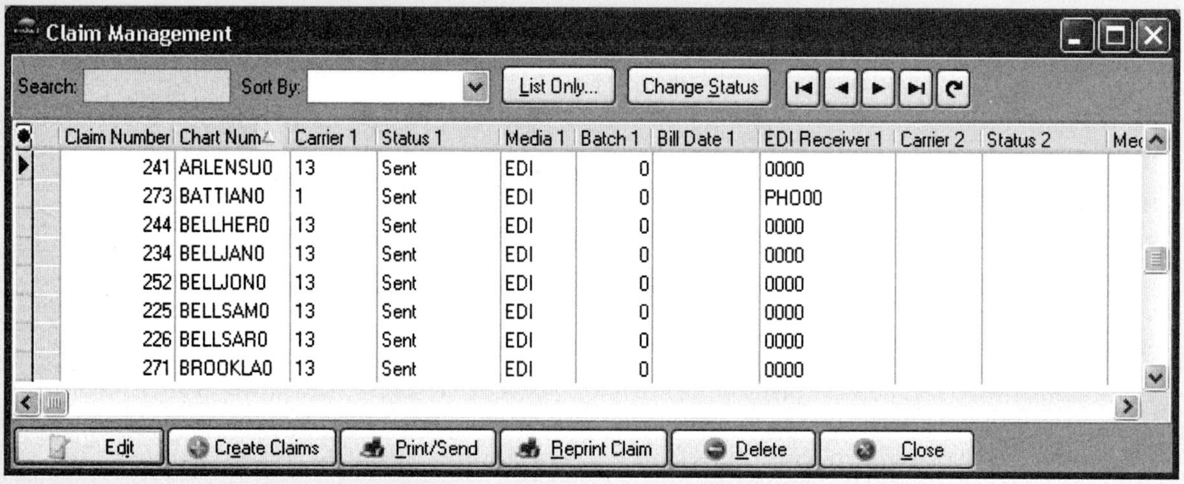

FIGURE 4 Claim Management Dialog Box

Appendix B

The Interactive Simulated CMS-1500 Form

This Appendix provides a brief introduction to the interactive simulated CMS-1500 form that was created for use with this text. The interactive version of the form is available at the book's Online Learning Center website, www.mhhe.com/newbycarr. Once you are at the website, click on the Student Edition link on the left. Under Course-wide content, you will then click on the CMS-1500 link.

On the website, you will find two versions of the electronic form—an HTML version and an Adobe version. Your Internet browser or operating system may affect the performance of these forms, so two claim completion options are being provided. You will need access to the Internet in order to get these forms.

HTML Version

This version should be completed directly in your Internet browser. When you click on the link for this version, a separate window will open. You can then type in all of the required information directly into the form. Once you are done, you will click the "I'm finished!" button at the very bottom of the form. This will activate two more buttons.

- "Save As PDF"—clicking this button will allow you to save the file as a PDF document to your computer.
- "Print"—clicking this button will allow you to print the file so that you have a hardcopy.

Now, you can either e-mail the PDF document to your instructor or hand in a hardcopy to your instructor. Please note that you will not be able to edit the form once you click the "I'm finished!" button, and will need to start the form over instead.

Adobe Version

This version uses Adobe Form Filler functionality, which requires access to Adobe Acrobat Reader. If you need the latest version of the free reader, you can download it from www.adobe.com. It is recommended that you do not try to complete the form within your browser. Instead, you will first save the file to your computer by clicking on the "Save a copy" icon. You can then type in all of the required information directly into the form. Once you are done, select "save as" from the File menu and re-name the file per your instructor's direction (or use this naming convention: lastname_firstname_chapter#.pdf) and then save it where you want to on your computer. You can then print the form (select the Print option on the File menu) or e-mail it to your instructor as required (select the Attach to Email option on the File menu). You can still make edits to this version of the form after you have saved it to your computer.

NAVIGATION TIPS

For either version of the form, you can click directly in the box where you want to type the needed information. You can also use the Tab key to move from box to box. In addition, you can use the scroll bar on the right side of the screen to move up and down in the form.

Professional Websites

Government Sites and Resources

CCI

Medicare Correct Coding Initiative automated edits are online, at www.cms.gov/NationalCorrectCodInitEd

CMS

Coverage of the Centers for Medicare and Medicaid Services: Medicare, Medicaid, CHIP, HIPAA, CLIA topics, www.cms.gov

Medicare Learning Network, cms.gov/mlngeninfo

Online Medicare manuals, cms.gov/manuals/IOM/list.asp

Medicare Physician Fee Schedule, cms.gov/PhysicianFeeSched

General information on Medicare, www.cms.gov/MLNGenInfo

Beneficiary Notices Initiative, www.cms.gov/BNI

Beneficiary Preventive Services Information, www.cms.gov/Outreach-and-Education/Medicare-Learning-Network-MLN/MLNProducts/PreventiveServices.html

CMS Manuals, www.cms.gov/manuals

Enforcement, www.cms.gov/Enforcement

Quarterly Provider Updates, www.cms.gov/QuarterlyProviderUpdates

Physician Quality Reporting System, www.cms.gov/PQRS

Medicare General Information, www.medicare.gov

Medicare Fee Schedule, www.cms.gov/PfsLookup

Medicare Physician Fee Schedule, www.cms.gov/PhysicianFeeSched

Medicare Contracting Reform, www.cms.gov/MedicareContractingReform

Medicare Coverage Database, www.cms.gov/mcd/overview.asp

Medicare Physician Website, www.cms.gov/center/physician.asp

Medicare FFS Provider Web Pages, www.cms.gov/Outreach-and-Education/Medicare-Learning-Network-MLN/MLNProducts/FFS_Provider_Web_Pages.html

Medicaid General Information, http://www.medicaid.gov/

Medicaid Integrity Program, www.cms.gov/MedicaidIntegrityProgram

Children's Health Insurance Program, http://www.medicaid.gov/CHIP/CHIP-Program-Information.html

Clinical Laboratory Improvement Amendments (CLIA), www.cms.gov/CLIA

CMS Consortia, www.cms.gov/consortia

POS Codes, www.cms.gov/Medicare/Coding/place-of-service-codes/

HAC/POA Fact Sheet, www.cms.gov/HospitalAcqCond/Downloads/HAC Factsheet.pdf

Recovery Audit Program, www.cms.gov/RAC

EBSA

General information on the EBSA, www.dol.gov/ebsa

FEHB

General information on the FEHB, www.opm.gov/insure/health/

HCPCS

General information on HCPCS, www.cms.gov/MedHCPCSGenInfo

Annual alphanumeric Healthcare Common Procedure Coding System file, www.cms.gov/HCPCSReleaseCodeSets

DME PDAC, www.dmepdac.com

Health Information Technology, U.S. Department of Health & Human Services (HHS) IT Initiatives, healthit.hhs.gov/

HIPAA

Home page, www.cms.gov/hipaageninfo

Questions and Answers on HIPAA Privacy Policies, www.hhs.gov/ocr/privacy

HIPAA Privacy Rule, "Standards for Privacy of Individually Identifiable Health Information; Final Rule." 45 CFR Parts 160 and 164. *Federal Register 65*, no. 250 (2000), www.hhs.gov/ocr/hipaa/finalreg.html

HHS Breach Notifications, www.hhs.gov/ocr/privacy/hipaa/administrative/breachnotificationrule/breachtool.html

HHS Health Data Privacy Policy Notice, http://www.hhs.gov/privacy.html

ICD

NCHS (National Center for Health Statistics) posts the ICD-9-CM addenda and guidelines, www.cdc.gov/nchs/icd.htm

ICD-10-CM, www.cdc.gov/nchs/icd/icd10.htm, www.cms.gov/ICD10

ICD-9-CM Official Guidelines for Coding and Reporting, www.cdc.gov/nchs/icd/icd9.htm

ICD-10-CM to ICD-9-CM conversion tool, www.aapc.com/icd-10/codes/index.aspx

NUBC

The National Uniform Billing Committee develops and maintains a standardized data set for use by institutional providers to transmit claim and encounter information. This group is in charge of the 837I and the CMS-1450 (UB 04) claim formats. Refer to the NUBC website, www.nubc.org

NUCC

The National Uniform Claim Committee develops and maintains a standardized data set for use by the noninstitutional health care community to transmit claim and encounter information. This group is in charge of the 837P and the CMS-1500 claim formats. Refer to the NUCC website, www.nucc.org

OCR

The Office of Civil Rights of the HHS enforces the HIPAA Privacy Rule; Privacy Fact Sheets are online, www.hhs.gov/ocr/hipaa

OIG

The Office of Inspector General of the HHA home page links to fraud and abuse, advisory opinions, exclusion list, and other topics, www.oig.hhs.gov

Model compliance programs, http://oig.hhs.gov/fraud/complianceguidance.asp

FECA Program Information, www.oig.dol.gov/fecaprogram.htm

TRICARE and CHAMPVA

General TRICARE information, www.tricare.mil

CHAMPVA Overview, www.va.gov/hac

TRICARE Allowable Charges, www.tricare.mil/allowablecharges

TRICARE Claims, www.tricare.mil/claims

TRICARE Fraud and Abuse, www.tricare.mil/fraud

USPSTF

The U.S. Preventive Services Task Force, www.uspreventiveservicestaskforce.org/

Workers' Compensation

General information on states' workers' compensation agencies, www.workerscompensation.com

WPC

Washington Publishing Company is the link for HIPAA Transaction and Code Sets implementation guides. It also assists in the maintenance and distribution of the following HIPAA-related code lists at www.wpc-edi.com:

- Provider Taxonomy Codes
- Claim Adjustment Reason Codes
- Claim Status Codes
- Claim Status Category Codes

- Health Care Services Decision Reason Codes
- Insurance Business Process Application Error Codes
- Remittance Remark Codes

Billing and Insurance

BlueCross BlueShield Association, www.bluecares.com

FAIR Health, Inc., www.fairhealthus.org

The Kaiser Family Foundation website provides in-depth information on key health policy issues such as Medicaid, Medicare, and prescription drugs. Refer to the website, www.kff.org

Various sites, such as www.benefitnews.com, www.erisaclaim.com, and www.erisa.com, cover EMTALA, ERISA regulations and updates concerning provider and patient appeals of managed care organizations.

State insurance commissioners, www.naic.org/state_web_map.htm

Electronic Medical Records

AHIMA Coverage of Related Topics Located Under the Practice Brief tab on the AHIMA Home Page, www.ahima.org

Maintaining a Legally Sound Health Record

The Legal Process and Electronic Health Records

Implementing Electronic Signatures

HIM Practice Transformation/EHR's Impact on HIM Functions

Core Data Sets for the Physician Practice Electronic Health Record

Associations

AAFP American Academy of Family Physicians, www.aafp.org

AAHAM American Association of Healthcare Administrative Management, www.aaham.org

AAMA American Association of Medical Assistants, www.aama-ntl.org

AAPC American Academy of Professional Coders, www.aapc.com

ABA American Bar Association, www.abanet.org/health

ACA International (formerly American Collectors Association), www.acainternational.org

ACHE American College of Healthcare Executives, www.ache.org

AHA American Hospital Association, www.aha.org

AHA Central Office, www.ahacentraloffice.org

AHDI Association for Healthcare Documentation Integrity, www.ahdionline.org

AHIMA American Health Information Management Association, www.ahima.org

AHIP America's Health Plans, www.ahip.org

AHLA American Health Lawyers Association, www.healthlawyers.org

AMA American Medical Association, www.ama-assn.org

AMBA American Medical Billing Association, www.ambanet.net/AMBA.htm

AMT American Medical Technologists, www.amt1.com

ANA American Nurses Association, www.ana.org

HBMA Healthcare Billing and Management Association, www.hbma.com

HFMA Healthcare Financial Management Association, www.hfma.org

MGMA Medical Group Management Association, www.mgma.org

PAHCOM Professional Association of Health Care Office Management, www.pahcom.com

Selected Professional Coding Resources

Note that many commercial vendors of the annual coding books offer package prices for the year's CPT, ICD-9-CM and/or ICD-10-CM, and HCPCS references. Professional organizations may also offer discounts.

AHA Online Store
155 N. Wacker Dr.
Chicago, IL 60606
800 424 4301
www.ahaonlinestore.com
Official Coding Guidelines for ICD-9-CM

AMA Press
800 621 8335
www.amapress.com
Annual Editions of CPT, ICD, and HCPCS
www.ama-assn.org/go/CPT
CPT Assistant and CPT Clinical Examples

American Academy of Professional Coders (AAPC)
2480 South 8350 West, Suite B
Salt Lake City, UT 84120
800 626 CODE
www.aapc.com
Certification courses/examinations and coding-related publications

American Association of Health Information Management (AHIMA)
233 North Michigan Avenue, 21st Floor
Chicago, IL 60601 5809
312 233 1100
www.ahima.org
Certification courses/examinations and coding-related publications

BC Advantage Magazine
877 700 3002
info@billing-coding.com
Medical billing and coding newsletter

Coding Strategies, Inc.
5401 Dallas Hwy, Suite 606
Powder Springs, GA 30127
877 6 CODING
www.codingstrategies.com
Medical coding education and specialty publications

Conomikes Associates, Inc.
990 Highland Drive, Suite 110A
San Diego, CA 92075
800 421 6512
www.conomikes.com
Newsletters and handbooks

Contexo Media
7440 Creek Road, Suite 401
Sandy, UT 84093
800 344 5724
www.codingbooks.com
Annual editions of ICD-9-CM and ICD-10-CM, CPT, and HCPCS books; seminars

DecisionHealth
Two Washingtonian Center
9737 Washingtonian Blvd., Suite 200
Gaithersburg, MD 20878-7364
www.decisionhealth.com
Newsletters and publications

HCPro, Inc.
75 Sylvan Street, Suite A-101
Danvers, MA 01923
800 650 6787
www.hcpro.com
Training materials and E-newsletters

InGauge Healthcare Solutions
5076 Winters Chapel Road
Atlanta, GA 30360
800 253 4945
Online resource for coding reference books
www.coderscentral.com

MedicalCodingBooks.com Inc.
7764 Belle Rose Circle
Roseville, CA 95678
866 900 8300
www.medicalcodingbooks.com
*Annual Editions of CPT, ICD-9-CM and ICD-10-CM, and HCPCS Code Books;
publications on practice management and coding reimbursement*
www.icd9coding.com
Online website for ICD and DRG codes

National Center for Health Statistics (NCHS)
3311 Toledo Road
Hyattsville, MD 20782
800 232 4636
www.cdc.gov/nchs/icd.htm
*ICD-9-CM and ICD-10-CM code sets, addenda, and coding guidelines available for
downloading*

OptumInsight
13625 Technology Drive
Eden Prairie, MN 55344
888 445 8745
www.optuminsight.com
*Annual editions of ICD-9-CM and ICD-10-CM, CPT, and HCPCS books; newsletters,
and electronic reference manuals*

The Coding Institute
2222 Sedwick Drive
Durham, NC 27713
800 508 2582
www.codinginstitute.com
Coding resources in medical specialties; seminars

United States Government Printing Office
www.gpo.gov
Federal Register

Appendix D

Forms

CMS-1500 (02/12)

DRAFT - NOT FOR OFFICIAL USE

HEALTH INSURANCE CLAIM FORM
APPROVED BY NATIONAL UNIFORM CLAIM COMMITTEE (NUCC) 02/12

☐☐ PICA   PICA ☐☐

| 1. MEDICARE ☐ (Medicare#) MEDICAID ☐ (Medicaid#) TRICARE ☐ (ID#/DoD#) CHAMPVA ☐ (Member ID#) GROUP HEALTH PLAN ☐ (ID#) FECA BLK LUNG ☐ (ID#) OTHER ☐ (ID#) | 1a. INSURED'S I.D. NUMBER (For Program in Item 1) |

2. PATIENT'S NAME (Last Name, First Name, Middle Initial)

3. PATIENT'S BIRTH DATE MM DD YY   SEX M ☐ F ☐

4. INSURED'S NAME (Last Name, First Name, Middle Initial)

5. PATIENT'S ADDRESS (No., Street)

6. PATIENT RELATIONSHIP TO INSURED Self ☐ Spouse ☐ Child ☐ Other ☐

7. INSURED'S ADDRESS (No., Street)

CITY   STATE

8. RESERVED FOR NUCC USE

CITY   STATE

ZIP CODE   TELEPHONE (Include Area Code) ( )

ZIP CODE   TELEPHONE (Include Area Code) ( )

9. OTHER INSURED'S NAME (Last Name, First Name, Middle Initial)

10. IS PATIENT'S CONDITION RELATED TO:

11. INSURED'S POLICY GROUP OR FECA NUMBER

a. OTHER INSURED'S POLICY OR GROUP NUMBER

a. EMPLOYMENT? (Current or Previous) YES ☐ NO ☐

a. INSURED'S DATE OF BIRTH MM DD YY   SEX M ☐ F ☐

b. RESERVED FOR NUCC USE

b. AUTO ACCIDENT? PLACE (State) YES ☐ NO ☐

b. OTHER CLAIM ID (Designated by NUCC)

c. RESERVED FOR NUCC USE

c. OTHER ACCIDENT? YES ☐ NO ☐

c. INSURANCE PLAN NAME OR PROGRAM NAME

d. INSURANCE PLAN NAME OR PROGRAM NAME

10d. CLAIM CODES (Designated by NUCC)

d. IS THERE ANOTHER HEALTH BENEFIT PLAN? YES ☐ NO ☐ *If yes*, complete items 9, 9a, and 9d.

READ BACK OF FORM BEFORE COMPLETING & SIGNING THIS FORM.
12. PATIENT'S OR AUTHORIZED PERSON'S SIGNATURE I authorize the release of any medical or other information necessary to process this claim. I also request payment of government benefits either to myself or to the party who accepts assignment below.

SIGNED _____ DATE _____

13. INSURED'S OR AUTHORIZED PERSON'S SIGNATURE I authorize payment of medical benefits to the undersigned physician or supplier for services described below.

SIGNED _____

14. DATE OF CURRENT ILLNESS, INJURY, or PREGNANCY (LMP) MM DD YY QUAL.

15. OTHER DATE QUAL. MM DD YY

16. DATES PATIENT UNABLE TO WORK IN CURRENT OCCUPATION FROM MM DD YY TO MM DD YY

17. NAME OF REFERRING PROVIDER OR OTHER SOURCE   17a.   17b. NPI

18. HOSPITALIZATION DATES RELATED TO CURRENT SERVICES FROM MM DD YY TO MM DD YY

19. ADDITIONAL CLAIM INFORMATION (Designated by NUCC)

20. OUTSIDE LAB? YES ☐ NO ☐ $ CHARGES

21. DIAGNOSIS OR NATURE OF ILLNESS OR INJURY Relate A-L to service line below (24E)   ICD Ind. |

A. |_____ B. |_____ C. |_____ D. |_____
E. |_____ F. |_____ G. |_____ H. |_____
I. |_____ J. |_____ K. |_____ L. |_____

22. RESUBMISSION CODE   ORIGINAL REF. NO.

23. PRIOR AUTHORIZATION NUMBER

24. A. DATE(S) OF SERVICE From MM DD YY To MM DD YY	B. PLACE OF SERVICE	C. EMG	D. PROCEDURES, SERVICES, OR SUPPLIES (Explain Unusual Circumstances) CPT/HCPCS | MODIFIER	E. DIAGNOSIS POINTER	F. $ CHARGES	G. DAYS OR UNITS	H. EPSDT Family Plan	I. ID. QUAL	J. RENDERING PROVIDER ID. #
1									NPI
2									NPI
3									NPI
4									NPI
5									NPI
6									NPI

25. FEDERAL TAX I.D. NUMBER   SSN EIN ☐ ☐

26. PATIENT'S ACCOUNT NO.

27. ACCEPT ASSIGNMENT? (For govt. claims, see back) YES ☐ NO ☐

28. TOTAL CHARGE $

29. AMOUNT PAID $

30. Rsvd for NUCC Use

31. SIGNATURE OF PHYSICIAN OR SUPPLIER INCLUDING DEGREES OR CREDENTIALS (I certify that the statements on the reverse apply to this bill and are made a part thereof.)

SIGNED _____ DATE _____

32. SERVICE FACILITY LOCATION INFORMATION

a. NPI   b.

33. BILLING PROVIDER INFO & PH # ( )

a. NPI   b.

NUCC Instruction Manual available at: www.nucc.org   *PLEASE PRINT OR TYPE*   OMB APPROVAL PENDING

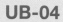

1		2		3a PAT. CNTL #		4 TYPE OF BILL
				b. MED. REC. #		
				5 FED. TAX NO.	6 STATEMENT COVERS PERIOD FROM THROUGH	7

8 PATIENT NAME a		9 PATIENT ADDRESS a			
b		b		c	d e

| 10 BIRTHDATE | 11 SEX | 12 DATE | ADMISSION 13 HR | 14 TYPE | 15 SRC | 16 DHR | 17 STAT | 18 | 19 | 20 | 21 | CONDITION CODES 22 23 24 25 26 27 28 | 29 ACDT STATE | 30 |

31 OCCURRENCE CODE DATE	32 OCCURRENCE CODE DATE	33 OCCURRENCE CODE DATE	34 OCCURRENCE CODE DATE	35 OCCURRENCE SPAN CODE FROM THROUGH	36 OCCURRENCE SPAN CODE FROM THROUGH	37
a						a
b						b

38		39 VALUE CODES CODE AMOUNT	40 VALUE CODES CODE AMOUNT	41 VALUE CODES CODE AMOUNT
		a		
		b		
		c		
		d		

42 REV. CD.	43 DESCRIPTION	44 HCPCS / RATE / HIPPS CODE	45 SERV. DATE	46 SERV. UNITS	47 TOTAL CHARGES	48 NON-COVERED CHARGES	49
1							1
2							2
3							3
4							4
5							5
6							6
7							7
8							8
9							9
10							10
11							11
12							12
13							13
14							14
15							15
16							16
17							17
18							18
19							19
20							20
21							21
22							22
23	PAGE ____ OF ____	CREATION DATE		TOTALS ➡			23

50 PAYER NAME	51 HEALTH PLAN ID	52 REL INFO	53 ASG. BEN.	54 PRIOR PAYMENTS	55 EST. AMOUNT DUE	56 NPI
A						57 OTHER PRV ID
B						
C						

58 INSURED'S NAME	59 P.REL	60 INSURED'S UNIQUE ID	61 GROUP NAME	62 INSURANCE GROUP NO.
A				
B				
C				

63 TREATMENT AUTHORIZATION CODES	64 DOCUMENT CONTROL NUMBER	65 EMPLOYER NAME
A		
B		
C		

66 DX	67	A	B	C	D	E	F	G	H	68
		I	J	K	L	M	N	O	P	Q

69 ADMIT DX	70 PATIENT REASON DX a b c	71 PPS CODE	72 ECI	73

74 PRINCIPAL PROCEDURE CODE DATE	a. OTHER PROCEDURE CODE DATE	b. OTHER PROCEDURE CODE DATE	75	76 ATTENDING NPI QUAL
				LAST FIRST
c. OTHER PROCEDURE CODE DATE	d. OTHER PROCEDURE CODE DATE	e. OTHER PROCEDURE CODE DATE		77 OPERATING NPI QUAL
				LAST FIRST
80 REMARKS		81CC a b c d		78 OTHER NPI QUAL
				LAST FIRST
				79 OTHER NPI QUAL
				LAST FIRST

UB-04 CMS-1450
© 2005 NUBC   OMB APPROVAL PENDING

NUBC National Uniform Billing Committee LIC9213257

THE CERTIFICATIONS ON THE REVERSE APPLY TO THIS BILL AND ARE MADE A PART HEREOF.

Abbreviations

AAMA	American Association of Medical Assistants
AAMT	American Association for Medical Transcription
AAPC	American Academy of Professional Coders
ABN	advance beneficiary notice
a.c.	before meals
ACO	accountable care organization
adm	admitted
AHIMA	American Health Information Management Association
AMA	American Medical Association
AMT	American Medical Technologists
ANSI	American National Standards Institute
AP	(1) accounts payable, (2) anterior-posterior
APC	ambulatory patient classification
A/R	accounts receivable
ASC	ambulatory surgical center
ASU	ambulatory surgical unit
AWV	Annual Wellness Visit
BCBS	Blue Cross and Blue Shield
b.i.d.	twice a day
BLK Lung	black lung
BMI	body mass index
BP	blood pressure
BUN	blood urea nitrogen
bx	biopsy
ca	cancer
CAGC	claim adjustment group code
CARC	claim adjustment reason code
C&S	culture and sensitivity
cc	cubic centimeter
CC	(1) physicians' records: chief complaint, (2) hospital documentation: comorbidities and complications
CCA	Certified Coding Associate
CCHIT	Certification Commission for Healthcare Information Technology
CCI	Correct Coding Initiative (national; Medicare)
CCS	Certified Coding Specialist
CCS-P	Certified Coding Specialist-Physician-Based
CCYY	year, indicates entry of four digits for the century (CC) and year (YY)
CDHP	consumer-driven health plan
CE	covered entity
CHAMPUS	Civilian Health and Medical Program of the Uniformed Services, now TRICARE
CHAMPVA	Civilian Health and Medical Program of the Department of Veterans Affairs
CLIA	Clinical Laboratory Improvement Amendment
cm	centimeter
CMA	Certified Medical Assistant
CMS	Centers for Medicare and Medicaid Services
CNS	central nervous system
COB	coordination of benefits

COBRA	Consolidated Omnibus Budget Reconciliation Act of 1985
COP	conditions of participation
CPC	Certified Professional Coder
CPC-H	Certified Professional Coder-Hospital Outpatient Facility
CPE	complete physical exam
CPT	*Current Procedural Terminology*
CSRS	Civil Service Retirement System
CV	cardiovascular
D&C	dilation and curettage
DD	day, indicates entry of two digits for the day
DEERS	Defense Enrollment Eligibility Reporting System
DME	durable medical equipment
DMEPOS	durable medical equipment, prosthetics, orthotics, and supplies
DOB	date of birth
DOJ	Department of Justice
DOS	date of service
DPT	diphtheria, pertussis, and tetanus
DRG	diagnosis-related group
DRS	designated record set
dx	diagnosis
EDI	electronic data interchange
EEG	electroencephalogram
EENT	eyes, ears, nose, and throat
EFT	electronic funds transfer
EHR	electronic health record
EIN	Employee Identification Number
EKG	electrocardiogram
EMC	electronic media claim
E/M code	Evaluation and Management code
EMG	emergency
EMR	electronic medical record
ENMT	ears, nose, mouth, and throat
ENT	ears, nose, and throat
EOB	explanation of benefits
EOC	episode of care
EP	established patient
EPSDT	Early and Periodic Screening, Diagnosis, and Treatment
ER	emergency room
ERISA	Employee Retirement Income Security Act of 1974
ETOH	alcohol
F	female
FCA	False Claims Act
FECA	Federal Employees' Compensation Act
FEHBP	Federal Employees Health Benefits Program
FERA	Fraud Enforcement and Recovery Act
FERS	Federal Employees Retirement System
FH	family history
FI	fiscal intermediary

FICA	Federal Insurance Contribution Act	mcg	microgram
FMAP	Federal Medicaid Assistance Percentage	MCM	*Medicare Carriers Manual*
F/U	follow-up	MCO	managed care organization
FUO	fever, unknown origin	MD	medical doctor
Fx	fracture	mEq	milliequivalent
g, gm	gram	MFS	Medicare Fee Schedule
GEM	general equivalence mappings	mg	milligram
GI	gastrointestinal	MIP	Medicare Integrity Program
GPCI	geographic practice cost index	mL	milliliter
gr	grain	MLN	Medicare Learning Network
GTIN	Global Trade Item Number	mm	millimeter
GU	genitourinary	MM	month, indicates entry of two digits for the month
GYN	gynecologic, gynecologist	MMA	Medicare Modernization Act
h	hour	MMR	measles, mumps, and rubella
H&P	history and physical	MRN	Medicare Remittance Notice, Medicare Redetermination Notice
HBA	health benefits adviser		
HCERA	Health Care and Education Reconciliation Act	MS	musculoskeletal
HCFA	Health Care Financing Administration, currently CMS	MSA	Medicare Savings Account
		MS-DRGs	Medicare-Severity DRGs
HCPCS	Healthcare Common Procedure Coding System	MSN	Medicare Summary Notice
HEDIS	Health Employer Data and Information Set	MTF	Military Treatment Facility
HEENT	head, eyes, ears, nose, and throat	MTS	Medicare Transaction System
HGB	hemoglobin	NCCI	National Correct Coding Initiative
HHA	home health agency	NCQA	National Committee for Quality Assurance
HHS	Department of Health and Human Services	NDC	National Drug Code
HiB	hemophilus influenza type B vaccine	NEC	not elsewhere classified
HIE	health information exchange	NEMB	notice of exclusion from Medicare benefits
HIM	health information management	Neuro	neurologic, neurological
HIPAA	Health Insurance Portability and Accountability Act	NO.	number
		nonPAR	nonparticipating
HIT	health information technology	NOS	not otherwise specified
HMO	health maintenance organization	NP	(1) new patient, (2) nurse-practitioner
HPI	history of present illness	NPI	National Provider Identifier
HS	hour of sleep	n.p.o.	nothing per os (by mouth)
hx	history	NPP	Notice of Privacy Practices
I&D	incision and drainage	NPPES	National Plan and Provider Enumerator System
ID, I.D.	identification	NSF	nonsufficient funds
ID #, I.D. #	identification number	NUCC	National Uniform Claim Committee
ICD-9-CM	*International Classification of Diseases*, Ninth Revision, *Clinical Modification*	OB	obstetrics
		OCR	Office of Civil Rights
ICD-10-CM	*International Classification of Diseases*, Tenth Revision, *Clinical Modification*	OESS	Office of E-Health Standards and Services
		OIG	Office of the Inspector General
ICD-10-PCS	*International Classification of Diseases*, Tenth Revision, *Procedure Coding System*	OMB	Office of Management and Budget
		op	operative
ICU	intensive care unit	opt	optional
IM	intramuscular	OSHA	Occupational Safety and Health Administration
INFO	information	OV	office visit
IPA	individual practice association	OWCP	Office of Workers' Compensation Programs
IV	intravenous	OZ	product number, Health Care Uniform Code Council
JCAHO	Joint Commission on Accreditation of Healthcare Organizations		
kg	kilogram	PA	physician assistant
L	liter	P&A	percussion and auscultation
LCD	local coverage determination	p.c.	after meals
LLQ	left lower quadrant	PCM	Primary Care Manager (TRICARE)
LMP	last menstrual period	PCP	primary care physician/provider
LPN	licensed practical nurse	PE	physical exam
LUQ	left upper quadrant	PECOS	Provider Enrollment Chain and Ownership System
m	meter	PH #	phone number
M	male	PHI	protected health information
MA	medical assistant		

PHR	personal health record	RVU	relative value unit
PIN	provider identifier number	Rx	prescription
PIP	personal injury protection	SCHIP	State Children's Health Insurance Program
PM/EHR	practice management/electronic health record	SDA	same-day appointment
PMH	past medical history	SDI	state disability insurance
PMP	practice management program	SH	social history
PMPM	per member per month	SNF	skilled nursing facility
po	postoperative	SOAP	subjective/objective/assessment/plan
p.o.	per os (by mouth)	SOF	signature on file
POA	present on admission	S/P	status post
POS	place of service	SSDI	Social Security Disability Insurance
POS	point-of-service option	SSI	Supplemental Security Income
PPACA	Patient Protection and Affordable Care Act	SSN	Social Security number
PPD	purified protein derivative of tuberculin test	stat, STAT	immediately
PPO	preferred provider organization	STD	sexually transmitted disease
PPS	Prospective Payment System	subq, subcu	subcutaneous
PQRS	Physician Quality Reporting System	T&A	tonsillectomy and adenoidectomy
PR	patient responsibility	TANF	Temporary Assistance for Needy Families
p.r.n.	as desired or as needed	TCS	(HIPAA Electronic) Transaction and Code Sets
PSA	prostate-specific antigen	temp	temperature
PSO	provider-sponsored organization	t.i.d.	three times a day
psych	psychiatric	TM	tympanic membrane
pt	patient	TPA	third-party claims administrator
q.	every	TPO	treatment, payment, and healthcare operations
q.d.	every day	TPR	temperature, pulse, and respirations
q.h.	every hour	UA	urinalysis
q.i.d.	four times a day	UC	urine culture
q.o.d.	every other day	UCR	usual, customary, and reasonable
QIO	quality improvement organization	UHDDS	Uniform Hospital Discharge Data Set
q.2h.	every two hours	UPC	Universal Product Code
QUAL.	qualifier	UPIN	Unique Physician Identification Number
RA	remittance advice	UR	utilization review
RAC	Recovery Audit Contractor	URI	upper respiratory infection
RARC	remittance advice remark code	USIN	Unique Supplier Identification Number
RBRVS	Resource-Based Relative Value Scale (Medicare)	USPSTF	United States Preventive Services Task Force
REF.	reference	UTI	urinary tract infection
Resp	respiratory	VD	venereal disease
RHIA	Registered Health Information Administration	VIS	vaccine information sheet
RHIT	Registered Health Information Technology	VP	Vendor Product Number
RLQ	right lower quadrant	VS	vital signs
RMA	Registered Medical Assistant	wbc	white blood cells
RN	registered nurse	WBC	white blood count
R/O	rule out	yo	year old
ROS	review of systems	YY	year, indicates entry of two digits for the year; may also be noted as CCYY, which allows for entry of four digits for the century (CC) and year (YY)
RTC	return to clinic		
RUG	Resource Utilization Group	ZPIC	Zone Program Integrity Contractor
RUQ	right upper quadrant		
RVS	relative value scale		

5010 format   The format for electronic claims.

837I   HIPAA-mandated format for claims for institutional services.

837P claim   The HIPAA-mandated electronic transaction for claims; also called the HIPAA claim.

A

abuse   Actions that improperly use another person's resources.

accept assignment   A participating physician's agreement to accept the allowed charge as payment in full.

accounts payable (AP)   The practice's operating expenses, such as overhead, salaries, supplies, and insurance.

accounts receivable (A/R)   Monies owed to a medical practice by its patients and third-party payers.

Acknowledgment of Receipt of Notice of Privacy Practices   Form accompanying a covered entity's Notice of Privacy Practices; covered entities must make a good-faith effort to have patients sign the acknowledgment.

add-on code   Procedure that is performed and reported only in addition to a primary procedure, indicated in CPT by a plus sign (+).

adjudication   The process followed by health plans to examine claims and determine benefits.

adjustment code   An administrative code used to explain an adjustment on the insured's account.

adjustment   A change to a patient's account, such as a returned check fee.

administrative code set   Under HIPAA, required codes for various data elements, such as taxonomy codes and place of service (POS) codes.

Admission of Liability   Carrier's determination that an employer is responsible for an employee's claim under workers' compensation.

admitting diagnosis (ADX)   The patient's condition determined by a physician at admission to an inpatient facility.

advance beneficiary notice of noncoverage (ABN)   Medicare form used to inform a patient that a service to be provided is not likely to be reimbursed by the program.

Affordable Care Act (ACA)   Health system reform legislation signed in 2010 that introduced a number of significant benefits for patients.

aging   Classification of accounts receivable by the length of time an account is due.

allowed charge   The maximum charge that a health plan pays for a specific service or procedure; also called allowable charge, maximum fee, and other terms.

Alphabetic Index   The section of the ICD-10-CM in which diseases and injuries with corresponding diagnosis codes are presented in alphabetical order.

ambulatory care   Outpatient care.

appeal   A request sent to a payer for reconsideration of a claim adjudication.

assignment of benefits   Authorization by a policyholder that allows a health plan to pay benefits directly to a provider.

attending physician   The clinician primarily responsible for the care of the patient from the beginning of a hospitalization.

audit   Methodical review; in medical insurance, a formal examination of a physician's accounting or patient medical records.

authorization   (1) Document signed by a patient to permit release of particular medical information under the stated specific conditions. (2) A health plan's system of approving payment of benefits for services that satisfy the plan's requirements; see *preauthorization*.

automobile insurance policy   A contract between an insurance company and an individual, under which the individual pays a premium in exchange for coverage of specified car-related financial losses.

autoposting   Software feature that enables automatic entry of payments on a remittance advice to credit an individual's account.

B

bad debt   An account deemed uncollectible.

balance billing   Collecting the difference between a provider's usual fee and a payer's lower allowed charge from the insured.

benefits   The amount of money a health plan pays for services covered in an insurance policy.

billing provider   The person or organization (often a clearinghouse or billing service) sending a HIPAA claim, as distinct from the pay-to provider who receives payment.

birthday rule   The guideline that determines which of two parents with medical coverage has the primary insurance for a child; the parent whose day of birth is earlier in the calendar year is considered primary.

BlueCard   A BCBS program that provides benefits for plan subscribers who are away from their local areas.

BlueCross BlueShield Association (BCBS)   The national licensing agency of BlueCross and BlueShield plans.

breach An impermissible use or disclosure under the Privacy Rule that compromises the security or privacy of PHI and also that could pose significant risk of financial, reputational, or other harm to the affected person.

breach notification The document notifying an individual of a breach.

bundled code The procedure code for a surgical package that covers a group of services that should not be listed individually.

bundled payment A single predetermined payment for an entire episode of care.

business associate (BA) A person or organization that performs a function or activity for a covered entity but is not part of its workforce.

C

cap rate The contractually set periodic prepayment to a provider for specified services to each enrolled plan member.

capitation Payment method in which a prepayment covers the provider's services to a plan member for a specified period of time.

carrier block Data entry area located in the upper right of the CMS-1500 that allows for a four-line address for the payer.

carve out A part of a standard health plan that is changed under a negotiated employer-sponsored plan; also refers to subcontracting of coverage by a health plan.

cash flow The movement of monies into or out of a business.

catastrophic cap The maximum annual amount a TRICARE beneficiary must pay for deductible and cost share.

catchment area Under TRICARE, a geographic area served by a hospital, clinic, or dental clinic and usually based on Zip codes to set an approximate 40-mile radius of military inpatient treatment facilities.

categorically needy A person who receives assistance from government programs such as Temporary Assistance for Needy Families (TANF).

category A three-character code used to classify a particular disease or injury.

Category I code Procedure codes found in the main body of CPT (Evaluation and Management, Anesthesia, Surgery, Pathology, and Laboratory, Radiology, and Medicine).

Category II code Optional CPT codes that track performance measures for a medical goal such as reducing tobacco use.

Category III code Temporary codes for emerging technology, services, and procedures that are used instead of unlisted codes when available.

CCI edits CPT code combinations that are used by computers in the Medicare system to check claims.

Centers for Medicare and Medicaid Services (CMS) Federal agency within the Department of Health and Human Services (HHS) that runs Medicare, Medicaid, clinical laboratories (under the CLIA program), and other government health programs.

certification number Identifying code assigned by a government program or health insurance plan when preauthorization is required; also called the prior authorization number.

certification The recognition of a person demonstrating a superior level of skill on a national test by an official organization.

charge capture Office procedures that ensure that billable services are recorded and reported for payment.

charge master (charge ticket) A hospital's list of the codes and charges for its services.

chart number A unique number that identifies a patient.

chief complaint (CC) A patient's description of the symptoms or other reasons for seeking medical care from a provider.

Children's Health Insurance Program (CHIP) Program offering health insurance coverage for uninsured children under Medicaid.

Civilian Health and Medical Program of the Department of Veterans Affairs (CHAMPVA) The Civilian Health and Medical Program of the Department of Veterans Affairs (previously known as the Veterans Administration) that shares health care costs for families of veterans with 100 percent service-connected disabilities and the surviving spouses and children of veterans who die from service-connected disabilities.

Civilian Health and Medical Program of the Uniformed Services (CHAMPUS) Now the TRICARE program; formerly the Civilian Health and Medical Program of the Uniformed Services (Army, Navy, Air Force, Marine Corps, Coast Guard, Public Health Service, and National Oceanic and Atmospheric Administration) that serves spouses and children of active-duty service members, military retirees and Civilian Health and Medical Program of the Department of Veterans Affairs.

claim attachment Documentation that a provider sends to a payer in support of a health care claim.

claim control number Unique number assigned to a health care claim by the sender.

claim filing indicator code Administrative code used to identify the type of health plan.

claim frequency code (claim submission reason code) Administrative code that identifies the claim as original, replacement, or void/cancel action.

clean claim A claim that is accepted by a health plan for adjudication.

clearinghouse A company (billing service, repricing company, or network) that converts nonstandard transactions into standard transactions and transmits the data to health plans; also handles the reverse process, changing standard transactions from health plans into nonstandard formats for providers.

CMS-1450 Paper claim for hospital services; also known as the UB-04.

CMS-1500 Paper claim for physician services.

CMS-1500 (02/12) The NUCC-revised paper claim with modified instructions.

code linkage The connection between a service and a patient's condition or illness; establishes the medical necessity of the procedure.

code set Alphabetic and/or numeric representations for data. Medical code sets are systems of medical terms that are required for HIPAA transactions. Administrative (nonmedical) code sets, such as taxonomy codes and ZIP codes, are also used in HIPAA transactions.

coding The process of translating a description of a diagnosis or procedure into a standardized code.

coinsurance The portion of charges that an insured person must pay for health care services after payment of the deductible amount; usually stated as a percentage.

collections A term that refers to all the activities that are related to patient accounts and follow-up.

combination code A single code that classifies both the etiology and the manifestation(s) of a particular condition.

comorbidities Admitted patient's coexisting conditions that affect the length of the hospital stay or the course of treatment.

compliance plan A medical practice's written plan for the following: the appointment of a compliance officer and committee; a code of conduct for physicians' business arrangements and employees' compliance; training plans; properly prepared and updated coding tools such as job reference aids, encounter forms, and documentation templates; rules for prompt identification and refunding of overpayments; and ongoing monitoring and auditing of claim preparation.

complications Conditions an admitted patient develops after surgery or treatment that affect the length of hospital stay or the course of further treatment.

condition code Two-digit numeric or alphanumeric codes used to report a special condition or unique circumstance about a claim.

Consolidated Omnibus Budget Reconciliation Act (COBRA) Federal law requiring employers with more than twenty employees to allow employees who have been terminated for reasons other than gross misconduct to pay for coverage under the employer's group health plan for eighteen months after termination.

consultation Service performed by a physician to advise a requesting physician about a patient's condition and care; the consultant does not assume responsibility for the patient's care and must send a written report back to the requestor.

consumer-driven health plan (CDHP) Type of medical insurance that combines a high-deductible health plan with a medical savings plan that covers some out-of-pocket expenses.

convention Typographic technique or standard practice that provides visual guidelines for understanding printed material.

conversion factor Dollar amount used to multiply a relative value unit to arrive at a charge.

coordination of benefits (COB) A clause in an insurance policy that explains how the policy will pay if more than one insurance policy applies to the claim.

copayment An amount that a health plan requires a beneficiary to pay at the time of service for each health care encounter.

Correct Coding Initiative (CCI) Computerized Medicare system to prevent overpayment for procedures.

cost-share Coinsurance for a TRICARE or CHAMPVA beneficiary.

covered entity (CE) Under HIPAA, a health plan, clearinghouse, or provider that transmits any health information in electronic form in connection with a HIPAA transaction; does not specifically include workers' compensation programs, property and casualty programs, or disability insurance programs.

covered services Medical procedures and treatments that are included as benefits under an insured's health plan.

credentialing Periodic verification that a provider or facility meets the professional standards of a certifying organization; physician credentialing involves screening and evaluating qualifications and other credentials, including licensure, required education, relevant training and experience, and current competence.

crossover claims Claims for a Medicare or Medicaid beneficiary; Medicare is the primary payer and automatically transmits claim information to Medicaid as the secondary payer.

***Current Procedural Terminology* (CPT)** Publication of the American Medical Association containing the HIPAA-mandated standardized classification system for reporting medical procedures and services performed by physicians.

cycle billing Type of billing in which patients with current balances are divided into groups to even out statement printing and mailing throughout a month, rather than mailing all statements once a month.

D

data element The smallest unit of information in a HIPAA transaction.

database A collection of related facts.

day sheet In a medical office, a report that summarizes the business day's charges and payments, drawn from all the patient ledgers for the day.

deductible An amount that an insured person must pay, usually on an annual basis, for health care services before a health plan's payment begins.

Defense Enrollment Eligibility Reporting System (DEERS) The worldwide database of TRICARE and CHAMPVA beneficiaries.

designated record set (DRS) A covered entity's records that contain protected health information (PHI); for providers, the designated record set is the medical/financial patient record.

destination payer In HIPAA claims, the health plan receiving the claim.

determination A payer's decision about the benefits due for a claim.

development Payer process of gathering information in order to adjudicate a claim.

diagnosis The physician's opinion of the nature of the patient's illness or injury.

diagnosis-related groups (DRGs) A system of analyzing conditions and treatments for similar groups of patients used to establish Medicare fees for hospital inpatient services.

diagnostic statement A physician's description of the main reason for a patient's encounter; may also describe related conditions or symptoms.

disability compensation programs Programs that provide partial reimbursement for lost income when a disability—whether work-related or not—prevents an individual from working.

discounted fee-for-service A negotiated payment schedule for health care services based on a reduced percentage of a provider's usual charges.

documentation The systematic, logical, and consistent recording of a patient's health status—history, examinations, tests, results of treatments, and observations—in chronological order in a patient medical record.

downcoding A payer's review and reduction of a procedure code (often an E/M code) to a lower level than reported by the provider.

E

E/M code Procedure codes that cover physicians' services performed to determine the optimum course for patient care; listed in the Evaluation and Management section of CPT.

Early and Periodic Screening, Diagnosis, and Treatment (EPSDT) Medicaid's prevention, early detection, and treatment program for eligible children under the age of twenty-one.

elective surgery Nonemergency surgical procedure that can be scheduled in advance.

electronic claim (e-claim) Health care claims that are sent electronically.

electronic data interchange (EDI) The system-to-system exchange of data in a standardized format.

electronic funds transfer (EFT) Electronic routing of funds between banks.

electronic health record (EHR) A computerized lifelong health care record with data from all sources.

electronic remittance advice (ERA) A transaction that explains a payer's payment decisions to the provider.

Employee Retirement Income Security Act of 1974 (ERISA) A federal law that provides incentives and protection against litigation for companies that set up employee health and pension plans.

encounter form A list of the diagnoses, procedures, and charges for a patient's visit; also called the superbill.

encounter An office visit between a patient and a medical professional.

encryption Encryption is a method of converting an original message of regular text into encoded text.

eponym A name or phrase that is formed from or based on a person's name; usually describes a condition or procedure associated with that person.

Equal Credit Opportunity Act (ECOA) Law which prohibits credit discrimination on the basis of race, color, religion, national origin, sex, marital status, age, or because a person receives public assistance.

established patient (EP) Patient who has received professional services from a provider (or another provider with the same specialty in the same practice) within the past three years.

etiology The cause or origin of a disease.

exclusion notes Entries in the Tabular List limiting applicability of particular codes to specified conditions.

explanation of benefits (EOB) Document sent by a payer to a patient that shows how the amount of a benefit was determined.

external cause code An ICD-10-CM code for an external cause of a disease or injury.

F

Fair Debt Collection Practices Act (FDCPA) of 1977 Laws regulating collection practices.

family deductible Fixed, periodic amount that must be met by the combination of payments for covered services to each individual of an insured/dependent group before benefits from a payer begin.

Federal Employees' Compensation Act (FECA) A federal law that provides workers' compensation insurance for civilian employees of the federal government.

Federal Employees Health Benefits (FEHB) Program The health insurance program that covers employees of the federal government.

Federal Insurance Contribution Act (FICA) The federal law that authorizes payroll deductions for the Social Security Disability Program.

Federal Medicaid Assistance Percentage (FMAP) Basis for federal government Medicaid allocations to individual states.

fee schedule A list of the usual fees a physician charges for procedures and services.

fee-for-service Method of charging under which a provider's payment is based on each service performed.

final report A report filed by the physician in a state workers' compensation case when the patient is discharged.

financial policy A practice's rules governing payment from patients for medical services.

first report of injury A report filed in state workers' compensation cases that contains the employer's name and address, employee's supervisor, date and time of accident, geographic location of injury, and patient's description of what happened.

fiscal agent An organization that processes claims for a government program, such as Medicaid.

Flexible Blue The BCBS consumer-driven health plan.

flexible savings account (FSA) Type of consumer-driven health plan funding option that has employer and employee contributions; funds left over revert to the employer.

formulary A list of a health plan's selected drugs and their proper dosages; often a plan pays only for the drugs it lists.

fraud Intentional deceptive act to obtain a benefit.

G

GEM Acronym for general equivalent mappings, reference tables of related ICD-10-CM and ICD-9-CM codes prepared by the federal government.

gender rule Coordination of benefits rule for a child insured under both parents' plans under which the father's insurance is primary.

global period The number of days surrounding a surgical procedure during which all services relating to the procedure—preoperative, during the surgery, and postoperative—are considered part of the surgical package and are not additionally reimbursed.

group health plan (GHP) Under HIPAA, a plan (including a self-insured plan) of an employer or employee organization to provide health care to the employees, former employees, or their families. Plans that are self-administered and have fewer than fifty participants are not group health plans.

guarantor billing Grouping patient billing under the insurance policyholder; the guarantor receives statements for all patients covered under the policy.

guarantor A person who is the insurance policyholder for a patient of the practice.

H

health care claim An electronic transaction or a paper document filed with a health plan to receive benefits.

Health Care Common Procedure Coding System (HCPCS) Procedure codes for Medicare claims, made up of CPT codes (Level I) and national codes (Level II).

health information technology (HIT) Computer hardware and software information systems that record, store, and manage patient information.

Health Information Technology for Economic and Clinical Health (HITECH) Act Law that guides the use of federal stimulus money to promote the adoption and meaningful use of health information technology, mainly using electronic health records.

health insurance claim number (HICN) A Medicare beneficiary's identification number; appears on the Medicare card.

Health Insurance Portability and Accountability Act (HIPAA) of 1996 Enacted by the U.S. Congress in 1996 to protect health insurance coverage for workers and their families when they change or lose their jobs; it also requires the establishment of national standards for electronic health care transactions and national identifiers for providers, health insurance plans, and employers.

health maintenance organization (HMO) A managed health care system in which providers agree to offer health care to the organization's members for fixed periodic payments from the plan; usually members must receive medical services only from the plan's providers.

health plan Under HIPAA, an individual or group plan that either provides or pays for the cost of medical care; includes group health plans, health insurance issuers; health maintenance organizations, Medicare Part A or B, Medicaid, TRICARE, and other government and nongovernment plans.

health reimbursement account (HRA) Type of consumer-driven health plan funding option under which an employer sets aside an annual amount an employee can use to pay for certain types of health care costs.

health savings account (HSA) Type of consumer-drive health plan funding option under which employers, employees, both employers and employees, or individuals set aside funds that can be used to pay for certain types of health care costs.

high-deductible health plan (HDHP) Type of health plan combining high-deductible insurance, usually a PPO with a relatively low premium, and a funding option to pay for patients' out-of-pocket expenses up to the deductible.

HIPAA claim The HIPAA-mandated electronic transaction for claims; also called the 837P claim.

HIPAA Coordination of Benefits The HIPAA AS-CX12N 837 transaction that is sent to a secondary or tertiary payer on a claim with the primary payer's remittance advice.

HIPAA Electronic Health Care Transactions and Code Sets (TCS) The HIPAA rule governing the electronic exchange of health information.

HIPAA Eligibility for a Health Plan The HIPAA X12N 270/217 transaction in which a provider asks a health plan for information on a patient's eligibility for benefits and receives an answer from the plan.

HIPAA Privacy Rule Law that regulates the use and disclosure of patients' protected health information (PHI).

HIPAA Referral Certification and Authorization The HIPAA X12N 278 transaction in which a provider asks a health plan for approval of a service and the health plan responds, providing a certification number for an approved request.

HIPAA Security Rule Law that requires covered entities to establish administrative, physical, and technical safeguards to protect the confidentiality, integrity, and availability of health information.

home plan A BCBS plan in the community where the subscriber has contracted for coverage.

host plan A participating provider's local BCBS plan.

I

ICD-10-CM Official Guidelines for Coding and Reporting The general rules, inpatient (hospital) coding guidance, and outpatient (physician office/clinic) coding guidance from the four cooperating parties (CMS advisers and participants from the AHA, AHIMA, and NCHS).

ICD-10-CM The HIPAA-mandated diagnosis code set as of October 1, 2014.

ICD-10-PCS The procedural coding system used to code procedures performed during hospitalization.

ICD-9-CM The previously HIPAA-mandated diagnosis code set.

inclusion notes Entries in the Tabular List addressing the applicability of certain codes to specified conditions.

indemnity plan An insurance company's agreement to reimburse a policyholder a predetermined amount for covered losses.

independent medical examination (IME) Examination by a physician to confirm that an individual is permanently disabled that is conducted at the request of a state workers' compensation office or an insurance carrier.

independent practice association (IPA) Type of health maintenance organization in which physicians are self-employed and provide services to both HMO members and nonmembers.

Index to External Causes Reference listing all the external causes of diseases and injuries that are listed in the related chapter of the Tabular List.

individual deductible Fixed amount that must be met periodically by each individual of an insured/dependent group before benefits from a payer begin.

individual health plan (IHP) Medical insurance plan purchased by an individual, rather than through a group affiliation.

individual relationship code Administrative code that specifies the patient's relationship to the subscriber (insured).

Inpatient Prospective Payment System (IPPS) Medicare payment system for hospital services; based on diagnosis-related groups (DRGs).

inpatient A person admitted to a medical facility for services that require an overnight stay.

insurance aging report A report grouping unpaid claims transmitted to payers by the length of time that they remain due, such as 30, 60, 90, or 120 days.

insured The policyholder or subscriber to a health plan or medical insurance policy; also known as a guarantor.

Internet-Only Manuals (IOM) Medicare's collection of manuals that have day-to-day operation instructions, policies, and procedures based on statutes and regulations.

K

key component Factor required to be documented for various levels of evaluation and management services.

L

late enrollee Category of enrollment in a commercial health plan that may have different eligibility requirements.

laterality The use of the ICD-10-CM classification system to capture the side of the body that is documented; the fourth, fifth, or sixth characters of a code specify the affected side(s).

level of service The amount of work, time, and decision making involved in an encounter.

lien A written, legal claim on property to secure the payment of a debt.

limiting charge In Medicare, the highest fee (115 percent of the Medicare Fee Schedule) that nonparticipating physicians may charge for a particular service.

line item control number On a HIPAA claim, the unique number assigned by the sender to each service line item reported.

local coverage determination (LCD) Notices sent to physicians that contain detailed and updated information about the coding and medical necessity of a specific Medicare service.

M

main number A five-digit number to which one or more two-digit CPT modifiers may be assigned.

main term The word that identifies a disease or condition in the Alphabetic Index.

managed care System that combines the financing and the delivery of appropriate, cost-effective health care services to its members.

managed care organization (MCO) Organization offering some type of managed health care plan.

manifestation Characteristic sign or symptom of a disease.

master patient index (MPI) Hospital's main patient database.

maximum benefit limit The amount an insurer agrees to pay for an insured's covered expenses over the course of the insured person's lifetime.

meaningful use The utilization of certified EHR technology to improve quality, efficiency, and patient safety in the health care system.

Medicaid Program that pays for health care services for people with incomes below the national poverty level.

medical assistant An administrative medical employee.

medical billing cycle A ten-step process that results in timely payment for medical services.

medical insurance Financial plan that covers the cost of hospital and medical care.

medical records Files that contain the documentation of a patient's medical history, record of care, progress notes, correspondence, and related billing/financial information.

Medical Savings Account (MSA) The Medicare health savings account program.

medical standards of care State-specified performance measures for the delivery of health care by medical professionals.

MediCal California's Medicaid program.

medical documentation and billing cycle A combination of the billing cycle and medical documentation cycle of a practice, which explains how using EHRs is integrated with practice management programs.

medically indigent Medicaid classification for people with high medical expenses and low financial resources, although not sufficiently low to receive cash assistance; medically needy.

medically necessary Medical treatment that is appropriate and rendered in accordance with generally accepted standards of medical practice; the place of service must also be appropriate for the diagnosis and care provided.

medically needy Medicaid classification for people with high medical expenses and low financial resources, although not sufficiently low to receive cash assistance; medically indigent.

medically unlikely edits (MUEs) CMS-established units of service edits used in order to lower the Medicare fee-for-service paid claims error rate.

Medicare The federal health insurance program for people who are sixty-five or older.

Medicare administrative contractor (MAC) The contractors who handle claims and related functions for both Medicare Parts A and B.

Medicare Advantage Medicare plans other than the Original Medicare Plan.

Medicare beneficiary A person who is covered by Medicare.

Medicare Integrity Program (MIP) A CMS program designed to identify and address fraud, waste, and abuse.

Medicare Learning Network (MLN) An online collection of articles that explain all Medicare topics.

Medicare Part A The part of the Medicare program that pays for hospitalization, care in a skilled nursing facility, home health care, and hospice care.

Medicare Part B The part of the Medicare program that pays for physician services, outpatient hospital services, durable medical equipment, and other services and supplies.

Medicare Part C Managed care health plans offered to Medicare beneficiaries under the Medicare Advantage program.

Medicare Part D Prescription drug reimbursement plans offered to Medicare beneficiaries.

Medicare Physician Fee Schedule (MPFS) The RBRVS-based allowed fees that are the basis for Medicare reimbursement.

Medicare Remittance Notice (MRN) The RA that the office receives from Medicare.

Medicare Secondary Payer (MSP) Federal law requiring private payers who provide general health insurance to Medicare beneficiaries to be the primary payers for beneficiaries' claims.

Medicare Summary Notice (MSN) Type of remittance advice from Medicare to beneficiaries to explain how benefits were determined.

Medicare-Severity DRGs (MS-DRGs) A new type of DRG adopted by Medicare in 2008 to better reflect the different severity of illness among patients who have the same basic diagnosis.

Medigap Insurance plan offered by a private insurance carrier to supplement Medicare Original Plan coverage.

Medi-Medi beneficiary Person who is eligible for both Medicare and Medicaid benefits.

Military Treatment Facility (MTF) Government facility providing medical services for members and dependents of the uniformed services.

minimum necessary standard Principle that individually identifiable health information should be disclosed only to the extent needed to support the purpose of the disclosure.

moderate sedation A moderate, drug-induced depression of consciousness during which patients can respond to verbal commands.

modifier A number that is appended to a code to report particular facts. CPT modifiers report special circumstances involved with a procedure or service.

monthly enrollment list Document of eligible members of a capitated plan registered with a particular PCP for a monthly period.

N

national coverage determination (NCD) Medicare policy stating whether and under what circumstances a service is covered by the Medicare program.

National Provider Identifier (NPI) Under HIPAA, unique ten-digit identifier assigned to each provider by the National Provider System.

National Uniform Claim Committee (NUCC) Organization responsible for the content of health care claims.

NEC (not elsewhere classified) An abbreviation indicating the code to be used when a disease or condition cannot be placed in any other category.

Neoplasm Table Reference that provides code numbers for neoplasms by anatomical site and divided by the description of the neoplasm.

network A group of providers in a managed care organization that allows patients to avoid paying higher charges.

new patient (NP) A patient who has not received professional services from a provider (or another provider with the same specialty in the same practice) within the past three years.

nonavailability statement (NAS) A form required for preauthorization when a TRICARE member seeks medical services in other than military treatment facilities.

noncovered (excluded) services Medical procedures that are not included in a plan's benefits.

nonessential modifier A supplementary word or phrase that helps define a code in ICD-10-CM.

nonparticipating provider (nonPAR) A provider who chooses not to join a particular government or other health plan.

NOS (not otherwise specified) An abbreviation indicating the code to be used when no information is available for assigning a disease or condition a more specific code.

Notice of Contest Carrier's determination to deny liability for an employee's workers' compensation claim.

Notice of Privacy Practices (NPP) A HIPAA-mandated description of a covered entity's principles and procedures related to the protection of patients' health information.

NSF checks Checks written from an account that does not have adequate funds (or has "nonsufficient funds") to cover the check, and are not honored by the bank; also referred to as "bounced" or "returned" checks.

O

occupational diseases or illnesses Conditions caused by the work environment over a period longer than one workday or shift; also known as nontraumatic injuries.

Occupational Safety and Health Administration (OSHA) A program created by Congress in 1970 to protect workers from health and safety risks on the job.

Office for Civil Rights (OCR) Government agency that enforces the HIPAA Privacy Act.

Office of E-Health Standards and Services (OESS) The part of CMS that enforces the other HIPAA standards.

Office of the Inspector General (OIG) Government agency that investigates and prosecutes fraud against government health care programs such as Medicare.

Office of Workers' Compensation Programs (OWCP) A part of the U.S. Department of Labor that administers programs to cover work-related illnesses or injuries suffered by civilian employees of federal agencies, including occupational diseases acquired by them.

open enrollment period Span of time during which a policyholder selects from an employer's offered benefits; often used to describe the fourth quarter of the year for employees in employer-sponsored health plans or the designated period for enrollment in a Medicare or Medigap plan.

Original Medicare Plan The Medicare fee-for-service plan.

out-of-network   A provider that does not have a participation agreement with a plan. Using out-of-network providers is more expensive for the plan's enrollees.

out-of-pocket   Expenses the insured must pay before benefits begin.

outpatient   A patient who receives health care in a hospital setting without admission; the length of stay is generally less than twenty-three hours.

Outpatient Prospective Payment System (OPPS)   The payment system for Medicare Part B services that facilities provide on an outpatient basis.

outside laboratory   Purchased laboratory services.

overpayment   From the payer's point of view, improper or excessive payment resulting from billing errors for which the provider owes a refund.

P

panel   In CPT, a single code grouping laboratory tests that are frequently done together.

partial payment   A patient payment made during the checkout process based on an estimate by the practice of what the patient will owe.

participating provider (PAR)   A provider who agrees to provide medical services to a payer's policyholders according to the terms of the plan's contract.

password   Confidential authentication information composed of a string of characters.

patient aging report   A report grouping unpaid patients' bills by the length of time that they remain due, such as 30, 60, 90, or 120 days.

patient information form   Form that includes a patient's personal, employment, and insurance company data needed to complete a health care claim; also known as a registration form.

patient ledger   The record of a patient's financial transactions.

patient refund   Money that is owed to a patient.

patient statement   A report that shows the services provided to a patient, total payments made, total charges, adjustments, and balance due.

payer of last resort   Regulation that Medicaid pays last on a claim when a patient has other insurance coverage.

pay-to provider   The person or organization that is to receive payment for services reported on a HIPAA claim; may be the same as or different from the billing provider.

per member per month (PMPM)   Periodic capitated prospective payment to a provider that covers only services listed on the schedule of benefits.

personal injury protection (PIP)   Insurance coverage for medical expenses and other expenses related to a motor vehicle accident.

physician of record   Provider under a workers' compensation claim who first treats the patient and assesses the level of disability.

Physician Quality Reporting System (PQRS)   A voluntary quality reporting program established by CMS in which physicians or other eligible professionals collect and report their practice data in relation to a set of patient-care performance measures that are established annually.

place of service (POS) code   HIPAA administrative code that indicates where medical services were provided.

placeholder character (x)   A character "x" that is inserted in a code to fill a blank space.

PM/EHR   Software program that combines both a PM and an EHR in a single product.

point-of-service (POS) plan   In HMOs, a plan that permits patients to receive medical services from non-network providers; this choice requires a larger patient payment than visits with network providers.

policyholder   Person who buys an insurance plan; the insured, subscriber, or guarantor.

practice management program (PMP)   Business software designed to organize and store a medical practice's financial information; often includes scheduling, billing, and electronic medical records features.

preauthorization   Prior authorization from a payer for services to be provided; if preauthorization is not received, the charge is usually not covered.

precertification   Generally, preauthorization for hospital admission or outpatient procedures.

preferred provider organization (PPO)   Managed care organization structured as a network of health care providers who agree to perform services for plan members at discounted fees; usually, plan members can receive services from non-network providers for a higher charge.

premium   Money the insured pays to a health plan for a health care policy.

present on admission (POA)   A code used in situations when a condition existed at the time the order for inpatient admission occurs.

Primary Care Manager (PCM)   Provider who coordinates and manages the care of TRICARE beneficiaries.

primary care physician (PCP)   A physician in a health maintenance organization who directs all aspects of a patient's care, including routine services, referrals to specialists within the system, and supervision of hospital admissions; also known as a gatekeeper.

primary insurance   Health plan that pays benefits first when a patient is covered by more than one plan.

primary procedure   The most resource-intensive (highest paid) CPT procedure done during a patient's encounter.

principal diagnosis (PDX)   The condition established after study to be chiefly responsible for the admission.

principal procedure   The procedure that is most closely related to the treatment of the principal diagnosis.

prior authorization number   Identifying code assigned by a government program or health insurance plan when preauthorization is required; also called the certification number.

procedure code   Code that identifies medical treatment or diagnostic services.

procedures   The services and treatments performed by a practice.

progress report   A report filed by the physician in state workers' compensation cases when a patient's medical condition or disability changes; also known as a supplemental report.

protected health information (PHI)   Individually identifiable health information that is transmitted or maintained by electronic media.

provider Person or entity that supplies medical or health services and bills for or is paid for the services in the normal course of business. A provider may be a professional member of the health care team, such as a physician, or a facility, such as a hospital or skilled nursing home.

Q

qualifier Two-digit code for a type of provider identification number other than the National Provider Identifier (NPI).

R

real-time claims adjudication (RTCA) A process used to generate the actual amount owed by a patient, as opposed to an estimate of that amount.

reconciliation Comparison of two numbers to determine whether they differ.

referral The transfer of patient care from one physician to another.

referral number Authorization number given by a referring physician to the referred physician.

referral waiver Document a patient is asked to sign guaranteeing payment when a required referral authorization is pending.

referring physician The physician who refers the patient to another physician for treatment.

registration Process of gathering personal and insurance information about a patient during admission to a hospital.

remittance advice (RA) Health plan document describing a payment resulting from a claim adjudication; also called an explanation of benefits (EOB).

rendering provider Term used to identify the physician or other medical professional who provides the procedure reported on a health care claim if other than the pay-to provider.

resequenced CPT procedure codes that have been reassigned to another sequence, or CPT range of codes.

resource-based relative value scale (RBRVS) The payment system used by Medicare to establish relative value units for services based on resources.

retention schedule A practice policy that governs which information from patients' medical records is to be stored, for how long it is to be retained, and the storage medium to be used.

revenue cycle management (RCM) All the actions that help to ensure that the provider receives maximum appropriate payment for services.

rider Document that modifies an insurance contract.

S

secondary claim Claims sent to a secondary payer reporting what the primary payer paid on the claim.

secondary insurance The health plan that pays benefits after the primary plan pays when a patient is covered by more than one plan.

section guidelines Usage notes provided at the beginnings of CPT sections.

self-insured health plan An organization that assumes the risks of paying for health insurance directly and sets up a fund from which to pay.

self-pay patient A patient who does not have insurance coverage.

separate procedure Descriptor used in the Surgery Section of CPT for a procedure that is usually part of a surgical package but may also be performed separately or for a different purpose, in which case it may be billed.

sequelae Problems that result from a previous disease or injury.

service line information On a HIPAA claim, information about the services being reported.

seventh-character extension The necessary assignment of a seventh character to a code; often for the sequence of an encounter.

Social Security Disability Insurance (SSDI) The federal disability compensation program for salaried and hourly wage earners, self-employed people who pay a special tax, and widows, widowers, and minor children with disabilities whose deceased spouse/parent would qualify for Social Security benefits if alive.

sponsor The uniformed service member in a family qualified for TRICARE or CHAMPVA.

statement A report that shows the services provided to a patient, total payments made, total charges, adjustments, and balance due.

stop-loss provision Protection against the risk of large losses or severely adverse claims experience; may be included in a participating provider's contract with a plan or bought by a self-funded plan.

subcategory A four- or five-character code number.

subscriber The insured.

subterm Word or phrase that describes a main term in the Alphabetic Index.

supplemental insurance Insurance plan, such as Medigap, that provides benefits for services that are not normally covered by a primary plan.

Supplemental Security Income (SSI) Government program that helps pay living expenses for low-income older people and those who are blind or have disabilities.

surgical package Combination of services included in a single procedure code for some surgical procedures in CPT.

T

Table of Drugs and Chemicals A reference in table format listing drugs and chemicals in the Tabular List.

Tabular List Part of ICD-10-CM in which diagnosis codes are listed in chapters alphanumerically.

taxonomy code Administrative code set under HIPAA used to report a physician's specialty when it affects payment.

Telephone Consumer Protection Act of 1991 Federal law that regulates consumer collections to ensure fair and ethical treatment of debtors; governs calling hours and methods.

Temporary Assistance for Needy Families (TANF) Government program that provides cash assistance for low-income families.

tertiary claim Claims sent to a tertiary payer reporting what the primary and secondary payers paid on the claim.

tertiary insurance The third payer on a claim.

third-party liability The obligation of a government program or insurance plan to pay all or part of a patient's medical costs.

third-party payer Private or government organization that insures or pays for health care on the behalf of beneficiaries; the insured person is the first party, the provider the second party, and the payer the third party.

timely filing The Medicare law requiring claims to be filed within one calendar year after the date of service.

trace number A number assigned to a HIPAA 270 electronic transaction sent to a health plan to inquire about patient eligibility for benefits.

transaction The electronic exchange of health care information.

treatment, payment, and operations (TPO) Under HIPAA, patients' protected health information may be shared without authorization for the purpose of treatment, payment and operations.

TRICARE Government health program that serves dependents of active-duty service members, military retirees and their families, some former spouses, and survivors of deceased military members; formerly called CHAMPUS.

TRICARE Extra TRICARE's managed care health plan that offers a network of civilian providers.

TRICARE for Life Program for beneficiaries who are both Medicare and TRICARE eligible.

TRICARE Prime The basic managed care health plan offered by TRICARE.

TRICARE Prime Remote Program that provides no-cost health care through civilian providers for service members and their families who are on remote assignment.

TRICARE Reserve Select (TRS) TRICARE coverage for reservists.

TRICARE Standard The fee-for-service health plan offered by TRICARE.

Truth in Lending Act Federal law requiring disclosure of finance charges and late fees for payment plans.

U

UB-04 Currently mandated paper claim for hospital billing.

UCR (usual, customary, reasonable) Setting fees by comparing the usual fee the provider charges for the service, the customary fee charged by most providers in the community, and the fee that is reasonable considering the circumstances.

unbundle The incorrect billing practice of breaking a panel or package of services/procedures into component parts and reporting them separately.

uncollectible account Money that cannot be collected from the practice's payers or patients and must be written off.

unlisted procedures Services that are not listed in CPT; they are reported with an unlisted procedure code and require a special report when used.

upcoding Use of a procedure code that provides a higher payment than the code for the service actually provided.

urgently needed care In Medicare, a beneficiary's unexpected illness or injury requiring immediate treatment; Medicare plans pay for this service even if it is provided outside the plan's service area.

utilization review The payer's process for determining medical necessity—whether the review is conducted before or after the services are provided.

utilization review organization (URO) An organization hired by the payer to evaluate the medical necessity of planned procedures.

V

vocational rehabilitation Retraining program covered by workers' compensation to prepare a patient for reentry into the workforce.

W

waiting period An amount of time that must pass before a newly hired employee or a dependent is eligible to enroll in a health plan.

walkout receipt Medical billing program report given to a patient that lists the diagnoses, services provided, fees, and payments received and due after an encounter.

Welfare Reform Act A 1996 law that established the Temporary Assistance for Needy Families program in place of the Aid to Families with Dependent Children program and that tightened Medicaid eligibility requirements.

write off To deduct an amount from a patient's account because of a contractual agreement to accept a payer's allowed charge or for other reasons.

Z

Z code The abbreviation for codes from the twentieth chapter of the ICD-10-CM that identify factors that influence health status and encounters that are not due to illness or injury.

Text References

Chapter 1

Page 16, Eight core functions of an EHR, from the Committee on Data Standards for Patient Safety, *Key Capabilities of an Electronic Health Record System: Letter Report.*

Figure 1.2, from Susan M. Sanderson, *Practice Management and EHR: A Total Patient Encounter for Medisoft® Clinical*, 1/e. © 2012 McGraw Hill Companies, Inc. Reprinted with permission.

Chapter 2

Figure 2.1, Figure 2.3 and Case 2.2 Figure, from Joanne D. Valerius et al., *Medical Insurance: An Integrated Claims Process Approach*, 5/e. © 2012 McGraw Hill Companies, Inc. Reprinted with permission.

Figure 2.2, source: Practice Partner® is a Registered Trademark of McKesson Corporation. Screen shots and material pertaining to Practice Partner® Software used with permission of MCKESSON Corporation. © 2010 MCKESSON Corporation. All rights reserved.

Chapter 3

Figure 3.1, Figure 3.3, Figure 3.4, Figure 3.5, Figure 3.6, Figure 3.7a, Figure 3.7b, and Figure 3.8 from Joanne D. Valerius et al., *Medical Insurance: An Integrated Claims Process Approach*, 5/e. © 2012 McGraw Hill Companies, Inc. Reprinted with permission.

Figure 3.2, from Susan M. Sanderson, *Practice Management and EHR: A Total Patient Encounter For Medisoft® Clinical*, 1/e. © 2012 McGraw Hill Companies, Inc. Reprinted with permission.

Chapter 4

Figure 4.3, from Cynthia Newby, *Medical Coding Workbook for Physician Practices and Facilities: ICD-10 Edition.* © 2012 McGraw Hill Companies, Inc. Reprinted with permission.

Chapter 5

Figure 5.2, Figure 5.3, and Table 5.1, from Joanne D. Valerius et al., *Medical Insurance: An Integrated Claims Process Approach*, 5/e. © 2012 McGraw Hill Companies, Inc. Reprinted with permission.

Chapter 6

Table 6.1, Table 6.2, Table 6.3, Figure 6.1, Figure 6.2, Figure on Estimating the Patient's Bill, Figure 6.3, and Figure 6.4, from Joanne D. Valerius et al., *Medical Insurance: An Integrated Claims Process Approach*, 5/e. © 2012 McGraw Hill Companies, Inc. Reprinted with permission.

Chapter 7

Table 7.4, Figure 7.4, Figure 7.5a, and Figure 7.5b, from Joanne D. Valerius et al., *Medical Insurance: An Integrated Claims Process Approach*, 5/e. © 2012 McGraw Hill Companies, Inc. Reprinted with permission.

Chapter 8

Figure 8.1, Figure 8.2, and Figure 8.3, from Joanne D. Valerius et al., *Medical Insurance: An Integrated Claims Process Approach*, 5/e. © 2012 McGraw Hill Companies, Inc. Reprinted with permission.

Chapter 9

Figure 9.1, from Joanne D. Valerius et al., *Medical Insurance: An Integrated Claims Process Approach*, 5/e. © 2012 McGraw Hill Companies, Inc. Reprinted with permission.

Chapter 10

Figure 10.2, from Joanne D. Valerius et al., *Medical Insurance: An Integrated Claims Process Approach*, 5/e. © 2012 McGraw Hill Companies, Inc. Reprinted with permission.

Chapter 11

Figure 11.1, from Joanne D. Valerius et al., *Medical Insurance: An Integrated Claims Process Approach*, 5/e. © 2012 McGraw Hill Companies, Inc. Reprinted with permission.

Chapter 13

Figure 13.1, Figure 13.2, Figure of Report for an Assigned Claim, Thinking It Through 13.2 Figure, Figure of Patient Statement, Figure 13.3a, Figure 13.3b, Figure 13.3c, Figure 13.4, Thinking It Through 13.5 Figure, Thinking It Through 13.6 Figure, from Joanne D. Valerius et al., *Medical Insurance: An Integrated Claims Process Approach*, 5/e. © 2012 McGraw Hill Companies, Inc. Reprinted with permission.

Chapter 14

Table 14.1 and Thinking It Through 14.5, from Joanne D. Valerius et al., *Medical Insurance: An Integrated Claims Process Approach*, 5/e. © 2012 McGraw Hill Companies, Inc. Reprinted with permission.